AF094704

Pathogenesis and Novel Therapeutics in Asthma

Pathogenesis and Novel Therapeutics in Asthma

Editor

Stanislawa Bazan-Socha

MDPI • Basel • Beijing • Wuhan • Barcelona • Belgrade • Manchester • Tokyo • Cluj • Tianjin

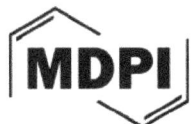

Editor
Stanislawa Bazan-Socha
Jagiellonian University
Medical College
Poland

Editorial Office
MDPI
St. Alban-Anlage 66
4052 Basel, Switzerland

This is a reprint of articles from the Special Issue published online in the open access journal *Biomedicines* (ISSN 2227-9059) (available at: https://www.mdpi.com/journal/biomedicines/special_issues/Asthma__).

For citation purposes, cite each article independently as indicated on the article page online and as indicated below:

LastName, A.A.; LastName, B.B.; LastName, C.C. Article Title. *Journal Name* **Year**, *Volume Number*, Page Range.

ISBN 978-3-0365-7842-2 (Hbk)
ISBN 978-3-0365-7843-9 (PDF)

© 2023 by the authors. Articles in this book are Open Access and distributed under the Creative Commons Attribution (CC BY) license, which allows users to download, copy and build upon published articles, as long as the author and publisher are properly credited, which ensures maximum dissemination and a wider impact of our publications.

The book as a whole is distributed by MDPI under the terms and conditions of the Creative Commons license CC BY-NC-ND.

Contents

About the Editor

Stanislawa Bazan-Socha

Stanislawa Bazan-Socha M.D., Ph.D., graduated from the Jagiellonian University Medical College in Krakow, Poland, in 1996. She is a specialist in internal medicine, allergy, and clinical immunology, and is currently employed as an Associate Professor at the Department of Internal Medicine, Jagiellonian University Medical College in Krakow, Poland. Her research is related to the pathology of asthma and autoimmune diseases and artificial intelligence methods in medical data analysis.

Main awards:

Young Scientists Scholarship from Foundation for Polish Science, Warsaw 2001;

Prime Minister's Award for the Ph.D. thesis, Warsaw 2002;

Aurelia Baczko Contest award for the best Ph.D. dissertation in medicine in 2002, awarded by the Society for the Promotion and Propagation of Sciences, Warsaw 2002;

First Award in the 22nd Annual Dr. Erwin Margulies Competition in Thrombosis Research, Sol Sherry Thrombosis Research Center, Temple University School of Medicine, Philadelphia PA, USA, 2002.

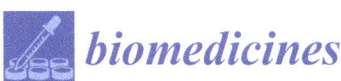 *biomedicines*

MDPI

Editorial

Editorial to the Special Issue "Pathogenesis and Novel Therapeutics in Asthma"

Stanisława Bazan-Socha * and Bogdan Jakieła

Department of Internal Medicine, Faculty of Medicine, Jagiellonian University Medical College,
31-008 Krakow, Poland
* Correspondence: stanislawa.bazan-socha@uj.edu.pl; Tel.: +48-12-400-34-72

Citation: Bazan-Socha, S.; Jakieła, B.
Editorial to the Special Issue
"Pathogenesis and Novel
Therapeutics in Asthma".
Biomedicines **2023**, *11*, 268.
https://doi.org/10.3390/
biomedicines11020268

Received: 12 January 2023
Accepted: 16 January 2023
Published: 19 January 2023

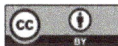

Copyright: © 2023 by the authors.
Licensee MDPI, Basel, Switzerland.
This article is an open access article
distributed under the terms and
conditions of the Creative Commons
Attribution (CC BY) license (https://
creativecommons.org/licenses/by/
4.0/).

In recent years, substantial progress has been made in our understanding of asthma pathomechanisms, especially phenotyping. However, asthma is a heterogeneous disease caused by a variety of inflammatory responses. Furthermore, the current pharmacotherapy mainly affects symptoms and does not modify the disease progression, including airway remodeling. Thus, further research on asthma is still of significant importance. In this Special Issue entitled "Pathogenesis and Novel Therapeutics in Asthma", we addressed various important aspects of asthma, such as disease phenotyping, novel biomarkers, and concepts of customized treatment.

This Special Issue contains seven original articles on the pathomechanism of asthma, including in vitro research investigating novel disease mechanisms and clinical studies on potential disease biomarkers. For example, in an interesting report, Schindler V. et al. [1] used the air−liquid interface culture of bronchial epithelial cells derived from asthma patients and control subjects to study the microRNA profile (miRNA) in released extracellular vesicles (EVs). The authors describe considerable differences in miRNA content, depending on the side of secretion. Over two hundred miRNAs were differentially expressed by comparing EVs isolated from the apical and basolateral cell sides. Interestingly, several miRNAs showed altered expression in cells derived from asthma patients (32 miRNAs in apical EVs, 23 in basolateral) in comparison to the controls. Furthermore, the study evaluated miRNA-associated functions and targets that confirmed differences that were dependent on the site of secretion. For example, apically released EVs contained miRNAs that regulate mammalian targets of rapamycin (mTOR) and mitogen-activated protein kinase (MAPK) signaling pathways, while miRNAs released basolaterally targeted, among others, T and B cell receptor signaling. In conclusion, the study confirms side-specific differences in the miRNA cargo of EVs released by airway epithelium, providing further evidence of the critical role these cells play in the regulation of the immune response in asthmatic airways.

Another original paper investigates the role of NF-κB activation in profibrotic signaling that contributes to airway remodeling in severe asthma. Ramakrishnan R. et al. [2] investigated whether Bcl10 protein, one of the upstream mediators of NF-κB activation, participates in profibrotic signaling in bronchial fibroblasts. The authors demonstrated increased Bcl10 protein expression in airway biopsies and fibroblasts isolated from severe asthma patients. They also confirmed that the selective inhibition of Bcl10 reduced the expression of profibrotic cytokines by activated fibroblasts. This study indicates that targeting Bcl10-associated signaling could be a novel therapeutic option for inhibiting airway inflammation and remodeling in severe asthma.

The study by Bazan-Socha S. et al. [3] documented an increased systemic oxidative stress response in the peripheral blood of asthmatic patients. The authors developed a real-time coumarin boric acid assay (CBA) that enabled a detailed analysis of the kinetics of protein hydroperoxide (HP) formation in serum samples. The study demonstrated increased systemic oxidative stress response in asthma. Furthermore, increased HP formation appeared to be inversely correlated with lung function, as well as being positively associated with inflammatory blood and airway biomarkers. The authors conclude that oxidative stress response is an important component of airway inflammation in asthma, and antioxidant supplementation may benefit asthma management. Interestingly, another study in this Special Issue analyzed whether OmeGo [4], an enzymatically liberated fish oil formulation with potent antioxidant functions, could indeed modify airway inflammation. Currie et al. [4] demonstrated how OmeGo supplementation significantly decreased airway inflammation and remodeling parameters in the murine model of allergic asthma. In many aspects, it showed a similar efficacy as pharmacologic inhibition of the type (T)2-inflammatory response. The data presented by Currie et al. [4] and Bazan-Socha et al. [3] support the need for future clinical studies to evaluate whether a similar approach aimed at reducing oxidative stress could be helpful in asthma.

Special attention must also be placed on the original report published by Ching-Hsiung Lin et al. [5]. These authors assessed the prevalence of fungal sensitization in asthma and checked whether it is associated with specific immune profiles and more severe disease outcomes. Interestingly, they found that about 90% of asthmatics in Taiwan population had fungi-specific IgE in serum, suggesting that this problem may be underestimated worldwide. Furthermore, the serum levels of IL-6 and IL-17A correlated positively with the severity of fungi sensitization; however, only IL-17A was associated with increased asthma-related emergency department visits in the past. Therefore, the Th17-mediated immune response related to fungal sensitization in asthma could be a potential therapeutic target for anti-IL17A therapy. In addition to the possible linkage with fungal allergy, IL-17A has been linked with neutrophilic inflammation in severe asthma [6]. Earlier studies confirmed that this particular inflammatory phenotype is also associated with the increased airway production of leukotriene B4 (LTB4), a lipid mediator acting as a potent chemoattractant for neutrophils. Here, Kwak D.W. et al. [7] used a murine model of steroid-resistant airway inflammation to show that the activation of an LTB4 receptor 2 (BLT2) upregulates granulocyte colony-stimulating factor (G-CSF) synthesis, contributing to the neutrophilic inflammatory response. Interestingly, G-CSF production and subsequent airway neutrophilia depended on the 12-lipoxygenase pathway, which catalyzes the synthesis of the BLT2 ligand, 12(S)-hydroxyeicosatetraenoic acid (HETE). The authors conclude that this pathway may serve as a potential target for treating severe neutrophilic asthma.

Finally, the clinical study by Mormile I. et al. [8] provides exciting data on the factors influential in predicting the response to allergen immunotherapy (AIT). The authors developed a novel rating system called the Predictive Response to Immunotherapy Score (PRIS), which combined both clinical and laboratory measures. This scoring system was next validated in a large cohort of 110 patients who were eligible for sublingual immunotherapy (SLIT) at baseline and at 12 and 24 months follow-up. PRIS was effective in predicting symptom response to SLIT. The parameters that significantly contributed to the scoring included, among others: patients' age, major disease features (e.g., rhinitis and asthma), and various clinical and laboratory parameters that reflect the severity of allergy (e.g., number of allergen sensitizations, levels of specific IgE). The results of this study suggest that initial PRIS scoring might be recommended as a valuable tool for clinicians to identify patients who may find AIT most beneficial.

Original research studies are followed by a comprehensive review paper by Patel K. and Stokes Peebles, Jr. [9], focusing on the role of PGI_2 (prostacyclin) in regulating the allergic inflammatory response. PGI_2 is a metabolic product of the cyclooxygenase pathway, which is constitutively expressed by many airway resident cells and induced during inflammatory conditions. It has been recognized as an effective vasodilator with anti-platelet aggregatory effects since its discovery in 1976 [10]. Furthermore, in vitro and in vivo studies demonstrated its potent anti-inflammatory functions. This review discusses pathways regulating PGI_2 production and signaling, including various immunomodulatory functions mediated by IP receptors and peroxisome proliferator-activated nuclear receptors.

Special attention was paid to cell-specific actions of PGI_2 and the perspectives of using this pathway in future treatments of allergic diseases and asthma.

This Special Issue ends with a systemic review by Calzetta L. et al. [11], seeking to assess the novel therapeutic agents for asthma therapy investigated in recent Phase I and II randomized controlled trials (RCTs). Based on the literature search and data retrieved from the ClinicalTrial.org database, the authors included 19 clinical trials that had been completed in the last five years (2017–2022). Next, they summarized the types of therapeutic interventions and outcomes, data quality, and potential bias. Overall, the authors identified sixteen classes of novel treatment options for asthma. Among those are anti-inflammatory compounds interfering with the T2 inflammatory response, such as an inhaled form of lipocalin-derived protein inhibiting α subunit of interleukin (IL)-4 receptor (AZD1402), and depemokimab, a long-acting monoclonal antibody (mAb) targeting IL-5. Preliminary RCTs also documented the effectiveness of mAbs against airway alarmins, e.g., those blocking IL-33 (itepekimab and etokimab) or the IL-33 receptor (melrilimab), as well as the mAb fragment against thymic stromal lymphopoietin (TSLP), administered via a dry powder inhaler (ecleralimab). An attractive therapeutic option in asthma, also mentioned by Calzetta et al. [11], could be the blocking of the actions of prostaglandin-D_2 (PGD_2), an important lipid mediator released by activated mast cells and eosinophils. Early data suggest the effectiveness of the DP2 receptor antagonist GB001, which was administered orally in improving asthma control, with better effects obtained in eosinophilic asthma.

The authors also discuss the potential treatments that may have wider application in severe asthma, including patients with non-T2 variants of the disease. For example, data on anti-IL-17A mAb (CJM1120) suggest it may improve symptom control in severe non-eosinophilic asthma. Another therapeutic option includes thyrosine kinase inhibitors, such as Bruton's tyrosine kinase inhibitor remibrutinib, and pan-JAK inhibitor TD-8236. By blocking the signaling associated with tyrosine kinase activity, these drugs have the potential to control overactivated inflammatory pathways in severe asthma. Particular attention should be given to velsecorat, a novel drug acting as a non-steroidal selective glucocorticoid receptor modulator (SGRM). This drug efficiently suppresses inflammation with fewer adverse effects, preferably acting as a transrepressor of steroid receptors. Another therapeutic option for asthma includes the inhalation of sodium channel inhibitor (BI443651), which may have beneficial effects by changing the mucus viscosity in the lower airways. The history of dexpramipexole, an oral drug initially investigated for the treatment of amyotrophic lateral sclerosis, is also interesting. Due to its potent eosinophil-reducing activity, this compound is currently being tested in hypereosinophilic syndrome and asthma. All the mentioned medications seem promising, although larger RCTs are needed to prove their efficiency and safety in asthma and allergy.

In conclusion, this Special Issue represents a novel and interesting view on asthma research. However, further studies elucidating the complex mechanisms of asthma (particularly non-T2) will be of great importance. Furthermore, the newly proposed asthma therapies require validation in different phenotypes and endotypes of the disease.

Author Contributions: Conceptualization, S.B.-S.; methodology, S.B.-S. and B.J.; writing—original draft preparation, S.B.-S.; writing—review and editing S.B.-S. and B.J.; supervision, S.B.-S. All authors have read and agreed to the published version of the manuscript.

Conflicts of Interest: The authors declare no conflict of interest.

References

1. Schindler, V.E.M.; Alhamdan, F.; Preußer, C.; Hintz, L.; Alhamwe, B.A.; Nist, A.; Stiewe, T.; von Strandmann, E.P.; Potaczek, D.P.; Thölken, C.; et al. Side-Directed Release of Differential Extracellular Vesicle-Associated MicroRNA Profiles from Bronchial Epithelial Cells of Healthy and Asthmatic Subjects. *Biomedicines* **2022**, *10*, 622. [CrossRef]
2. Ramakrishnan, R.K.; Bajbouj, K.; Guimei, M.; Rawat, S.S.; Kalaji, Z.; Hachim, M.Y.; Mahboub, B.; Ibrahim, S.M.; Hamoudi, R.; Halwani, R.; et al. Bcl10 Regulates Lipopolysaccharide-Induced Pro-Fibrotic Signaling in Bronchial Fibroblasts from Severe Asthma Patients. *Biomedicines* **2022**, *10*, 1716. [CrossRef] [PubMed]

3. Bazan-Socha, S.; Wójcik, K.; Olchawa, M.; Sarna, T.; Pięta, J.; Jakieła, B.; Soja, J.; Okoń, K.; Zarychta, J.; Zaręba, L.; et al. Increased Oxidative Stress in Asthma—Relation to Inflammatory Blood and Lung Biomarkers and Airway Remodeling Indices. *Biomedicines* **2022**, *10*, 1499. [CrossRef] [PubMed]
4. Currie, C.; Framroze, B.; Singh, D.; Lea, S.; Bjerknes, C.; Hermansen, E. Assessing the Anti-Inflammatory Effects of an Orally Dosed Enzymatically Liberated Fish Oil in a House Dust Model of Allergic Asthma. *Biomedicines* **2022**, *10*, 2574. [CrossRef] [PubMed]
5. Lin, C.H.; Li, Y.R.; Kor, C.T.; Lin, S.H.; Ji, B.C.; Lin, M.T.; Chai, W.H. The Mediating Effect of Cytokines on the Association between Fungal Sensitization and Poor Clinical Outcome in Asthma. *Biomedicines* **2022**, *10*, 1452. [CrossRef]
6. Nakagome, K.; Matsushita, S.; Nagata, M. Neutrophilic Inflammation in Severe Asthma. *Int. Arch. Allergy Immunol.* **2012**, *158* (Suppl. S1), 96–102. [CrossRef]
7. Kwak, D.-W.; Park, D.; Kim, J.-H. Leukotriene B4 Receptor 2 Mediates the Production of G-CSF That Plays a Critical Role in Steroid-Resistant Neutrophilic Airway Inflammation. *Biomedicines* **2022**, *10*, 2979. [CrossRef]
8. Mormile, I.; Granata, F.; Detoraki, A.; Pacella, D.; Della Casa, F.; De Rosa, F.; Romano, A.; de Paulis, A.; Rossi, F.W. Predictive Response to Immunotherapy Score: A Useful Tool for Identifying Eligible Patients for Allergen Immunotherapy. *Biomedicines* **2022**, *10*, 971. [CrossRef] [PubMed]
9. Patel, K.; Peebles, R.S. Prostacyclin Regulation of Allergic Inflammation. *Biomedicines* **2022**, *10*, 2862. [CrossRef] [PubMed]
10. Moncada, S.; Gryglewski, R.; Bunting, S.; Vane, J.R. An Enzyme Isolated from Arteries Transforms Prostaglandin Endoperoxides to an Unstable Substance That Inhibits Platelet Aggregation. *Nature* **1976**, *263*, 663–665. [CrossRef] [PubMed]
11. Calzetta, L.; Aiello, M.; Frizzelli, A.; Pistocchini, E.; Ritondo, B.L.; Rogliani, P.; Chetta, A. Investigational Treatments in Phase I and II Clinical Trials: A Systematic Review in Asthma. *Biomedicines* **2022**, *10*, 2330. [CrossRef] [PubMed]

Disclaimer/Publisher's Note: The statements, opinions and data contained in all publications are solely those of the individual author(s) and contributor(s) and not of MDPI and/or the editor(s). MDPI and/or the editor(s) disclaim responsibility for any injury to people or property resulting from any ideas, methods, instructions or products referred to in the content.

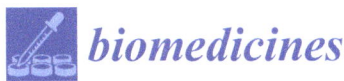 *biomedicines*

Systematic Review

Investigational Treatments in Phase I and II Clinical Trials: A Systematic Review in Asthma

Luigino Calzetta [1,*], Marina Aiello [1], Annalisa Frizzelli [1], Elena Pistocchini [2], Beatrice Ludovica Ritondo [2], Paola Rogliani [2] and Alfredo Chetta [1]

[1] Respiratory Disease and Lung Function Unit, Department of Medicine and Surgery, University of Parma, 43126 Parma, Italy
[2] Unit of Respiratory Medicine, Department of Experimental Medicine, University of Rome "Tor Vergata", 00133 Rome, Italy
* Correspondence: luigino.calzetta@unipr.it

Citation: Calzetta, L.; Aiello, M.; Frizzelli, A.; Pistocchini, E.; Ritondo, B.L.; Rogliani, P.; Chetta, A. Investigational Treatments in Phase I and II Clinical Trials: A Systematic Review in Asthma. *Biomedicines* **2022**, *10*, 2330. https://doi.org/10.3390/biomedicines10092330

Academic Editor: Stanislawa Bazan-Socha

Received: 27 July 2022
Accepted: 14 September 2022
Published: 19 September 2022

Publisher's Note: MDPI stays neutral with regard to jurisdictional claims in published maps and institutional affiliations.

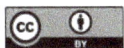

Copyright: © 2022 by the authors. Licensee MDPI, Basel, Switzerland. This article is an open access article distributed under the terms and conditions of the Creative Commons Attribution (CC BY) license (https://creativecommons.org/licenses/by/4.0/).

Abstract: Inhaled corticosteroids (ICS) remain the mainstay of asthma treatment, along with bronchodilators serving as control agents in combination with ICS or reliever therapy. Although current pharmacological treatments improve symptom control, health status, and the frequency and severity of exacerbations, they do not really change the natural course of asthma, including disease remission. Considering the highly heterogeneous nature of asthma, there is a strong need for innovative medications that selectively target components of the inflammatory cascade. The aim of this review was to systematically assess current investigational agents in Phase I and II randomised controlled trials (RCTs) over the last five years. Sixteen classes of novel therapeutic options were identified from 19 RCTs. Drugs belonging to different classes, such as the anti-interleukin (IL)-4Rα inhibitors, anti-IL-5 monoclonal antibodies (mAbs), anti-IL-17A mAbs, anti-thymic stromal lymphopoietin (TSLP) mAbs, epithelial sodium channel (ENaC) inhibitors, bifunctional M_3 receptor muscarinic antagonists/β_2-adrenoceptor agonists (MABAs), and anti-Fel d 1 mAbs, were found to be effective in the treatment of asthma, with lung function being the main assessed outcome across the RCTs. Several novel investigational molecules, particularly biologics, seem promising as future disease-modifying agents; nevertheless, further larger studies are required to confirm positive results from Phase I and II RCTs.

Keywords: asthma; efficacy; investigational; Phase I; Phase II; RCT

1. Introduction

The 2022 Global Initiative for Asthma (GINA) report [1] describes asthma as a heterogeneous disease, often characterised by chronic airway inflammation, with a history of respiratory symptoms, including wheeze, shortness of breath, chest tightness, and cough that vary over time and in intensity, along with variable expiratory airflow limitation.

The long-term goals of asthma management are to achieve symptom control, reduce the risk of exacerbations and mortality, preserve lung function, and minimise drug-related side effects [1]. The stepwise approach used for pharmacological treatment in asthma mandates an iterative cycle of assessment, adjustment of pharmacological and nonpharmacological treatment, and review of the therapeutic response [1].

Over the last 30 years, inhaled corticosteroids (ICS) have been the mainstay of asthma treatment, with the long-acting β_2-adrenoceptor agonist (LABA) formoterol/ICS combination serving as the preferred controller and/or reliever therapy, depending on asthma severity [2]. Nevertheless, this therapeutic option has become increasingly unattractive due to its inability to alter the natural course of the disease, including asthma progression [3]. Although ICS are clinically efficacious in most asthmatics, a considerable subset of patients (3–10%) remain uncontrolled despite optimal therapeutic adherence and proper inhaler technique [4]. Even after using the highest dosage of ICS, such individuals do not achieve control over their symptoms, and often need to step up to treatment with oral corticosteroids (OCS) in order to avert future episodes of life-threatening exacerbations [5].

This variability in the therapeutic response is the result of the highly heterogeneous nature of asthma [6] in terms of pathogenesis, disease severity, and outcomes [7]. Asthma is nowadays referred to as an umbrella diagnosis encompassing a plethora of endotypes and clinical phenotypes that vary from mild to severe forms [8].

More recently, the management of asthma has evolved from a blockbuster approach of "one size fits all" to a more personalised one, which treats the patient rather than the disease. In the early 2000s, the introduction of biological therapies directed towards specific inflammatory pathways advanced the improvement of asthma outcomes, initially with the anti-IgE monoclonal antibody (mAb) omalizumab [9], followed 10 years later by the approval of the mAbs anti-interleukin (IL)-5 mepolizumab and reslizumab, and the anti-IL-5Rα benralizumab [10]. The newest treatment options for severe uncontrolled asthma include the mAbs anti-IL-4/IL-13 dupilumab [11] and the anti-thymic stromal lymphopoietin (TSLP) tezepelumab [12]. Such mAbs have noteworthy properties, reducing asthma exacerbations with an OCS sparing effect [10].

In recent years, a lot of effort has been put into the development of a more personalised approach [13]. The ability to target specific inflammatory mediators and cellular pathways via highly selective therapeutic agents has progressively revolutionised the treatment of a complex, heterogeneous disorder such as asthma [14]. Although current medications may improve symptom control, QoL, and the frequency and severity of exacerbations, they do not really induce asthma remission [3].

Therefore, the aim of this review was to systematically assess the investigational agents in Phase I and II under development in the last five years, in order to understand whether there is some emerging drug and/or formulation that might be developed in the future for effective treatment of asthmatic patients.

2. Materials and Methods

2.1. Review Question

The question of this systematic review was to assess whether some of the current investigational agents in Phase I and II clinical trials (CTs) might be suitable for effective treatment of asthmatic patients.

2.2. Search Strategy

The protocol of this synthesis of the current literature has been registered to the international prospective register of systematic reviews (PROSPERO, Protocol ID: CRD42022336605), and performed in agreement with the Preferred Reporting Items for Systematic Reviews and Meta-Analyses Protocols (PRISMA-P) [15], with the relative flow diagram reported in Figure 1. This study satisfied all the recommended items reported by the PRISMA 2020 checklist [16].

The PICO (Patient problem, Intervention, Comparison, and Outcome) framework was applied to develop the literature search strategy and question, as previously reported [17]. Namely, the "Patient problem" included asthmatic patients; the "Intervention" regarded investigational agents in Phase I and II CTs; the "Comparison" was performed with respect to placebo (PCB) and/or active comparators; the assessed "Outcomes" were lung function, symptoms control, blood eosinophil count (BEC), fractioned exhaled nitric oxide (FENO), exacerbations and hospitalisations, the use of rescue medications, and quality of life (QoL).

A comprehensive literature search was performed for Phase I and II CTs, written in English and investigating the impact of investigational treatments in patients with asthma. The search was performed in ClinicalTrials.gov in order to provide relevant studies available within the past 5 years (from May 2017 to May 2022).

The term "asthma" was searched for the disease, "Interventional Studies (Clinical Trials)" was selected for the study type, "Terminated" and "Completed" were chosen for the recruitment status, and "Early Phase I", "Phase I", and "Phase II" were selected in the Additional Criteria of the Advanced Search in the ClinicalTrials.org database.

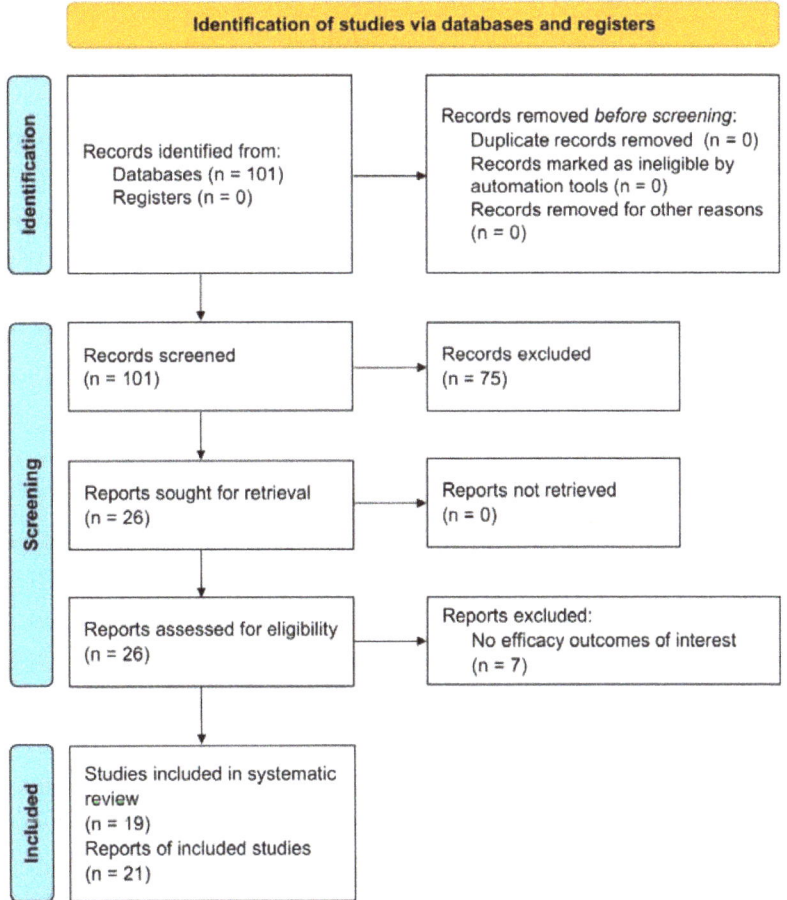

Figure 1. PRISMA 2020 flow diagram for the identification of the RCTs included in the qualitative and quantitative syntheses. PRISMA: Preferred Reporting Items for Systematic Reviews and Meta-Analyses; RCT: randomised controlled trial.

2.3. Study Selection

Randomised controlled trials (RCTs) reporting results concerning the efficacy profile of investigational treatments vs. PCB and/or active comparators were included in the systematic review.

Two reviewers independently checked the relevant studies identified from ClinicalTrials.gov. The studies were selected in agreement with previously mentioned criteria, and any difference in opinion regarding eligibility was resolved by consensus.

2.4. Data Extraction

Data from included studies were extracted and checked for study references, a NCT number identifier, study duration, treatments and comparators with doses and regimen of administration, number and characteristics of analysed patients, age, gender, smoking habit, forced expiratory volume in 1 s (FEV_1), peak expiratory flow (PEF), Asthma Control

Questionnaire (ACQ) score and other outcomes related to the impact on symptoms, BEC, FENO, asthma exacerbations, hospital admissions, rescue medication use, Asthma QoL Questionnaire (AQLQ) score, St George's Respiratory Questionnaire (SGRQ) score, and study quality assessment via the Jadad Score [18] and Cochrane Risk of Bias 2 (RoB 2) [19].

2.5. Endpoints

The co-primary endpoints of this systematic review were the impact of investigational treatments on lung function and symptoms control.

The secondary endpoints were the impact of investigational treatments on blood eosinophil count, FENO, exacerbations and hospitalisations, the use of rescue medications, and QoL.

2.6. Strategy for Data Synthesis

Data from original papers were extracted and reported via qualitative synthesis, and the statistical significance was set at $p < 0.05$.

2.7. Quality Score

The summary of the risk of bias for each included randomised trial was analysed via the Jadad score [18] and Cochrane RoB 2 [19]. The weighted assessment of the overall risk of bias was analysed via the Cochrane RoB 2 [19] using the robvis visualisation software [20,21]. The Jadad score, with a scale of 1–5 (with a score of 5 being the best quality), was used to assess the quality of the papers concerning the likelihood of bias related with randomisation, double blinding, withdrawals, and dropouts [18]. Studies were considered of low quality at Jadad score < 3, of medium quality at Jadad score = 3, and of high quality at Jadad score > 3. The weighted assessment of the risk of bias was analysed via the Cochrane RoB 2 tool [19] by using the robvis visualisation software [20,21].

Two reviewers independently assessed the quality of individual studies, and any difference in opinion about the quality score was resolved by consensus.

3. Results

3.1. Study Characteristics

Of the 101 records identified in the ClinicalTrials.gov database, 75 documents were excluded due to inconsistency between the study title and the PICO framework or because no results were available. Among the remaining CTs, 19 RCTs were deemed eligible for the systematic review.

Study results for seven RCTs [22–29] were retrieved from ClinicalTrials.gov, results for five RCTs [30–39] were published in full text articles, and data for two RCTs [40–43] were obtained through the European Union (EU) Clinical Trial Register. Results for two RCTs [44–47] were available only from conference abstracts or posters, data for one RCT [48–50] were retrieved from both the EU Clinical Trial Register and abstract, and for another RCT, they were retrieved from both ClinicalTrials.gov and the abstract [51,52]. Results for one RCT [53,54] were provided on the pharmaceutical company's website. The main characteristics of the studies included in the systematic review are reported in Table 1.

Table 1. Characteristics of the studies included in the systematic review.

Study and Year	ClinicalTrials.gov Identifier and/or Company ID	Class of Drug	Study Characteristics	Treatment Duration (wks)	Number of Analysed Patients	Drugs, Doses, and Regimen of Administration	Comparator	Route of Administration	Inhaler Device (Brand)	Patients' Characteristics	Age (Years)	Male (%)	Current Smokers (%)	Post Bronchodilator FEV$_1$ (% Predicted)	Investigated Outcome	Jadad Score
Moss et al., 2022 LEDA [...]	NCT03608576	DP$_2$ antagonist	Phase IIb, multicentre, randomised, PCB-controlled, double-blind parallel-group study	24	481	Standard of care treatment + GB001 20 mg, 40 mg, 60 mg QD	Standard of care treatment + PCB	GB001 and PCB PO	NA	Moderate to severe eosinophilic asthma (pre-bronchodilator FEV$_1$ ≤ 85% predicted and airway reversibility or AHR; peripheral blood eosinophil count > 250 cells/μL)	51.8	35.8	0.0	NA	FEV$_1$, PEF, ACQ, symptoms control, and exacerbations	3
Singh et al., 2022 [...]	NCT03287310	Anti-IL-5 mAb	Phase I, multicentre, randomised, PCB-controlled, double-blind parallel-group study	1 day	48	As-needed SABA and stable low to moderate dose of ICS or ICS/LABA + single dose of depemokimab (GSK3511294) 2 mg, 10 mg, 30 mg, 100, 300 mg	As-needed SABA and stable low-to-moderate dose of ICS or stable low-to-moderate dose of ICS/LABA + PCB	SABA, ICS/LABA, ICS-oral inhalation; depemokimab: SC	NA	Mild to moderate asthma (pre-bronchodilator FEV$_1$ ≥ 60% predicted, ACT score ≥19, and blood eosinophil count of ≥200 cells/μL)	44.0	95.8	0.0	81.0	FEV$_1$ and eosinophil count	5
Cass et al., 2021 [...]	NCT02715570	Antifungal triazole	Phase I, single centre, two-part randomised, PCB-controlled, single-blind crossover study	1 day	9	Single dose of PC945 5 mg	PCB	Oral inhalation	NA	Mild asthma	37.7	66.7	NA	NA	FEV$_1$	2
Chupp et al., 2021 GRANIT [...]	NCT03622112	ScRM	Phase IIb, multicentre, randomised, PCB-controlled, double-blind parallel-group study	12	805	Velsecorat (AZD7594) 50 μg, 90 μg, 180 μg, 360 μg, 720 μg QD	FF (100 μg QD); PCB	Oral inhalation	DPI (NA)	Asthma (patients who remain symptomatic on low dose BUD [200 μg BID in Europe and 180 μg BID in US]	53.2	42.0	NA	NA	FEV$_1$, PEF, ACQ, symptoms control, F$_E$NO, rescue medication use, and exacerbations	3
De Gaix et al., 2021 [...]	NCT03838731	Anti-Fel d 1 mAb cocktail	Phase II, single-centre, randomised, PCB-controlled, parallel-group study	1 day	56	Single dose of REGN1908-1909 600 mg	PCB	SC	NA	Mild asthma with cat allergy	29.3	37.5	NA	NA	FEV$_1$	3
Siddiqui et al., 2021 EXHALE [...]	NCT04046939	Synthetic aminobenzothiazole	Phase II, multicentre, randomised, PCB-controlled, double-blind parallel-group study	12	103	Dexpramipexole (KNS-760704) 37.5 mg, 75 mg, 150 mg BID	PCB	PO	NA	Moderate to severe eosinophilic asthma (FEV$_1$ ≤ 80% predicted and bronchodilator FEV$_1$ reversibility ≥ 12% and ≥200 mL)	45.3	47.6	0.0	NA	FEV$_1$, ACQ, eosinophilic count, F$_E$NO, and AQLQ	3

Table 1. Cont.

Study and Year	ClinicalTrials.gov Identifier and/or Company ID	Study Characteristics	Treatment Duration (wks)	Number of Analysed Patients	Drugs, Doses, and Regimen of Administration	Comparator	Route of Administration	Inhaler Device (Brand)	Patients' Characteristics	Age (Years)	Male (%)	Current Smokers (%)	Post Bronchodilator FEV$_1$ (% Predicted)	Investigated Outcome	Jadad Score
Wechsler et al., 2021 [..]	NCT03387852	Phase II, multicentre, randomised, PCB-controlled, double-blind parallel-group study	12	296	Progressive withdrawal of background medication with medium-to-high dose FP/LABA + itepekimab (SAR440340/REGN3500) 300 mg Q2W with or without dupilumab 300 mg Q2W	Progressive withdrawal of background medication with medium-to-high dose FP/LABA + PCB or dupilumab	FP/LABA: oral inhalation; itepekimab and dupilumab: SC	NA	Moderate to severe asthma (pre-bronchodilator FEV$_1$ ≥ 50% and <85% predicted and bronchodilator FEV$_1$ reversibility ≥ 12% and >200 mL; ≥1 severe exacerbation within 12 months prior to screening; FEV$_1$ ≥ 20% reduction in response to a provocative concentration of inhaled methacholine of <8 mg/mL within 12 months prior to screening)	49.1	36.0	0.0	NA	FEV$_1$, ACQ, symptoms control, eosinophil count, and F$_E$NO	3
Miller et al., 2020 [..]	NCT03257995	Phase II, multicentre, three-period complete block, randomised, PCB-controlled, double-blind crossover study	2	54	Background ICS medication and SABA + indacaterol maleate 150 μg QD	Background ICS medication and SABA + indacaterol acetate 150 μg QD; PCB	Oral inhalation	DPI (Breezhaler)	Asthma (pre-bronchodilator FEV$_1$ ≥ 50% and ≤90% predicted normal, increase in FEV$_1$ ≥ 12% and ≥ 200 mL within 30 min after administration of salbutamol 400 μg/albuterol 360 μg or equivalent dose)	48.0	33.3	0.0	86.0	FEV$_1$, PEF, and rescue medication use	3
Moermans et al., 2020 [..]	NCT03341403	Phase II/III, single-centre, randomised, PCB-controlled, double-blind parallel-group study	12	46	Stable asthma treatment + Probiotical® TID (containing Lactobacillus, Bifidobacterium, and Streptococcus thermophilus, 18 billion bacteria per pill)	Stable asthma treatment + PCB	PO	NA	Severe uncontrolled asthma (ACQ score > 1.5)	18.0–75.0	NA	NA	NA	ACQ and eosinophil count	3
NA, 2019 [.]	NCT03944707	Phase II, multicentre, randomised, PCB-controlled, subject- and investigator-blinded parallel-group study	12	76	BUD/FOR 160/9 μg BID + remibrutinib (LOU064) 100 mg QD	BUD/FOR 160/9 μg BID + PCB	BUD/FOR: oral inhalation; LOU064 and PCB: PO	BUD/FOR: DPI (NA)	Inadequately controlled asthma	50.7	34.2	NA	NA	FEV$_1$, PEF, ACQ, rescue medication use, and symptoms control	3
NA, 2019 [.]	NCT04150341	Phase II, multicentre, randomised, PCB-controlled, double-blind crossover study	2	24	TD-8236 150 μg, 1500 μg QD	PCB	Oral inhalation	DPI (NA)	Mild asthma with a known response to an allergen challenge (pre-bronchodilator FEV$_1$ ≥ 70% predicted)	42.0	70.8	NA	NA	FEV$_1$	3

Table 1. *Cont.*

Study and Year	ClinicalTrials.gov Identifier and/or Company ID	Class of Drug	Study Characteristics	Treatment Duration (wks)	Number of Analysed Patients	Drugs, Doses, and Regimen of Administration	Comparator	Route of Administration	Inhaler Device (Brand)	Patients' Characteristics	Age (Years)	Male (%)	Current Smokers (%)	Post Bronchodilator FEV$_1$ (% Predicted)	Investigated Outcome	Jadd Score
Brus et al., 2019 [..]	NCT03574805	IL-4Rα inhibitor	Phase I, multicentre, randomised, PCB-controlled, single-blind parallel-group study	≈1.4	42	AZD1402 (PRS-060) 2 mg, 6 mg, 20 mg, 60 mg BID	PCB	Oral inhalation	Nebuliser (InnoSpire Go)	Mild asthma (pre-bronchodilator FEV$_1$ ≥ 70% predicted and FEV$_1$/FVC ≥ 0.7)	28.4	88.1	0.0	NA	F$_E$NO	2
NA, 2018 [..]	NCT03393806	Anti-IL-33R mAb	Phase II, single-centre, randomised, PCB-controlled, double-blind parallel-group study	12	17	Standard of care treatment + melrilimab (GSK3772847/ CNTO7160) 10 mg/kg Q4W	Standard of care treatment + PCB	Melrilimab and PCB IV	NA	Moderate to severe asthma with allergic fungal airway disease	56.9	70.6	0.0	NA	FEV$_1$, ACQ, eosinophil count, F$_E$NO, and AQUQ	3
NA, 2018 [..]	NCT03469934	Anti-IL-33 mAb	Phase II, multicentre, randomised, PCB-controlled, parallel-group study	≈18	25	Background medication with high dose ICS/LABA + single dose of etokimab (ANB020) 300mg/100 mL	Background medication with high dose ICS/LABA + PCB	ICS/LABA oral inhalation; etokimab and PCB IV	NA	Severe eosinophilic asthma	38.5	72.0	NA	NA	FEV$_1$, eosinophil count, F$_E$NO, and exacerbations	3
NA, 2017 [..]	NCT02999686	anti-IL-17A mAb	Phase II, multicentre, randomised, PCB-controlled, subject- and investigator-blinded parallel-group study	12	118	Standard care of treatment + CJM112 200 mg QW for 4 wks, then QZW up to 12 wks	Standard care of treatment + PCB	CJM112 and PCB SC	NA	Inadequately controlled moderate to severe asthma (FEV$_1$ ≥ 40% and ≤90% predicted; ACQ score ≥ 1.5; total serum IgE <150 IU/mL; peripheral blood eosinophils < 300/μL)	56.6	39.8	NA	NA	FEV$_1$ and ACQ	3
NA, 2017 [..]	NCT02207243	Anti-IL-33R mAb	Phase IIa, multicentre, randomised, PCB-controlled, double-blind parallel-group study	16	165	FP/SAL 500/50 μg BID for 2 wks, then switch to FP 500 μg BID for 2 wks, then FP dose reduction by 50%-Q2W until discontinuation + melrilimab (GSK3772847/ CNTO7160) 10 mg/kg Q4W	FP/SAL (500/50 μg, BID) for 2 wks, then switch to FP (500 μg BID) for 2 wks, then FP dose reduction by 50%-Q2W until discontinuation + PCB	FP/SAL, FP: oral inhalation; melrilimab and PCB IV	FP/SAL, FP: DPI (Diskus)	Moderately severe asthma (bronchodilator FEV$_1$ reversibility > 12% and ≥200 mL; ACQ score ≥ 1.0 and <4.0)	52.9	28.5	0.0	NA	FEV$_1$, PEF, ACQ, symptoms control, rescue eosinophil count, F$_E$NO, exacerbations and hospitalisations, and SGRQ	3
NA, 2017 [..]	NCT03138811	Anti-TSLP mAb fragment	Phase I, multicentre, randomised, PCB-controlled, double-blind parallel-group study	12	28	Eceralimab (CSJ117) .. mg QD	PCB	Oral inhalation	DPI (PulmoSol)	Mild atopic asthma with an early and late response to a common inhaled allergen challenge	34.1	39.3	NA	NA	FEV$_1$	3

Table 1. *Cont.*

Study and Year	Class of Drug	ClinicalTrials.gov Identifier and/or Company ID	Study Characteristics	Treatment Duration (wks)	Number of Analysed Patients	Drugs, Doses, and Regimen of Administration	Comparator	Route of Administration	Inhaler Device (Brand)	Patients' Characteristics	Age (Years)	Male (%)	Current Smokers (%)	Post Bronchodilator FEV_1 (% Predicted)	Investigated Outcome	Jadad Score
NA, 2017 [..]	ENaC inhibitor	NCT02135899	Phase I, single-centre, randomised, PCB-controlled, double-blind, double-dummy crossover study	2 days	37	BI 443651 100 µg, 400 µg, 1200 µg, thrice 12 h apart	PCB	Oral inhalation	SMI (Respimat)	Mild asthma upon methacholine challenge (pre-bronchodilator $FEV_1 \geq 70\%$ predicted; $FEV_1 \geq 20\%$ reduction in response to a provocative concentration of inhaled methacholine of ≤1 mg; ACQ score < 1.5)	37.4	91.9	0.0	NA	FEV_1	3
NA, 2017 [..]	MABA	NCT03378648	Phase I/II, single-centre, randomised, PCB-controlled, double-blind, parallel-group study	1	48	CHF6366 40 µg, 80 µg, 160 µg, 240 µg QD	PCB	Oral inhalation	NA	Asthma (bronchodilator FEV_1 reversibility ≥ 12% and ≥200 mL)	38.1	64.6	NA	NA	FEV_1	3

ACQ: asthma control questionnaire; ACT: asthma control test; AHR: airway hyperresponsiveness; AQLQ: asthma quality of life questionnaire; BID: bis in die, twice daily; BTK: Bruton's tyrosine kinase; BUD: budesonide; DP2: prostaglandin D2 receptor; DPI: dry powder inhaler; ENaC: epithelial sodium channel; FENO: fractional exhaled nitric oxide; FEV_1: forced expiratory volume in the 1st second; FP: fluticasone propionate; FVC: forced vital capacity; ICS: inhaled corticosteroid; IL-n: interleukin-n; IL-nR: interleukin-n receptor; IV: intravenous; JAK: Janus kinase; LABA: long-acting β2 adrenoceptor agonist; mAb: monoclonal antibody; MABA: M₃ receptor muscarinic antagonists/β2-adrenoceptor agonist; NA: not available; PCB: placebo; PEF: peak expiratory flow; PO: oral; QD: quaque die, once daily; Q4W: once every 4 weeks; SABA: short-acting β2 agonist; SC: subcutaneous; SGRM: selective glucocorticoid receptor modulators; SMI: soft mist inhaler; SGRQ: St. George's Respiratory Questionnaire; TSLP: thymic stromal lymphopoietin; wks: weeks.

3.2. IL-4Rα Inhibitor

Antagonising the IL-4 receptor α subunit (IL-4Rα) interferes with the downstream IL-4/IL-13 signalling, which is central to the pathogenesis of asthma [55]. As a matter of fact, IL-4 regulates the proliferation and survival of T helper 2 (Th2) cells as well as immunoglobulin E (IgE) synthesis, while IL-13 is implicated as a key effector in AHR, mucus hypersecretion, ASM alterations, and subepithelial fibrosis [56].

In a Phase I RCT [46,47], mildly asthmatic patients received nebuliser treatment with the IL-4Rα inhibitor AZD1402 (PRS-060) at delivered doses of 2–60 mg twice daily (BID) to establish its efficacy profile. After a single administration, AZD1402 induced a rapid decrease in the FENO level, with a significant ($p < 0.05$) percentage reduction vs. PCB between 24.0% (95%CI 1.8–41.0) and 36.4% (95%CI 22.0–48.0) across all doses. No data are available for lung function and symptoms control [46,47].

3.3. Anti-IL-5 mAbs

Targeting BEC reduction through the inhibition of IL-5 represents an established therapeutic option in severe asthma [57]. Depemokimab (GSK3511294) is a subcutaneously administered anti-IL-5 mAb, designed for improved affinity and long-acting IL-5 suppression compared to the currently approved anti-IL-5 mAbs, and it has been evaluated in a first-in-human Phase I RCT [30,31] enrolling mild to moderate asthmatic patients with BEC $\geq$ 200 cells/µL at screening.

A single administration of depemokimab generally improved lung function parameters with an increase in the dose from 2 mg to 300 mg. Depemokimab 300 mg induced a greater improvement from baseline in FEV_1 (240 mL (95%CI 68–412)) vs. PCB (105 mL (95%CI not calculated)) and in percent predicted normal FEV_1 (7.65% (95%CI 1.76–13.54)) vs. PCB (3.85% (95%CI not calculated)). No data are available for symptoms control [30,31].

Across all doses, depemokimab markedly decreased the circulating BEC by >48.0% 24 h post-dose, and reductions of 54.0% and 53.0% were observed in patients treated, respectively, with depemokimab 100 mg and 300 mg. The duration of such marked suppression of BEC was dose dependent, and thus was maintained for longer with the increasing dose. Six months after the single-dose administration, depemokimab induced reductions in BEC of 31.0% (2 mg), 41.0% (10 mg), 72.0% (30 mg), 82.0% (100 mg), and 83.0% (300 mg) vs. PCB [30,31].

3.4. Anti-IL-17A mAbs

Increased expression of the Th17-derived cytokine IL-17A has been observed in sputum, airway tissue biopsies, and serum from asthmatic patients [58–62] and was positively associated with a more severe asthma phenotype [59,63,64] and neutrophilic inflammation [65]. Considering that Th17-high patients are less sensitive or even unresponsive to ICS [59,66] and that asthma progression differs from more treatable Th2 types of the disease [67], developing an effective therapy targeting Th17/IL-17A axis would overcome a major unmet need in severe asthma.

A Phase II RCT [22] investigated the subcutaneously administered anti-IL-17A mAb CJM112 300 mg when added to existing therapy in patients with inadequately controlled moderate to severe asthma, with low serum IgE and BEC. The effect of CJM112 treatment on trough FEV_1 was not different from PCB, but a significant ($p < 0.05$) improvement was observed in the ACQ6 score (mean difference (MD) −0.22 units (80%CI −0.41−−0.04)) and the ACQ7 score (MD −0.23 units (80%CI −0.40 to −0.06)) vs. PCB. A higher proportion of patients receiving CJM112 had a decrease of $\geq$0.5 units in the ACQ7 score compared with PCB (71.7% vs. 52.8%) [22].

3.5. Anti-IL-33 mAbs

Upon cellular damage or allergen exposure, interleukin (IL)-33 is released as an alarmin by airway epithelial cells, airway smooth muscle (ASM) cells (ASMCs), and endothelium to trigger innate and adaptive immune responses [68]. In patients affected by severe asthma refractory to steroids, IL-33 activates type 2 innate lymphoid cells (ILC2s), which may promote persistent airway eosinophilia [69]. Targeted inhibition of IL-33 receptor (IL-33R) signalling may prevent downstream production of type 2 cytokines and chemokines [70].

Two RCTs [32,33,40,41] investigated the anti-IL-33 mAbs itepekimab (SAR440340/ REGN3500) and etokimab (ANB020), and two other RCTs [23,24] assessed the efficacy of the anti-IL-33R mAb melrilimab (GSK3772847/CNTO7160).

A Phase II RCT [32,33] investigated the efficacy of subcutaneous itepekimab 300 mg administered alone or in combination with dupilumab 300 mg to patients with moderate to severe asthma, who progressively reduced and discontinued background therapy of inhaled corticosteroid/long-acting β2 adrenoceptor agonist (ICS/LABA) over 12 weeks. Itepekimab significantly ($p < 0.05$) improved trough FEV_1 compared to PCB (MD 140 mL (95%CI 10–270)) and it was as effective as dupilumab, but no improvement was seen upon treatment with the combination therapy. Itepekimab did not increase post-bronchodilator FEV_1 vs. PCB, but when combined with dupilmab, the improvement was significant ($p < 0.05$) (MD 130 mL (95%CI 10–250)) and comparable to that of dupilumab administered alone [32,33].

The percentage of patients with an event indicating a loss of asthma control was lower in the itepekimab (22.0%) and combination therapy (27.0%) groups vs. PCB (41.0%). The corresponding odds ratio (OR) for the comparison of itepekimab vs. PCB was significant ($p < 0.05$) (OR 0.42 (95%CI 0.20–0.88)) and similar to the OR for dupilumab vs. PCB; no difference was detected in the ORs for the comparison between combination therapy and PCB, itepekimab monotherapy, and dupilumab monotherapy. Itepekimab alone and combined with dupilumab significantly ($p < 0.05$) improved ACQ5 score vs. PCB (MD −0.42 units (95%CI −0.73−−0.12) and MD −0.32 units (95%CI −0.63−−0.01), respectively), and the effect was similar to that observed with dupilumab [32,33].

The BEC significantly ($p < 0.05$) decreased upon treatment with itepekimab administered alone or combined with dupilumab vs. PCB, and the effect was significantly ($p < 0.05$) different from that induced by dupilumab monotherapy, which, as expected [32], transiently induced blood eosinophilia. The FENO level was significantly ($p < 0.05$) lowered in the itepekimab group, although the magnitude of reduction was lower than that observed in the combination therapy and dupilumab groups. Patients treated with itepekimab administered alone or combined with dupilumab showed a significant ($p < 0.05$) improvement in their AQLQ score vs. PCB (MD 0.45 units (95% CI 0.14–0.77) and MD 0.43 units (95% CI 0.11–0.75), respectively), with an effect comparable to that of dupilumab [32,33].

In a Phase II RCT [40,41], a single dose of etokimab administered at 300 mg/100 mL via intravenous infusion did not improve FEV_1 compared to PCB in severe eosinophilic asthma; no data are available for symptoms control.

The reduction in peripheral BEC following etokimab treatment was similar to that observed with PCB, and no difference was detected in FENO levels. The number of asthma exacerbations experienced by patients treated with etokimab was no different from those treated with PCB [40,41].

A Phase II RCT [23] reported that intravenously administering melrilimab 10 mg/kg to patients with moderate to severe asthma and allergic fungal airway disease for 12 weeks did not improve their FEV_1 and ACQ5 score compared to PCB. No differences between melrilimab and PCB were observed with respect to the change from baseline in BEC, FENO level, and AQLQ score [23].

Another Phase II RCT [24] showed that melrilimab 10 mg/kg administered for 16 weeks to moderately severe asthmatic patients who gradually reduced and discontinued background therapy with fluticasone propionate/salmeterol (FP/SAL) 500/50 µg, did not improve trough FEV_1 and morning and evening PEF vs. PCB. The reduction in ACQ5 score was similar with both melrilimab and PCB, but the percentage of patients who experienced loss of asthma control was lower in the group treated with melrilimab (67.0%) than with PCB (81.0%). No differences between the two treatment groups were observed in the percentage of night-time awakenings due to asthma symptoms requiring rescue medication use and in the daytime asthma symptom score [24].

The effect induced on BEC and FENO level was similar in the melrilimab and PCB groups. The percentage of patients with an asthma exacerbation requiring OCS and/or hospitalisation was higher with melrilimab (13.0%) than with PCB (7.0%). No differences between the two groups were observed in terms of daily use of rescue medications and SGRQ total score [24].

3.6. Anti-TSLP mAbs

Similar to IL-33, TSLP is mainly an epithelium-derived alarmin, which plays an upstream role in the initiation of type-2-driven immune responses [71]. In asthma, the number of cells expressing TSLP messenger ribonucleic acid (mRNA) within the airway epithelium and submucosa is markedly increased compared to healthy controls [72]. In a subset of patients with severe asthma, TSLP expression remained enhanced, independent of treatment with high-dose ICS or OCS [73]. Therefore, targeting TSLP signalling represents an intriguing therapeutic strategy in asthma [74].

In a Phase I RCT [53,54] the anti-TSLP mAb fragment ecleralimab (CSJ117) 4 mg was administered via a dry powder inhaler (DPI) for 12 weeks to patients with mild atopic asthma, who exhibited an early asthmatic response (EAR) and late asthmatic response (LAR) to a common inhaled allergen. Ecleralimab did not induce an attenuation in the EAR, as documented by the maximum percentage fall in FEV_1 or as time-adjusted area under the curve (AUC), and numerically increased the minimum of the absolute in FEV_1 compared to PCB. During the LAR, ecleralimab significantly ($p < 0.05$) reduced the maximum percentage decrease in FEV_1 (MD -8.42% (90%CI -15.66---1.18)) from pre-allergen inhalation challenge and the time-adjusted AUC fall in FEV_1 (MD -7.18% (90%CI -11.92---2.44)), compared to PCB. Patients in the ecleralimab group showed a strong trend towards a significant ($p = 0.05$) increase in the minimum absolute FEV_1 during LAR vs. PCB (MD 0.27% (90%CI 0.00–0.55)) [53,54]. No data are available for symptoms control [53,54].

3.7. LABAs

The latest GINA report recommends treating patients with inadequately controlled asthma with a triple combination of indacaterol acetate/glycopyrronium bromide/mometasone [1]. Several studies provided evidence that indacaterol maleate is potent and safe in asthmatic patients [75–78].

A Phase I RCT [34,35] compared the efficacy of the maleate salt with the acetate salt of indacaterol 150 μg vs. PCB in patients with asthma. Indacaterol maleate significantly ($p < 0.001$) improved trough FEV_1 of 186.0 mL (95%CI 129.0–243.0), FEV_1 AUC0-4h by 248.0 mL (95%CI 186.0–310.0), and PEF of 33.0 L/min (95%CI 25.6–40.3) vs. PCB, and it was as effective as indacaterol acetate. No data are available for symptoms control. Rescue medication use was significantly ($p < 0.01$) reduced with both indacaterol salts of 0.42 puffs/day vs. PCB [34,35].

3.8. SGRMs

Compared to conventional glucocorticoids, nonsteroidal, selective glucocorticoid receptor modulators (SGRM) preferentially favour transrepression over transactivation [79]. SGRM are designed to activate the GC receptor and suppress inflammation by inhibiting nuclear factor-kappa B (NF-kB) and activator protein 1 (AP-1), whilst inducing less GC response element (GRE)-driven adverse effects [80].

Phase IIb GRANIT RCT [48–50] enrolled patients with inadequately controlled asthma on low-dose BUD to orally receive the SGRM velsecorat (AZD7594) 50–720 μg vs. PCB or open-label fluticasone furoate (FF) 100 μg over 12 weeks. Velsecorat dose-dependently improved trough FEV_1 over the entire treatment period. When administered at doses of 320 μg and 720 μg, velsecorat induced a trend towards a significant improvement in trough FEV_1 compared to PCB, which was numerically lower compared to the effect of

FF vs. PCB. Velsecorat 180–720 μg significantly ($p < 0.05$) improved morning PEF vs. PCB from 9.12 L/min (95%CI 0.20–18.05) to 16.60 L/min (95%CI 8.03–25.17)). Evening PEF was significantly ($p < 0.05$) increased with velsecorat 360 μg and 720 μg vs. PCB, respectively, by 10.26 L/min (95%CI 1.46–19.06) and 11.99 L/min (95%CI 3.57–20.42). The effect of velsecorat on PEF was comparable to that induced by FF vs. PCB [48–50].

Velsecorat administered at doses 90–720 μg significantly ($p < 0.05$) improved the ACQ5 score vs. PCB, by inducing a reduction between −0.19 units (95%CI −0.37–−0.02) and −0.27 units (95%CI −0.43–−0.10), and it was as effective as FF vs. PCB. Velsecorat 50 μg and 180–720 μg significantly ($p < 0.05$) reduced the daily asthma symptom score between −0.14 units (95%CI −0.26 ¬− −0.02) and −0.23 units (95%CI −0.35–−0.11) and improved the percentage of symptom-free days between 8.61% (95%CI 0.30–16.91) and 11.34% (95%CI 2.77–19.91) vs. PCB, to a similar extent as FF. The percentage of asthma control days significantly ($p < 0.05$) increased with velsecorat 50 μg, 360 μg, and 720 μg over the treatment period between 8.62% (95%CI 0.49–16.75) and 10.07% (95%CI 1.46–18.67), similar to FF [48–50].

At doses 50–180 μg, the effect of velsecorat on FENO values was not different to PCB, but when administered at 360 μg and 720 μg, the improvement was significant ($p < 0.05$) vs. PCB (MD 0.81 ppb (95%CI 0.69–0.95) and 0.65 ppb (95%CI 0.56–0.76), respectively), and comparable to that induced by FF vs. PCB [48–50].

Only velsecorat 360 μg significantly ($p < 0.05$) increased the percentage of rescue-free days by 11.79% (95%CI 1.49–22.09) vs. PCB, an effect that was superior to that of FF vs. PCB. Rescue medication use was significantly ($p < 0.05$) lowered with velsecorat 50 μg, 360 μg, and 720 μg vs. PCB (MD between −0.24 puffs (95%CI −0.43–−0.05) and −0.31 puffs (95%CI −0.49–−0.13), an effect similar to that induced by FF vs. PCB [48–50].

Velsecorat 50–720 μg significantly ($p < 0.05$) delayed the time to recurrent CompEx event (a composite endpoint combining severe asthma exacerbations and diary events) vs. PCB (hazard ratio (HR) between 0.20 (95%CI 0.100.38) and 0.58 (95%CI 0.26–0.95)). When administered at doses of 50 μg, 180 μg, 360 μg, and 720 μg, velsecorat significantly ($p < 0.05$) reduced the annualised CompEx event rate vs. PCB (MD between 0.11 (95%CI 0.04–0.25) and 0.44 (95%CI 0.20–0.94)), while at 90 μg, velsecorat induced a strong trend towards a significant reduction in the rate vs. PCB. Overall, no comparative analysis has been performed in the study between velsecorat and FF [48–50].

3.9. MABAs

Bifunctional M_3 receptor muscarinic antagonists/β_2-adrenoceptor agonists (MABAs) are dimeric molecules that simultaneously block M_3 muscarinic receptors while activating β2 receptors, and thus may be readily co-formulated with anti-inflammatory agents [81,82], simplifying dosing schedules and improving patient adherence to medication. A Phase I/II RCT [42,43] reported that in asthmatic patients, the inhaled MABA CHF6366 significantly ($p < 0.05$) improved the change from pre-dose in FEV_1 on day 1 when administered at 160 μg, but not at 40 μg, 80 μg, and 240 μg, compared to the effect induced by PCB, while no difference was detected in the change from pre-dose in FEV_1 on day 7; no data are available for symptoms control [42,43].

3.10. DP$_2$ Antagonists

Evidence suggests that preventing the activation of the prostaglandin D2 receptor (DP2) pathway improves symptoms of asthma and pulmonary function, and impairs any change in eosinophil shape, while indirectly inducing a reduction in the number of exacerbations in severe asthmatic patients [83].

The LEDA Phase IIb RCT [36,37] demonstrated that the DP2 antagonist GB001 given orally at 20 mg, 40 mg, and 60 mg, in addition to the standard of care therapy, induced an effect on FEV_1, PEF, and ACQ5 that was comparable to PCB in moderate to severe asthmatic patients with a BEC of ≥250 cells/μL. Across all doses, GB001 numerically reduced the odds of asthma worsening vs. PCB, with no dose–response effect; subgroup analysis based on baseline BEC and/or FENO did not indicate greater treatment efficacy with higher values. GB001 20 mg and 60 mg induced a significant ($p < 0.05$) delay in the time to first asthma worsening compared to PCB (HR 0.72 (95% CI 0.52–0.995) and HR 0.70 (95% CI, 0.51–0.97), respectively), while GB001 40 mg induced a numerical delay vs. PCB. Treatment with GB001 20 mg, 40 mg, and 60 mg significantly ($p < 0.05$) reduced the annualised rate of asthma worsening vs. PCB (RR 0.56 (95% CI 0.39–0.80), RR 0.65 (95% CI 0.46–0.93), and RR 0.68 (95% CI 0.48–0.96), respectively) [36,37].

There was a numerical reduction in the annualised rate of severe asthma exacerbations compared to PCB [36,37].

3.11. Selective BTK Inhibitors

Bruton's tyrosine kinase (BTK) is a member of the Tec family of tyrosine kinases involved in the high-affinity receptor for IgE (FcεRI)-dependent mast cell production of cytokines and degranulation [84,85], and in the IgE-mediated activation of human basophils [86]. BTK inhibitors could be useful to treat pathological mast cell responses of asthma [87].

A Phase II RCT [25] reported that orally administering remibrutinib (LOU064) 100 mg to inadequately controlled asthmatic patients did not induce an improvement in trough FEV_1 and in morning and evening PEF compared to PCB. Changes in the ACQ5 score, in the asthma symptom score, and in the number of puffs of SABA taken daily were not different between remibrutinib and PCB groups [25].

3.12. ENaC Inhibitors

An imbalance in ion transport across the airway epithelium has been implicated in asthma pathogenesis. Dysfunctions in the cystic fibrosis transmembrane conductance regulator and epithelial sodium channel (ENaC) cause changes in the airway surface liquid permeation, leading to modifications of mucus rheological properties and impairment. Blocking ENaC may reduce airway water reabsorption and increase mucus moist, therefore it is considered a potential target for the treatment of asthma [88].

A Phase I RCT [26] investigated the ENaC inhibitor BI 443651 100 μg, 400 μg, and 1200 μg administered via soft mist inhaler (SMI) to patients with mild asthma following a bolus methacholine (MCh) challenge. In the single-blind, double-dummy Part 1 of the RCT, no difference was detected between BI 443651 and PCB in terms of absolute change from baseline in maximum FEV_1 reduction. In the double-blind, double-dummy Part 2 of the RCT, only BI 443651 administered at 1200 μg significantly ($p < 0.05$) improved the maximum FEV_1 reduction vs. PCB (MD −157 mL (90%CI −266–−47)). No data are available for symptoms control [26].

3.13. Pan-JAK Inhibitors

According to in vitro studies performed on inflammatory cells isolated from asthmatic patients, pan-JAK inhibitors reduced cytokine levels and showed an additive effect on lymphocyte inhibition when combined with ICS [89]. Lung inflammation was improved upon treatment with pan-JAK inhibitors in animal models of airway inflammation [90–92].

A Phase II RCT [27] reported that the pan-JAK inhibitor TD-8236 administered at 150 μg and 1500 μg via DPI did not improve the FEV_1 AUC from 3 to 8 h and the maximum percentage decline in FEV_1 from 3 to 8 h following inhaled allergen challenge compared to PCB. No data are available for symptoms control [27].

3.14. Anti-Fel d 1 mAbs

The secretoglobulin Fel d 1 is the major cat allergen, eliciting IgE-mediated allergic symptoms in up to 95% of individuals with a cat allergy [93,94], such as sneezing, runny nose, nasal obstruction, conjunctivitis, and/or asthma [95]. REGN1908-1909 is an anti-Fel d 1 cocktail of two IgG4 mAbs, REGN1908 and REGN1909, with a high affinity for and noncompetitive binding to distinct epitopes of Fel d 1, which prevents the allergen cross-linking of IgE-FcεRI complexes on mast cells and basophils and the consequent degranulation and release of inflammatory mediators [96,97].

A Phase II RCT [51,52] investigated whether a single dose of the subcutaneously administered REGN1908-1909 600 mg effectively reduced bronchoconstriction in mild asthmatic patients with a cat allergy for up to 3 months following cat-allergen exposure. REGN1908-1909 significantly ($p < 0.05$) increased the median time to EAR (defined as the time leading to a $\geq 20\%$ reduction in FEV_1) vs. PCB on day 8 (HR 0.36 (95%CI 0.17–0.77)), day 29 (HR 0.24 (95%CI 0.12–0.48)), day 57 (HR 0.45 (95%CI 0.22–0.89)), and day 85 (HR 0.27 (95%CI 0.13–0.56)). REGN1908-1909 significantly ($p < 0.05$) improved FEV_1 AUC from 0 to 2 h vs. PCB at day 8 (MD 13.56% (95%CI 6.35–20.77)), at day 29 (MD 16.21% (95%CI 6.18–26.24)), at day 57 (MD 12.30% (95%CI 2.40–22.20)), and day 85 (MD 12.54% (95%CI 3.43–21.65)). No data are available for symptoms control [51,52].

3.15. Synthetic Amino-Benzothiazoles

The synthetic amino-benzothiazole dexpramipexole was first developed as a treatment for amyotrophic lateral sclerosis (ALS) and during the development program, a marked targeted depletion of BEC was observed in ALS patients; therefore, dexpramipexole holds promise for asthma and eosinophil-associated diseases [98].

In the EXHALE Phase II RCT [28,29], dexpramipexole (KNS-760704) orally administered at 37.5 mg, 75 mg, and 150 mg BID for 12 weeks was investigated in patients with poorly controlled moderate to severe eosinophilic asthma with an absolute BEC of ≥ 300 cells/μL. No differences were observed between dexpramipexole 37.5 mg and 75 mg and PCB in trough FEV_1 and post-bronchodilator FEV_1, while dexpramipexole 150 mg showed a numerical improvement in both outcomes vs. PCB at the end of the treatment period, and a significant increase in trough FEV_1 at weeks 16/18 vs. PCB. The effect of treatment on the ACQ6 score was similar to that observed in the PCB group [28,29].

Dexpramipexole 37.5 mg, 75 mg, and 150 mg significantly ($p < 0.05$) reduced BEC vs. PCB (ratio to PCB of 0.45 (95%CI 0.23–0.87), 0.34 (95%CI 0.18–0.65), and 0.23 (95%CI 0.120.43), respectively). The FENO level numerically reduced upon treatment with dexpramipexole vs. PCB across all doses. No differences were observed between the treatment and PCB groups in terms of a change in AQLQ score [28,29]

3.16. Antifungal Triazoles

Respiratory fungal infections complicate lung diseases and, particularly in severe asthma, up to 70.0% of patients are sensitised to at least one fungal allergen [5,99,100]. In a Phase I RCT [38,39], a single dose of inhaled PC945 5 mg did not induce a change in FEV_1 (defined as >15.0% change from baseline, measured 10 min after receiving PCB) in mild asthmatic patients, and no acute bronchospasm was observed.

3.17. Probiotics

Probiotics exhibited anti-inflammatory properties to modulate immune functions and were characterised by good tolerance and safety [44]. According to preliminary results of a Phase II/III RCT [44,45] in severe uncontrolled asthma, a change from baseline in ACQ score was similar in patients receiving the orally administered Probiotical® and PCB; no data are available on lung function. A significant ($p < 0.05$) reduction in the percentage of sputum eosinophils was observed between baseline and after 3 months of therapy in the Probiotical® group (0.5% (95%CI 0.0–2.3) vs. 0.1% (95%CI 0.0–0.5)) compared to the PCB group (4.5% (95%CI 1.5–9.3) vs. 2.4% (95%CI 1.2–9.4)) [44,45].

3.18. Risk of Bias

The traffic light plot for the assessment of each included RCT is reported in Figure 2A, and the weighted plot for the assessment of the overall risk of bias by domains is shown in Figure 2B.

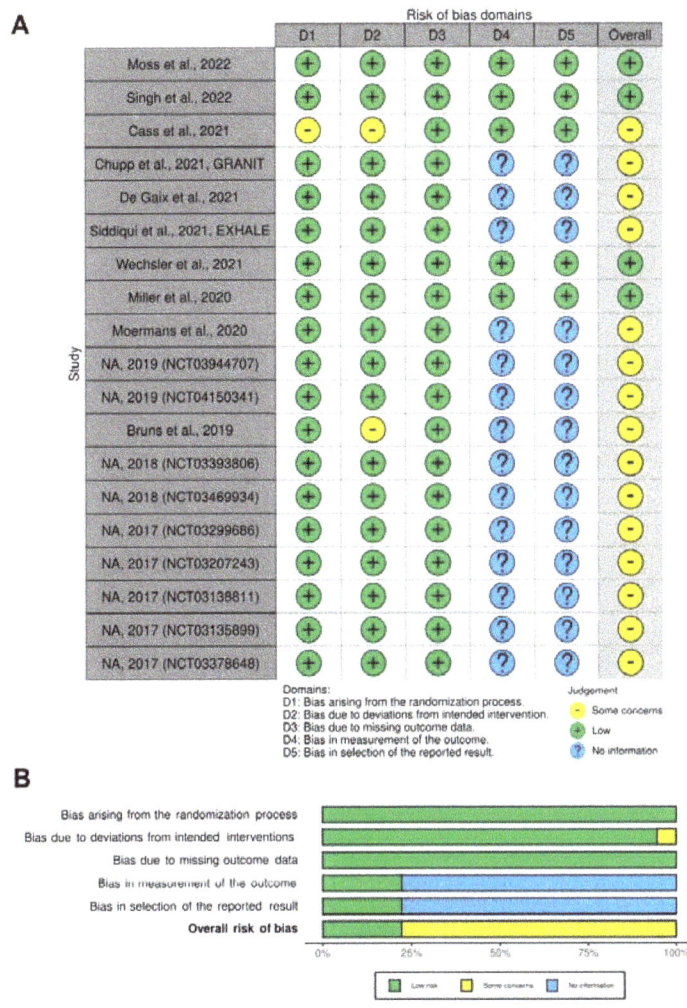

Figure 2. Assessment of the risk of bias via the Cochrane RoB 2 tool displayed by means of a traffic light plot of the risk of bias of the included RCTs (**A**), and weighted plot for the distribution of the overall risk of bias within each bias domain via the Cochrane RoB 2 tool (**B**) (n = 18 RCTs). Traffic light plot reports five risk of bias domains: D1, bias arising from the randomisation process; D2, bias due to deviations from intended intervention; D3, bias due to missing outcome data; D4, bias in measurement of the outcome; D5, bias in selection of the reported result. Yellow circle indicates some concerns on the risk of bias, green circle represents low risk of bias, and blue circle indicates no information. NA: not available; RCT: randomised controlled trial; RoB: risk of bias.

All of the included RCTs (100.0%) had a low risk of bias in missing outcome data. For 18 RCTs (94.7%), there was a low risk of bias for the randomisation process, and for 17 RCTs (89.5%), the bias due to deviations from intended intervention was low. For two RCTs (10.5%), there were some concerns in the domain of bias due to deviations from intended intervention, and for one RCT (5.3%) there were some concerns for the randomisation process.

For 14 RCTs (73.7%), no information was available with regard to the risk of bias in the measurement of the outcome and selection of the reported results, as no full text articles concerning the studies have been published yet.

4. Discussion

An investigational medication is defined as a drug and/or formulation that has been approved for clinical testing by either the U.S. Food and Drug Administration (FDA) or the European Medicines Agency (EMA), but has not gained marketing authorisation yet [101,102]. Over the last five years, results from 19 Phase I and II RCTs on investigational agents for the treatment of asthma reported data from sixteen classes of investigational agents. Specifically, these investigational drugs included AZD1402, BI 443651, CHF6366, CJM112, depemokimab, dexpramipexole, ecleralimab, etokimab, GB001, itepekimab, melrilimab, PC945, REGN1908-1909, remibrutinib, TD-8236, velsecorat, indacaterol acetate, and a probiotic. Overall, the quality of the studies was good, although often data were not published in full text articles; thus, scarce information was available to adequately perform the RoB assessment.

The investigational anti-IL-4Rα inhibitor AZD1402, the anti-IL-5 mAb depemokimab, the anti-IL-17A mAb CJM112, the anti-TSLP mAb ecleralimab, the ENaC inhibitor BI 443651, the MABA CHF6366, and the anti-Fel d 1 mAb REGN1908-1909 were proven effective in the treatment of asthma, although data almost exclusively regarded the assessment of lung function, and thus did not allow conclusions regarding symptoms control and the secondary endpoints of this systematic review. The effectiveness of the LABA indacaterol was confirmed even when delivered using the formulation with maleate salt, which demonstrated an effect that was comparable to the currently marketed indacaterol acetate on FEV_1, PEF, and rescue medication use reduction. Among the investigational anti-IL-33 mAbs, only itepekimab, but not etokimab and melrilimab, effectively improved asthma outcomes compared to PCB, but generally there was no further improvement observed when itepekimab was combined with dupilumab. Treatment with the SGRM velsecorat was generally superior to PCB when administered at higher doses.

Overall, investigational agents did not show superiority to active controls, with the exception of itepekimab, which significantly reduced BEC compared to dupilumab monotherapy, and velsecorat, which induced a significantly greater improvement in FEV_1 vs. PCB compared to that produced by FF vs. PCB.

The main efficacy outcome assessed by the RCTs included in this systematic review was FEV_1. In this respect, BI 443651, depemokimab, ecleralimab, indacaterol maleate, itepekimab, REGN1908-1909, and velsecorat produced a statistically significant improvement in lung function compared to PCB, thus representing promising add-on therapies for asthma in the future. It is also worth mentioning the synthetic amino-benzothiazole dexpramipexole, which was found to markedly reduce BEC across all the administered doses in patients with moderate to severe eosinophilic asthma, despite no significant improvement in lung function, relative to PCB [28,29].

The anti-IL-33 mAbs etokimab and melrilimab, the DP2 antagonist GB001, the selective BTK inhibitor remibrutinib, the pan-JAK inhibitor TD-8236, and the antifungal triazole PC945 induced an effect on lung function that was similar to PCB.

Although FEV_1 is generally recognised by the research community and regulatory agencies to be a suitable variable for airflow obstruction assessment [103], it is not the most relevant endpoint for testing investigational anti-inflammatory agents, including the DP2 antagonist GB001 and the pan-JAK inhibitor TD-8236, particularly for short-term assessment. Thus, for such treatments, other efficacy endpoints should be considered in future studies. Although probiotics utilised in dietary supplements reside in a sub-category under the general umbrella term of "foods" rather than drugs, according to both the FDA [104] and the European Food Safety Authority (EFSA) [105], the probiotic Probiotical® investigated in a Phase II RCT (NCT03341403) [44,45] for uncontrolled severe asthma was included in this systematic review and was treated as investigational agent. The hypothesis of such RCT [44,45] was that Probiotical® could have an impact in asthmatic patients who were not optimally controlled, reducing the local and systemic inflammatory state and then improving QoL and asthma control [44,45]. This hypothesis was also supported by the evidence that certain probiotic strains have anti-inflammatory and immunomodulatory effects in pre-clinical models of asthma [106,107] and RCTs of adult asthma [108,109]. Interestingly, although dietary supplements are not subjected to the pre-market approval requirement for drugs, an investigational new drug application must be submitted to the FDA if the clinical investigation is intended to evaluate whether a dietary supplement is useful in diagnosing, curing, mitigating, treating, or preventing a disease, under the Code of Federal Regulations Part 312 [110]. In contrast, in the EU, there is still no specific regulation covering probiotics, pre-biotics, synbiotics, or postbiotics, but as suggested by The International Scientific Association of Probiotics and Prebiotics consensus statement, the definition of such products requires a health benefit; thus, it is expected that the use of any of these terms would require a health claim approval [111].

In any case, the daily administration of Probiotical® showed some improvement in sputum eosinophil count after 3 months of therapy, but in agreement with the current scientific evidence, the use of probiotics as adjuvant therapy for asthma is not yet conclusive [112]. Three meta-analyses carried out to explore the potential effects of probiotics in preventing allergic diseases and asthma led to conflicting outcomes due to a high degree of heterogeneity among the studies, mostly concerning the design, the characteristics of included patients, the analysed variables, and the used probiotic strains [113–115].

The assessment of efficacy outcomes reported by the RCTs included in this systematic review indicates that not only were some of the investigational agents superior to PCB from a statistical point of view, but they also elicited clinically relevant effects compared to PCB in asthmatic patients, as reported in Table 2. As a matter of fact, itepekimab 300 mg Q2W, indacaterol maleate 150 µg QD, and velsecorat 720 µg QD overcame the Minimal Clinical Important Difference (MCID) [103] threshold for trough FEV_1 or risk of asthma exacerbation. Interestingly, velsecorat 720 µg QD, itepekimab 300 mg Q2W, and itepekimab 300 mg Q2W + dupilumab 300 mg Q2W were borderline to reach the MCID threshold for ACQ or AQLQ. Indeed, these promising results need to be confirmed by Phase III studies.

A main limitation of this systematic review is that most of the included studies (11 RCT, 57.9%) had a registry record on ClinicalTrials.gov and/or EU Clinical Trial Register but no associated publication, and thus, sponsors and principal investigators are exclusively responsible for the scientific accuracy of the provided results, which may be inconsistent across all the provided studies.

Additionally, findings for three RCT of the included studies were retrieved from grey literature which were not formally and rigorously peer reviewed, and thus should be carefully interpreted due to potential publication bias [116].

There is a strong pharmacological need to look beyond current therapeutic strategies and consider further promising biological drugs for asthma that are under development and for which results have not been posted on clinical trial registries and are not available in current literature.

Asthma remission is a complex condition that can be clinically defined as a sustained absence of symptoms, optimisation or stabilisation of lung function, and no use of OCS for exacerbation treatment [117], but controversy remains regarding the threshold of each item used to assess the asthma remission itself [118]. Although these terms do not necessarily imply the absence of airway pathology, a recent point of view suggested that asthma remission may be an achievable goal, at least in asthmatic patients with the T2 phenotype [117].

In conclusion, novel investigational agents, such as biologics, may have the potential to promote disease modification. Clearly, further larger studies are needed to confirm positive results from Phase I and II RCTs. So far, most of the investigated therapies have been evaluated as add-on options to current treatment, but it would be extremely advantageous for new therapies to be effective enough to replace current pharmaceutical options in order to simplify regimens of administration.

Table 2. Clinical effect of investigational agents currently evaluated in Phase I and II RCTs for the treatment of asthma compared to PCB on efficacy outcomes for which the MCID values are currently available. The investigational agents reported in this table also elicited statistically significant improvement vs. PCB ($p < 0.05$).

Outcome	Treatment	Drug Class	Delta Effect	Suggested MCID [103]	Beneficial Clinically Relevant Effect
Trough FEV$_1$	Itepekimab 300 mg Q2W	Anti-IL-33 mAb	140 mL (10–270)	>100 mL	Yes
	Indacaterol maleate 150 µg QD	LABA	186 mL (129–243)	>100 mL	Yes
Peak FEV$_1$	Itepekimab 300 mg Q2W + dupilumab 300 Q2W	Anti-IL-33 mAb + anti IL-4/IL-13 mAb	130 mL (10–250)	≥12% and ≥200 mL	No
PEF	Indacaterol maleate 150 µg QD	LABA	33.00 L/min (25.60–40.30)	>5.39%	?
Morning PEF	Velsecorat 720 µg QD	SGRM	16.60 L/min (8.03–25.17)	>5.39%	?
Evening PEF	Velsecorat 720 µg QD	SGRM	11.99 L/min (3.57–20.42)	>5.39%	?
	Itepekimab 300 mg Q2W	Anti-IL-33 mAb	−0.42 points (−0.73—−0.12)	>0.5 points	Borderline
ACQ	Itepekimab 300 mg Q2W + dupilumab 300 mg Q2W	Anti-IL-33 mAb + anti IL-4/IL-13 mAb	−0.32 points (−0.63—−0.01)	>0.5 points	No
	Velsecorat 720 µg QD	SGRM	−0.27 points (−0.43—−0.10)	>0.5 points	No
	CJM112 300 mg QW	IL-17A mAb	−0.23 points (−0.40—−0.06) *	>0.5 points	No
Exacerbations	Velsecorat 720 µg QD	SGRM	0.11 rate (0.04–0.25)	>−20% rate	Yes
AQLQ	Itepekimab 300 mg Q2W	Anti-IL-33 mAb	0.45 points (0.14–0.77)	>0.5 points	Borderline
	Itepekimab 300 mg Q2W + dupilumab 300 mg Q2W	Anti-IL-33 mAb + anti IL-4/IL-13 mAb	0.43 points (0.11–0.75)	>0.5 points	Borderline

* 80% Confidence Interval. ACQ: asthma control questionnaire; AQLQ: asthma quality of life questionnaire; FEV$_1$: forced expiratory volume in the 1st second; IL-n: interleukin-n; LABA: long-acting β$_2$-adrenoceptor agonist; mAb: monoclonal antibody; MCID: Minimal Clinical Important Difference; NA: not available; PCB: placebo; PEF: peak expiratory flow; Q2W: once every 2 weeks; QD: *quaque die*, once daily; RCT: randomised controlled trial; SGRM: selective glucocorticoid receptor modulator; TSLP: thymic stromal lymphopoietin.

Author Contributions: All the authors (L.C., M.A., A.F., E.P., B.L.R., P.R. and A.C.) made substantial contributions to the conception or design of the work; the acquisition, analysis, or interpretation of data; or the creation of new software used in the work; or have drafted the work or substantively revised it; all the authors (L.C., M.A., A.F., E.P., B.L.R., P.R. and A.C.) approved the submitted version; all the authors (L.C., M.A., A.F., E.P., B.L.R., P.R. and A.C.) agreed to be personally accountable for their own contributions and for ensuring that questions related to the accuracy or integrity of any part of the work, even ones in which the author was not personally involved, are appropriately investigated, resolved, and documented in the literature. All authors have read and agreed to the published version of the manuscript.

Funding: This research received no external funding.

Institutional Review Board Statement: Not applicable.

Informed Consent Statement: Not applicable.

Data Availability Statement: The data presented in this study are available in the article.

Conflicts of Interest: L.C. reports grants and personal fees from Boehringer Ingelheim, grants and personal fees from Novartis, nonfinancial support from AstraZeneca, grants from Chiesi Farmaceutici, grants from Almirall, personal fees from ABC Farmaceutici, personal fees from Edmond Pharma, grants and personal fees from Zambon, personal fees from Verona Pharma, personal fees from Ockham Biotech. M.A. has no conflicts of interest to declare. A.F. has no conflicts of interest to declare. E.P. has no conflicts of interest to declare. B.L.R. has no conflicts of interest to declare. P.R. reports grants and personal fees from Boehringer Ingelheim, grants and personal fees from Novartis, personal fees from AstraZeneca, grants and personal fees from Chiesi Farmaceutici, grants and personal fees from Almirall, grants from Zambon, personal fees from Biofutura, personal fees from GlaxoSmithKline, personal fees from Menarini, and personal fees from Mundipharma. A.C. received grants from Menarini and Astra Zeneca and a personal fee from Chiesi.

References

1. GINA Main Report—Global Initiative for Asthma, 2021 (n.d.). Available online: https://ginasthma.org/wp-content/uploads/20 21/05/GINA-Main-Report-2021-V2-WMS.pdf (accessed on 11 June 2021).
2. Singh, D.; Garcia, G.; Maneechotesuwan, K.; Daley-Yates, P.; Irusen, E.; Aggarwal, B.; Boucot, I.; Berend, N. New Versus Old: The Impact of Changing Patterns of Inhaled Corticosteroid Prescribing and Dosing Regimens in Asthma Management. *Adv. Ther.* **2022**, *39*, 1895–1914. [CrossRef] [PubMed]
3. Ray, A.; Singh, S.; Dutta, J.; Mabalirajan, U. Targeting molecular and cellular mechanisms in asthma. In *Targeting Cellular Signalling Pathways in Lung Diseases*, Springer: Singapore, 2021; pp. 27–51.
4. Hekking, P.P.W.; Wener, R.R.; Amelink, M.; Zwinderman, A.H.; Bouvy, M.L.; Bel, E.H. The prevalence of severe refractory asthma. *J. Allergy Clin. Immunol.* **2015**, *135*, 896–902. [CrossRef] [PubMed]
5. Chung, K.F.; Wenzel, S.E.; Brozek, J.L.; Bush, A.; Castro, M.; Sterk, P.J.; Adcock, I.M.; Bateman, E.D.; Bel, E.H.; Bleecker, E.R.; et al. International ERS/ATS guidelines on definition, evaluation and treatment of severe asthma. *Eur. Respir. J.* **2014**, *43*, 343–373. [CrossRef] [PubMed]
6. Kuruvilla, M.E.; Lee, F.E.H.; Lee, G.B. Understanding Asthma Phenotypes, Endotypes, and Mechanisms of Disease. *Clin. Rev. Allergy Immunol.* **2018**, *56*, 219–233. [CrossRef] [PubMed]
7. Sterk, P.J. Chronic diseases like asthma and COPD: Do they truly exist? *Eur. Respir. J.* **2016**, *47*, 359–361. [CrossRef]
8. Wenzel, S.E. Asthma phenotypes: The evolution from clinical to molecular approaches. *Nat. Med.* **2012**, *18*, 716–725. [CrossRef]
9. Pelaia, C.; Calabrese, C.; Terracciano, R.; de Blasio, F.; Vatrella, A.; Pelaia, G. Omalizumab, the first available antibody for biological treatment of severe asthma: More than a decade of real-life effectiveness. *Ther. Adv. Respir. Dis.* **2018**, *12*, 1753466618810192. [CrossRef]
10. Menzies-Gow, A.; Szefler, S.J.; Busse, W.W. The Relationship of Asthma Biologics to Remission for Asthma. *J. Allergy Clin. Immunol. Pract.* **2020**, *9*, 1090–1098. [CrossRef]
11. Moran, A.; Pavord, I.D. Anti-IL-4/IL-13 for the treatment of asthma: The story so far. *Expert Opin. Biol. Ther.* **2020**, *20*, 283–294. [CrossRef]
12. Hoy, S.M. Tezepelumab: First Approval. *Drugs* **2022**, *82*, 461–468. [CrossRef]
13. Cazzola, M.; Ora, J.; Cavalli, F.; Rogliani, P.; Matera, M.G. Treatable Mechanisms in Asthma. *Mol. Diagn. Ther.* **2021**, *25*, 111–121. [CrossRef] [PubMed]
14. Cazzola, M.; Rogliani, P.; Naviglio, S.; Calzetta, L.; Matera, M.G. An update on the currently available and emerging synthetic pharmacotherapy for uncontrolled asthma. *Expert Opin. Pharmacother.* **2022**, *23*, 1205–1216. [CrossRef] [PubMed]
15. Moher, D.; Shamseer, L.; Clarke, M.; Ghersi, D.; Liberati, A.; Petticrew, M.; Shekelle, P.; Stewart, L.A.; Prisma-P Group. Preferred reporting items for systematic review and meta-analysis protocols (PRISMA-P) 2015 statement. *Syst. Rev.* **2015**, *4*, 1. [CrossRef]

16. Page, M.J.; McKenzie, J.E.; Bossuyt, P.M.; Boutron, I.; Hoffmann, T.C.; Mulrow, C.D.; Shamseer, L.; Tetzlaff, J.M.; Akl, E.A.; Brennan, S.E.; et al. The PRISMA 2020 statement: An updated guideline for reporting systematic reviews. *BMJ.* **2021**, *372*, n71. [CrossRef]

17. Schardt, C.; Adams, M.B.; Owens, T.; Keitz, S.; Fontelo, P. Utilization of the PICO framework to improve searching PubMed for clinical questions. *BMC Med. Inf. Decis. Mak.* **2007**, *7*, 16. [CrossRef] [PubMed]

18. Jadad, A.R.; Moore, R.A.; Carroll, D.; Jenkinson, C.; Reynolds, D.J.; Gavaghan, D.J.; McQuay, H.J. Assessing the quality of reports of randomized clinical trials: Is blinding necessary? *Control Clin. Trials* **1996**, *17*, 1–12. [CrossRef]

19. Higgins, J.P.T.; Savović, J.; Page, M.J.; Elbers, R.G.; Sterne, J.A.C. Chapter 8: Assessing Risk of bias in a randomized trial. In *Cochrane Handbook for Systematic Reviews of Interventions Version 6.0 (Updated July 2019)*; John Wiley & Sons: Chichester, UK, 2019; pp. 205–228. Available online: https://training.cochrane.org/handbook (accessed on 1 June 2022).

20. Sterne, J.A.C.; Savovic, J.; Page, M.J.; Elbers, R.G.; Blencowe, N.S.; Boutron, I.; Cates, C.J.; Cheng, H.Y.; Corbett, M.S.; Eldridge, S.M.; et al. RoB 2: A revised tool for assessing risk of bias in randomised trials. *BMJ* **2019**, *366*, l4898. [CrossRef] [PubMed]

21. McGuinness, L.A. robvis: An R package and web application for visualising risk-of-bias assessments. *Res. Synth. Methods* **2021**, *12*, 55–61. [CrossRef]

22. *NCT03299686*; Study to Assess the Efficacy and Safety of CJM112 in Patients with Inadequately Controlled Severe Asthma. 2017. Available online: https://clinicaltrials.gov/ct2/show/NCT03299686 (accessed on 1 June 2022).

23. *NCT03393806*; Repeat Dose Study of GSK3772847 in Participants with Moderate to Severe Asthma with Allergic Fungal Airway Disease (AFAD). 2018. Available online: https://clinicaltrials.gov/ct2/show/NCT03393806 (accessed on 1 June 2022).

24. *NCT03207243*; Efficacy and Safety Study of GSK3772847 in Subjects with Moderately Severe Asthma. 2017. Available online: https://clinicaltrials.gov/ct2/show/NCT03207243 (accessed on 1 June 2022).

25. *NCT03944707*; Study of Efficacy and Safety of LOU064 in Inadequately Controlled Asthma Patients. 2019. Available online: https://www.clinicaltrials.gov/ct2/show/NCT03944707 (accessed on 1 June 2022).

26. *NCT03135899*; BI 443651 Methacholine Challenge. 2017. Available online: https://clinicaltrials.gov/ct2/show/NCT03135899 (accessed on 1 June 2022).

27. *NCT04150341*; Effect of Inhaled TD-8236 on Allergen-induced Asthmatic Response. 2019. Available online: https://clinicaltrials.gov/ct2/show/NCT04150341 (accessed on 1 June 2022).

28. Siddiqui, S.; Bozik, M.; Archibald, D.; Dworetzky, S.; Mather, J.; Killingsworth, R.; Ochkur, S.; Jacobsen, E.; Panettieri, R.; Prussin, C. Late Breaking Abstract—Phase 2 trial evaluating the effects of dexpramipexole on blood eosinophils, lung function, and airway biomarkers in eosinophilic asthma. *Eur. Respir. J.* **2021**, *58*, RCT2900. [CrossRef]

29. *NCT04046939*; Dexpramipexole Dose-Ranging Biomarker Study in Subjects with Eosinophilic Asthma (AS201). 2019. Available online: https://clinicaltrials.gov/ct2/show/NCT04046939 (accessed on 1 June 2022).

30. Singh, S.; Fuhr, R.; Bird, N.P.; Mole, S.; Hardes, K.; Man, Y.L.; Cahn, A.; Yancey, S.W.; Pouliquen, I.J. A Phase 1 study of the long-acting anti-IL-5 monoclonal antibody GSK3511294 in patients with asthma. *Br. J. Clin. Pharmacol.* **2022**, *88*, 702–712. [CrossRef]

31. *NCT03287310*; First Time in Human (FTIH) Study to Evaluate Safety, Tolerability, Immunogenicity, Pharmacokinetics (PK) and Pharmacodynamics (PD) of GSK3511294 Administered Subcutaneously (SC) in Subjects with Mild to Moderate Asthma. 2017. Available online: https://clinicaltrials.gov/ct2/show/NCT03287310 (accessed on 1 June 2022).

32. Wechsler, M.E.; Ruddy, M.K.; Pavord, I.D.; Israel, E.; Rabe, K.F.; Ford, L.B.; Maspero, J.F.; Abdulai, R.M.; Hu, C.-C.; Martincova, R.; et al. Efficacy and Safety of Itepekimab in Patients with Moderate-to-Severe Asthma. *N. Engl. J. Med.* **2021**, *385*, 1656–1668. [CrossRef] [PubMed]

33. *NCT03387852*; Evaluation of SAR440340 and as Combination Therapy with Dupilumab in Moderate-to-Severe Asthma Participants. 2018. Available online: https://clinicaltrials.gov/ct2/show/NCT03387852 (accessed on 1 June 2022).

34. Miller, D.; Vaidya, S.; Jauernig, J.; Ethell, B.; Wagner, K.; Radhakrishnan, R.; Tillmann, H.C. Lung function, pharmacokinetics, and tolerability of inhaled indacaterol maleate and acetate in asthma patients. *Respir. Res.* **2020**, *21*, 120. [CrossRef] [PubMed]

35. *NCT03257996*; Pharmacodynamics, Safety, Tolerability, and Pharmacokinetics of Two Orally Inhaled Indacaterol Salts in Adult Subjects with Asthma. 2017. Available online: https://clinicaltrials.gov/ct2/show/NCT03257995 (accessed on 1 June 2022).

36. Moss, M.H.; Lugogo, N.L.; Castro, M.; Hanania, N.A.; Ludwig-Sengpiel, A.; Saralaya, D.; Dobek, R.; Ojanguren, I.; Vyshnyvetskyy, I.; Bruey, J.-M.; et al. Results of a Phase 2b Trial with GB001, a Prostaglandin D2 Receptor 2 Antagonist, in Moderate to Severe Eosinophilic Asthma. *Chest* **2022**, *162*, 297–308. [CrossRef] [PubMed]

37. *NCT03683576*; GB001 in Adult Subjects with Moderate to Severe Asthma. 2018. Available online: https://clinicaltrials.gov/ct2/show/NCT03683576 (accessed on 1 June 2022).

38. Cass, L.; Murray, A.; Davis, A.; Woodward, K.; Albayaty, M.; Ito, K.; Strong, P.; Ayrton, J.; Brindley, C.; Prosser, J.; et al. Safety and nonclinical and clinical pharmacokinetics of PC945, a novel inhaled triazole antifungal agent. *Pharmacol. Res. Perspect.* **2021**, *9*, e00690. [CrossRef] [PubMed]

39. *NCT02715570*; A Study to Investigate the Safety, Tolerability and Pharmacokinetics of Single and Repeat Doses of PC945. 2017. Available online: https://clinicaltrials.gov/ct2/show/NCT02715570 (accessed on 3 June 2022).

40. *NCT03469934*; Proof of Concept Study to Investigate ANB020 Activity in Adult Patients with Severe Eosinophilic Asthma. 2018. Available online: https://clinicaltrials.gov/ct2/show/NCT03469934 (accessed on 3 June 2022).

41. *EudraCT Number 2017-000647-40*; Placebo-Controlled Proof of Concept Study to Investigate ANB020 Activity in Adult Patients with Severe Eosinophilic Asthma. 2018. Available online: https://www.clinicaltrialsregister.eu/ctr-search/trial/2017-000647-40/results (accessed on 3 June 2022).
42. *NCT03378648*; A Study to Investigate Safety, Tolerability, Pharmacokinetics and Pharmacodynamics of Single Dose in Healthy Volunteers, Repeat Doses in Asthmatic Patients and of Single Dose in COPD Patients of CHF6366. 2017. Available online: https://clinicaltrials.gov/ct2/show/NCT03378648 (accessed on 6 June 2022).
43. *EudraCT Number 2015-005551-27*; A FIRST in Human Randomised, Double-Blind, Placebo-Controlled Study of Single Ascending Doses in Healthy Male Volunteers and Repeated Ascending Dose in Asthmatic Patients Followed by a 3-Way Cross-Over, Placebo-Controlled, Single-Dose in COPD Patients to Investigate the Safety, Tolerability, Pharmacokinetics, and Pharmacodynamics of CHF6366. 2019. Available online: https://www.clinicaltrialsregister.eu/ctr-search/trial/2015-005551-27/results (accessed on 6 June 2022).
44. Moermans, C.; Graff, S.; Medard, L.; Schleich, F.; Paulus, V.; Guissard, F.; Henket, M.; Louis, R. Clinical trial: Impact of Probiotical® on asthma control and inflammation. *Eur. Respir. J.* **2020**, *56*, 5281. [CrossRef]
45. *NCT03341403*; Effect of a Synbiotic "Probiotical®" in Asthma. 2017. Available online: https://clinicaltrials.gov/ct2/show/NCT03341403 (accessed on 6 June 2022).
46. Bruns, I.; Fitzgerald, M.; Mensing, G.; Tsung, M.; Pardali, K.; Gardiner, P.; Keeling, D.; Axelsson, L.; Olsson, M.; Ghobadi, C.; et al. Late Breaking Abstract—Multiple ascending dose study of the inhaled IL-4Ra antagonist, AZD1402/PRS-060, in mild asthmatics demonstrates robust FeNO reduction and a promising clinical profile for the treatment of asthma. *Eur. Respir. J.* **2019**, *54*, PA3709. [CrossRef]
47. *NCT03574805*; Study of Multiple Doses of PRS-060 Administered by Oral Inhalation in Subjects with Mild Asthma. 2018. Available online: https://clinicaltrials.gov/ct2/show/NCT03574805 (accessed on 6 June 2022).
48. Chupp, G.L.; Beeh, K.M.; Jauhiainen, A.; Necander, S.; Brown, M.N.; Hamrén, U.W.; Forsman, H.; Kurdyukova, Y.; Steele, J.; Astbury, C.; et al. Results of a Phase 2a Dose Finding Study of Velsecorat, an Inhaled Non-Steroidal, Selective Glucocorticoid Receptor Modulator in Asthma (GRANIT). *Am. Thorac. Soc. Int. Conf. Meet. Abstr.* **2021**, *203*, A1202. [CrossRef]
49. *NCT03622112*; A Study to Assess the Efficacy and Safety of Multiple Dose Levels of AZD7594 Administered Once Daily by Inhalation in Asthmatic Subjects. 2018. Available online: https://clinicaltrials.gov/ct2/show/NCT03622112 (accessed on 6 June 2022).
50. *EudraCT Number 2017-002483-40*; A Phase 2b Randomised, Double-Blind, Placebo-Controlled, Parallel Arm, Multi-Centre Study to Assess Efficacy and Safety of Multiple Dose Levels of AZD7594 DPI Given Once Daily for Twelve Weeks, Compared to Placebo, in Asthmatics Symptomatic on Low Dose ICS. 2020. Available online: https://www.clinicaltrialsregister.eu/ctr-search/trial/2017-002483-40/results (accessed on 6 June 2022).
51. De Gaix, F.D.B.; Gherasim, A.; Domis, N.; Meier, P.; Shawki, F.; DeVeaux, M.; Ramesh, D.; Perlee, L.; Herman, G.; Weinreich, D.; et al. A Single-Dose of REGN1908-1909 Reduced Bronchoconstriction in Cat-Allergic Subjects with Mild Asthma for up to 3 months following a controlled cat allergen challenge: A Phase 2, Randomized, Double-Blind, Placebo-Controlled Study. *J. Allergy Clin. Immunol.* **2021**, *147*, AB158. [CrossRef]
52. *NCT03838731*; Study in Cat-Allergic Patients with Asthma to Evaluate the Efficacy of a Single Dose of REGN1908-1909 to Reduce Bronchoconstriction Upon Cat Allergen Challenge. 2019. Available online: https://clinicaltrials.gov/ct2/show/NCT03838731 (accessed on 6 June 2022).
53. *NCT03138811*; A Bronchoprovocation Study to Assess the Safety, Tolerability, Pharmacokinetics and Pharmacodynamics of CSJ117 in Adult Subjects with Mild Atopic Asthma. 2017. Available online: https://clinicaltrials.gov/ct2/show/NCT03138811 (accessed on 6 June 2022).
54. Novartis Pharmaceuticals. A randomized, subject and investigator-blinded, placebo-controlled, parallel-design, broncho-provocation study to evaluate the safety, tolerability, pharmacokinetics and pharmacodynamics of multiple doses of inhaled CSJ117 in adult subjects with mild atopic asthma. 2020. Available online: https://www.novctrd.com/ctrdweb/trialresult/trialresults/pdf?trialResultId=17681 (accessed on 6 June 2022).
55. Vatrella, A.; Fabozzi, I.; Calabrese, C.; Maselli, R.; Pelaia, G. Dupilumab: A novel treatment for asthma. *J. Asthma Allergy* **2014**, *7*, 123–130. [CrossRef]
56. Gour, N.; Wills-Karp, M. IL-4 and IL-13 signaling in allergic airway disease. *Cytokine* **2015**, *75*, 68–78. [CrossRef]
57. Legrand, F.; Klion, A.D. Biologic Therapies Targeting Eosinophils: Current Status and Future Prospects. *J. Allergy Clin. Immunol. Pract.* **2015**, *3*, 167–174. [CrossRef] [PubMed]
58. Molet, S.; Hamid, Q.; Davoine, F.; Nutku, E.; Taha, R.; Pagé, N.; Olivenstein, R.; Elias, J.; Chakir, J. IL-17 is increased in asthmatic airways and induces human bronchial fibroblasts to produce cytokines. *J. Allergy Clin. Immunol.* **2001**, *108*, 430–438. [CrossRef] [PubMed]
59. Chakir, J.; Shannon, J.; Molet, S.; Fukakusa, M.; Elias, J.; Laviolette, M.; Boulet, L.P.; Hamid, Q. Airway remodeling-associated mediators in moderate to severe asthma: Effect of steroids on TGF-β, IL-11, IL-17, and type I and type III collagen expression. *J. Allergy Clin. Immunol.* **2003**, *111*, 1293–1298. [CrossRef] [PubMed]
60. Bullens, D.M.A.; Truyen, E.; Coteur, L.; Dilissen, E.; Hellings, P.W.; Dupont, L.J.; Ceuppens, J.L. IL-17 mRNA in sputum of asthmatic patients: Linking T cell driven inflammation and granulocytic influx? *Respir. Res.* **2006**, *7*, 135. [CrossRef]

61. Zheng, R.; Wang, F.; Huang, Y.; Xiang, Q.; Dai, H.; Zhang, W. Elevated Th17 cell frequencies and Th17/Treg ratio are associated with airway hyperresponsiveness in asthmatic children. *J. Asthma* **2020**, *58*, 707–716. [CrossRef]
62. Doe, C.; Bafadhel, M.; Siddiqui, S.; Desai, D.; Mistry, V.; Rugman, P.; McCormick, M.; Woods, J.; May, R.; Sleeman, M.A.; et al. Expression of the T helper 17-associated cytokines IL-17A and IL-17F in asthma and COPD. *Chest* **2010**, *138*, 1140–1147. [CrossRef]
63. Agache, I.; Ciobanu, C.; Agache, C.; Anghel, M. Increased serum IL-17 is an independent risk factor for severe asthma. *Respir. Med.* **2010**, *104*, 1131–1137. [CrossRef]
64. Al-Ramli, W.; Préfontaine, D.; Chouiali, F.; Martin, J.G.; Olivenstein, R.; Lemière, C.; Hamid, Q. TH17-associated cytokines (IL-17A and IL-17F) in severe asthma. *J. Allergy Clin. Immunol.* **2009**, *123*, 1185–1187. [CrossRef]
65. Chesné, J.; Braza, F.; Mahay, G.; Brouard, S.; Aronica, M.; Magnan, A. IL-17 in severe asthma: Where do we stand? *Am. J. Respir. Crit. Care Med.* **2014**, *190*, 1094–1101. [CrossRef]
66. Chambers, E.S.; Nanzer, A.M.; Pfeffer, P.E.; Richards, D.F.; Timms, P.M.; Martineau, A.R.; Griffiths, C.J.; Corrigan, C.J.; Hawry-lowicz, C.M. Distinct endotypes of steroid-resistant asthma characterized by IL-17Ahigh and IFN-γhigh immunophenotypes: Potential benefits of calcitriol. *J. Allergy Clin. Immunol.* **2015**, *136*, 628–637.e4. [CrossRef]
67. Rahmawati, S.F.; Velde, M.t.; Kerstjens, H.A.M.; Dömling, A.S.S.; Groves, M.R.; Gosens, R. Pharmacological Rationale for Targeting IL-17 in Asthma. *Front. Allergy* **2021**, *2*, 694514. [CrossRef]
68. Mitchell, P.D.; O'Byrne, P.M. Epithelial-Derived Cytokines in Asthma. *Chest* **2017**, *151*, 1338–1344. [CrossRef]
69. Smith, S.G.; Chen, R.; Kjarsgaard, M.; Huang, C.; Oliveria, J.P.; O'Byrne, P.M.; Gauvreau, G.M.; Boulet, L.P.; Lemiere, C.; Martin, J.; et al. Increased numbers of activated group 2 innate lymphoid cells in the airways of patients with severe asthma and persistent airway eosinophilia. *J. Allergy Clin. Immunol.* **2016**, *137*, 75–86.e8. [CrossRef]
70. Bartemes, K.R.; Iijima, K.; Kobayashi, T.; Kephart, G.M.; McKenzie, A.N.; Kita, H. IL-33-responsive lineage-CD25+ CD44(hi) lymphoid cells mediate innate type 2 immunity and allergic inflammation in the lungs. *J. Immunol.* **2012**, *188*, 1503–1513. [CrossRef] [PubMed]
71. Kabata, H.; Flamar, A.L.; Mahlakõiv, T.; Moriyama, S.; Rodewald, H.R.; Ziegler, S.F.; Artis, D. Targeted deletion of the TSLP receptor reveals cellular mechanisms that promote type 2 airway inflammation. *Mucosal Immunol.* **2020**, *13*, 626–636. [CrossRef] [PubMed]
72. Ying, S.; O'Connor, B.; Ratoff, J.; Meng, Q.; Mallett, K.; Cousins, D.; Robinson, D.; Zhang, G.; Zhao, J.; Lee, T.H.; et al. Thymic Stromal Lymphopoietin Expression Is Increased in Asthmatic Airways and Correlates with Expression of Th2-Attracting Chemokines and Disease Severity. *J. Immunol.* **2005**, *174*, 8183–8190. [CrossRef] [PubMed]
73. Shikotra, A.; Choy, D.F.; Ohri, C.M.; Doran, E.; Butler, C.; Hargadon, B.; Shelley, M.; Abbas, A.R.; Austin, C.D.; Jackman, J.; et al. Increased expression of immunoreactive thymic stromal lymphopoietin in patients with severe asthma. *J. Allergy Clin. Immunol.* **2012**, *129*, 104–111.e9. [CrossRef]
74. Park, S.; Park, Y.; Son, S.H.; Lee, K.; Jung, Y.W.; Lee, K.Y.; Jeon, Y.H.; Byun, Y. Synthesis and biological evaluation of peptide-derived TSLP inhibitors. *Bioorg. Med. Chem. Lett.* **2017**, *27*, 4710–4713. [CrossRef]
75. Chuchalin, A.G.; Tsoi, A.N.; Richter, K.; Krug, N.; Dahl, R.; Luursema, P.B.; Cameron, R.; Bao, W.; Higgins, M.; Woessner, R.; et al. Safety and tolerability of indacaterol in asthma: A randomized, placebo-controlled 28-day study. *Respir. Med.* **2007**, *101*, 2065–2075. [CrossRef]
76. Beasley, R.W.; Donohue, J.F.; Mehta, R.; Nelson, H.S.; Clay, M.; Moton, A.; Kim, H.J.; Hederer, B.M. Effect of once-daily indacaterol maleate/mometasone furoate on exacerbation risk in adolescent and adult asthma: A double-blind randomised controlled trial. *BMJ Open* **2015**, *5*, e006131. [CrossRef]
77. Kanniess, F.; Boulet, L.P.; Pierzchala, W.; Cameron, R.; Owen, R.; Higgins, M. Efficacy and safety of indacaterol, a new 24-hour β2-agonist, in patients with asthma: A dose-ranging study. *J. Asthma* **2008**, *45*, 887–892. [CrossRef] [PubMed]
78. Yang, W.H.; Martinot, J.B.; Pohunek, P.; Beier, J.; Magula, D.; Cameron, R.; Owen, R.; Higgins, M. Tolerability of indacaterol, a novel once-daily beta2-agonist, in patients with asthma: A randomized, placebo-controlled, 28-day safety study. *Ann. Allergy Asthma Immunol.* **2007**, *99*, 555–561. [CrossRef]
79. Sedwick, C. Wanted: A New Model for Glucocorticoid Receptor Transactivation and Transrepression. *PLoS Biol.* **2014**, *12*, e1001814. [CrossRef] [PubMed]
80. Van Moortel, L.; Gevaert, K.; de Bosscher, K. Improved Glucocorticoid Receptor Ligands: Fantastic Beasts, but How to Find Them? *Front. Endocrinol.* **2020**, *11*, 712. [CrossRef]
81. Cazzola, M.; Lopez-Campos, J.L.; Puente-Maestu, L. The MABA approach: A new option to improve bronchodilator therapy. *Eur. Respir. J.* **2013**, *42*, 885–887. [CrossRef]
82. de Miguel-Díez, J.; Jiménez-García, R. Considerations for new dual-acting bronchodilator treatments for chronic obstructive pulmonary disease. *Expert Opin. Investig. Drugs* **2014**, *23*, 453–456. [CrossRef]
83. Domingo, C.; Palomares, O.; Sandham, D.A.; Erpenbeck, V.J.; Altman, P. The prostaglandin D2 receptor 2 pathway in asthma: A key player in airway inflammation 11 Medical and Health Sciences 1107 Immunology 11 Medical and Health Sciences 1102 Cardiorespiratory Medicine and Haematology. *Respir. Res.* **2018**, *19*, 189. [CrossRef]
84. Hata, D.; Kawakami, Y.; Inagaki, N.; Lantz, C.S.; Kitamura, T.; Khan, W.N.; Maeda-Yamamoto, M.; Miura, T.; Han, W.; Hartman, S.E.; et al. Involvement of Bruton's tyrosine kinase in FcepsilonRI-dependent mast cell degranulation and cytokine production. *J. Exp. Med.* **1998**, *187*, 1235–1247. [CrossRef]

85. Iyer, A.S.; Morales, J.L.; Huang, W.; Ojo, F.; Ning, G.; Wills, E.; Baines, J.D.; August, A. Absence of Tec family kinases interleukin-2 inducible T cell kinase (Itk) and Bruton's tyrosine kinase (Btk) severely impairs Fc epsilonRI-dependent mast cell responses. *J. Biol. Chem.* **2011**, *286*, 9503–9513. [CrossRef]

86. MacGlashan, D.; Honigberg, L.A.; Smith, A.; Buggy, J.; Schroeder, J.T. Inhibition of IgE-mediated secretion from human basophils with a highly selective Bruton's tyrosine kinase, Btk, inhibitor. *Int. Immunopharmacol.* **2011**, *11*, 475–479. [CrossRef]

87. Phillips, J.E.; Renteria, L.; Burns, L.; Harris, P.; Peng, R.; Bauer, C.M.T.; Laine, D.; Stevenson, C.S. Btk Inhibitor RN983 Delivered by Dry Powder Nose-only Aerosol Inhalation Inhibits Bronchoconstriction and Pulmonary Inflammation in the Ovalbumin Allergic Mouse Model of Asthma. *J. Aerosol. Med. Pulm. Drug Deliv.* **2016**, *29*, 233–241. [CrossRef] [PubMed]

88. Wang, W.; Ji, H.L. Epithelial sodium and chloride channels and asthma. *Chin. Med. J.* **2015**, *128*, 2242–2249. [CrossRef] [PubMed]

89. Southworth, T.; Plumb, J.; Gupta, V.; Pearson, J.; Ramis, I.; Lehner, M.D.; Miralpeix, M.; Singh, D. Anti-inflammatory potential of PI3Kδ and JAK inhibitors in asthma patients. *Respir. Res.* **2016**, *17*, 124. [CrossRef] [PubMed]

90. Ashino, S.; Takeda, K.; Li, H.; Taylor, V.; Joetham, A.; Pine, P.R.; Gelfand, E.W. Janus kinase 1/3 signaling pathways are key initiators of TH2 differentiation and lung allergic responses. *J. Allergy Clin. Immunol.* **2013**, *133*, 1162–1174.e4. [CrossRef]

91. Calama, E.; Ramis, I.; Domènech, A.; Carreño, C.; de Alba, J.; Prats, N.; Miralpeix, M. Tofacitinib ameliorates inflammation in a rat model of airway neutrophilia induced by inhaled LPS. *Pulm. Pharmacol. Ther.* **2017**, *43*, 60–67. [CrossRef]

92. Calbet, M.; Ramis, I.; Calama, E.; Carreño, C.; Paris, S.; Maldonado, M.; Orellana, A.; Calaf, E.; Pauta, M.; de Alba, J.; et al. Novel inhaled pan-JAK inhibitor, LAS194046, reduces allergen-induced airway inflammation, late asthmatic response, and PSTAT activation in brown Norway rats. *J. Pharmacol. Exp. Ther.* **2019**, *370*, 137–147. [CrossRef]

93. van Ree, R.; van Leeuwen, W.A.; Bulder, I.; Bond, J.; Aalberse, R.C. Purified natural and recombinant Fel d 1 and cat albumin in in vitro diagnostics for cat allergy. *J. Allergy Clin. Immunol.* **1999**, *104*, 1223–1230. [CrossRef]

94. Grönlund, H.; Saarne, T.; Gafvelin, G.; van Hage, M. The major cat allergen, fel d 1, in diagnosis and therapy. *Int. Arch. Allergy Immunol.* **2010**, *151*, 265–274. [CrossRef]

95. Kamal, M.A.; Dingman, R.; Wang, C.Q.; Lai, C.H.; Rajadhyaksha, M.; DeVeaux, M.; Orengo, J.M.; Radin, A.; Davis, J.D. REGN1908-1909 monoclonal antibodies block Fel d 1 in cat allergic subjects: Translational pharmacokinetics and pharmacodynamics. *Clin. Transl. Sci.* **2021**, *14*, 2440–2449. [CrossRef]

96. Orengo, J.M.; Radin, A.R.; Kamat, V.; Badithe, A.; Ben, L.H.; Bennett, B.L.; Zhong, S.; Birchard, D.; Limnander, A.; Rafique, A.; et al. Treating cat allergy with monoclonal IgG antibodies that bind allergen and prevent IgE engagement. *Nat. Commun.* **2018**, *14*, 2440–2449. [CrossRef]

97. Shamji, M.H.; Singh, I.; Layhadi, J.A.; Ito, C.; Karamani, A.; Kouser, L.; Sharif, H.; Tang, J.; Handijiev, S.; Parkin, R.V.; et al. Passive prophylactic administration with a single dose of Anti–Fel d 1 monoclonal antibodies REGN1908–1909 in cat allergen–induced allergic rhinitis: A randomized, double-blind, placebo-controlled clinical trial. *Am. J. Respir. Crit. Care Med.* **2021**, *204*, 23–33. [CrossRef] [PubMed]

98. Knopp Biosciences. Dexpramipexole Targets Eosinophilic Inflammation, (n.d.). Available online: https://www.nature.com/articles/d43747-020-01157-2 (accessed on 6 June 2022).

99. Denning, D.W.; O'Driscoll, B.R.; Hogaboam, C.M.; Bowyer, P.; Niven, R.M. The link between fungi and severe asthma: A summary of the evidence. *Eur. Respir. J.* **2006**, *27*, 615–626. [CrossRef] [PubMed]

100. Denning, D.W.; Pashley, C.; Hartl, D.; Wardlaw, A.; Godet, C.; del Giacco, S.; Delhaes, L.; Sergejeva, S. Fungal allergy in asthma-state of the art and research needs. *Clin. Transl. Allergy* **2014**, *4*, 14. [CrossRef]

101. Van Norman, G.A. Drugs and Devices: Comparison of European and U.S. Approval Processes. *JACC Basic Transl. Sci.* **2016**, *1*, 399–412. [CrossRef] [PubMed]

102. European Medicines Agency. *Guideline for Good Clinical Practice E6(R2)*; European Medicines Agency: Amsterdam, The Netherlands, 2016.

103. Rogliani, P.; Calzetta, L. Clinical Interpretation of Efficacy Outcomes in Pharmacological Studies on Triple Fixed-Dose Combination Therapy for Uncontrolled Asthma: Assessment of IRIDIUM and ARGON Studies. *J. Exp. Pharmacol.* **2022**, *14*, 1–5. [CrossRef]

104. FDA. *Dietary Supplements: Questions and Answers*; FDA: Silver Spring, MD, USA, 2015.

105. European Food Safety Authority (EFSA). *Food Supplements, (n.d.)*; EFSA: Parma, Italy, 2006.

106. Jang, S.O.; Kim, H.J.; Kim, Y.J.; Kang, M.J.; Kwon, J.W.; Seo, J.H.; Kim, H.Y.; Kim, B.J.; Yu, J.; Hong, S.J. Asthma prevention by Lactobacillus rhamnosus in a mouse model is associated with CD4 +CD25 +Foxp3 +T cells, Allergy. *Asthma Immunol. Res.* **2012**, *4*, 150–156. [CrossRef]

107. Feleszko, W.; Jaworska, J.; Rha, R.D.; Steinhausen, S.; Avagyan, A.; Jaudszus, A.; Ahrens, B.; Groneberg, D.A.; Wahn, U.; Hamelmann, E. Probiotic-induced suppression of allergic sensitization and airway inflammation is associated with an increase of T regulatory-dependent mechanisms in a murine model of asthma. *Clin. Exp. Allergy* **2006**, *37*, 498–505. [CrossRef]

108. Drago, L.; de Vecchi, E.; Gabrieli, A.; de Grandi, R.; Toscano, M. Immunomodulatory effects of Lactobacillus salivarius LS01 and Bifidobacterium breve BR03, alone and in combination, on peripheral blood mononuclear cells of allergic asthmatics, Allergy. *Asthma Immunol. Res.* **2015**, *7*, 409–413. [CrossRef]

109. Liu, A.; Ma, T.; Xu, N.; Jin, H.; Zhao, F.; Kwok, L.-Y.; Zhang, H.; Zhang, S.; Sun, Z. Adjunctive Probiotics Alleviates Asthmatic Symptoms via Modulating the Gut Microbiome and Serum Metabolome. *Microbiol. Spectr.* **2021**, *9*, e0085921. [CrossRef]

110. Food and Drug Administration (FDA). *Investigational New Drug Applications (INDs)—Determining Whether Human Research Studies Can Be Conducted without an IND | FDA*; FDA: Silver Spring, MD, USA, 2013.

111. Salminen, S.; Collado, M.C.; Endo, A.; Hill, C.; Lebeer, S.; Quigley, E.M.M.; Sanders, M.E.; Shamir, R.; Swann, J.R.; Szajewska, H.; et al. The International Scientific Association of Probiotics and Prebiotics (ISAPP) consensus statement on the definition and scope of postbiotics. *Nat. Rev. Gastroenterol. Hepatol.* **2021**, *18*, 649–667. [CrossRef]
112. Chiu, C.J.; Huang, M.T. Asthma in the precision medicine era: Biologics and probiotics. *Int. J. Mol. Sci.* **2021**, *22*, 4528. [CrossRef] [PubMed]
113. Lin, J.; Zhang, Y.; He, C.; Dai, J. Probiotics supplementation in children with asthma: A systematic review and meta-analysis. *J. Paediatr. Child Health* **2018**, *54*, 953–961. [CrossRef] [PubMed]
114. Du, X.; Wang, L.; Wu, S.; Yuan, L.; Tang, S.; Xiang, Y.; Qu, X.; Liu, H.; Qin, X.; Liu, C. Efficacy of probiotic supplementary therapy for asthma, allergic rhinitis, and wheeze: A meta-analysis of randomized controlled trials. *Allergy Asthma Proc.* **2019**, *40*, 250–260. [CrossRef] [PubMed]
115. Wei, X.; Jiang, P.; Liu, J.; Sun, R.; Zhu, L. Association between probiotic supplementation and asthma incidence in infants: A meta-analysis of randomized controlled trials. *J. Asthma.* **2020**, *57*, 167–178. [CrossRef]
116. Haddaway, N.R.; Collins, A.M.; Coughlin, D.; Kirk, S. The role of google scholar in evidence reviews and its applicability to grey literature searching. *PLoS ONE* **2015**, *10*, e0138237. [CrossRef]
117. Lommatzsch, M.; Brusselle, G.G.; Canonica, G.W.; Jackson, D.J.; Nair, P.; Buhl, R.; Virchow, J.C. Disease-Modifying Anti-Asthmatic Drugs. *Lancet* **2022**, *399*, 1664–1668. [CrossRef]
118. Calzetta, L.; Rogliani, P. Letter to the Editor Regarding "Clinical Remission in Severe Asthma: A Pooled Post Hoc Analysis of the Patient Journey with Benralizumab". *Adv. Ther.* **2022**, *39*, 3857–3861. [CrossRef]

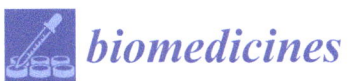

MDPI

Review

Prostacyclin Regulation of Allergic Inflammation

Kunj Patel [1,2] and R. Stokes Peebles, Jr. [1,3,4,*]

1 Division of Allergy, Pulmonary, and Critical Care Medicine, Vanderbilt University Medical Center, Nashville, TN 37232-2650, USA
2 Department of Pathology, Microbiology, and Immunology, Vanderbilt University School of Medicine, Nashville, TN 37232-2650, USA
3 United States Department of Veterans Affairs, Nashville, TN 37232-2650, USA
4 T-1218 MCN, Vanderbilt University Medical Center, 1161 21st Avenue South, Nashville, TN 37232-2650, USA
* Correspondence: stokes.peebles@vanderbilt.edu; Tel.: +1-615-322-3412; Fax: +1-615-343-7448

Abstract: Prostacyclin is a metabolic product of the cyclooxygenase pathway that is constitutively expressed and can be induced during inflammatory conditions. While prostacyclin and its analogs have historically been considered effective vasodilators and used in treating pulmonary hypertension, prostacyclin has demonstrated potent anti-inflammatory effects in animal models of allergic airway inflammation. In vitro studies reveal that prostacyclin directly inhibits type 2 cytokine production from CD4+ Th2 cells and ILC2 and reduces the ability of dendritic cells to generate Th2 cytokine production from CD4+ T cells in an antigen-specific manner. Thus, there is strong evidence that prostacyclin may be an additional therapeutic target for treating allergic inflammation and asthma in human subjects.

Keywords: prostacyclin; allergic inflammation; airway remodeling; proinflammatory; anti-inflammatory; cytokines

Citation: Patel, K.; Peebles, R.S., Jr. Prostacyclin Regulation of Allergic Inflammation. *Biomedicines* **2022**, *10*, 2862. https://doi.org/10.3390/biomedicines10112862

Academic Editor: Stanisława Bazan-Socha

Received: 30 September 2022
Accepted: 4 November 2022
Published: 9 November 2022

Publisher's Note: MDPI stays neutral with regard to jurisdictional claims in published maps and institutional affiliations.

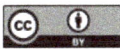

Copyright: © 2022 by the authors. Licensee MDPI, Basel, Switzerland. This article is an open access article distributed under the terms and conditions of the Creative Commons Attribution (CC BY) license (https://creativecommons.org/licenses/by/4.0/).

1. Introduction

Allergic inflammation arises from both innate and adaptive immune responses that are characterized by an increase in the production of type 2 cytokines, such as interleukin (IL)-4, IL-5, IL-9, and IL-13 [1,2]. These cytokines are important in the pathogenesis of allergic diseases such as asthma, atopic dermatitis, allergic rhinitis, and food allergy. IL-4 can cause isotype switching of B cells to IgE production and drives naïve CD4+ T cells to a Th2 phenotype. IL-5 is the most important cytokine in eosinophil differentiation, migration, and survival, which is significant because eosinophils are critical in allergic inflammation pathogenesis. IL-9 has important effects on mast cell development, while IL-13 is a central mediator of airway responsiveness and mucus production, both cardinal features of asthma. An increased understanding of allergen-induced inflammation over the past decade reveals that activated CD4+ Th2 cells alone are not solely responsible for propagating allergic disease. In addition to CD4+ Th2 cells, group 2 innate lymphoid cells (ILC2) also produce IL-5, IL-9, and IL-13 and, in special circumstances, may also secrete IL-4 [3]. Importantly, ILC2 produces IL-5 at a significantly greater level than even CD4+ Th2 cells [4]. In patients with severe asthma, Th1, Th17, and CD8+ cytotoxic lymphocytes and neutrophils may even be observed [5].

In this review, we will focus on the role of prostaglandin (PG)I$_2$ in regulating the allergic inflammatory pathway detailed in the preceding paragraph. As we will discuss, endogenous PGI$_2$ restrains allergen-induced inflammatory responses, and both in vivo and in vitro studies in mice suggest that exogenous PGI$_2$ may be a target for the treatment of allergic diseases such as asthma. PGI$_2$ is one of the five primary prostaglandins. Prostaglandins are eicosanoids, active lipid compounds that are produced through arachidonic acid metabolism via the cyclooxygenase (COX) pathway. The sequential metabolism of arachidonic acid leading to prostaglandin production may be constitutive or induced in response to pathophysiological conditions, such as inflammation [6]. Arachidonic acid is released from the nuclear and cytoplasmic plasma membrane via the action of phospholipase A_2 (PLA_2). COX-1 and COX-2 convert arachidonic acid to an unstable intermediary, PGG_2, which can then be converted to PGH_2 by COX and peroxidase activity [7]. Tissue-specific enzymes and isomerases convert PGH_2 into the five primary prostanoids, which include PGE_2, PGD_2, $PGF_{2\alpha}$, PGI_2, and thromboxane A_2. Whether a specific prostaglandin is produced or not is dependent upon the expression of the synthase for that prostaglandin in that tissue.

PGI_2 is most commonly referred to as prostacyclin, and we will use this terminology in this review. Prostacyclin was discovered in 1976 by Vane and Moncada [8]. Prostacyclin is generated by PGI synthase (PGIS) converting PGH_2 into PGI_2, and PGIS is primarily, but not exclusively, localized in endothelial cells, where it is most abundantly expressed (Figure 1) [7]. Traditionally, prostacyclin has been recognized as an effective vasodilator within both systemic and pulmonary circulations, as it elicits smooth muscle relaxation and has been observed to have anti-platelet aggregatory effects [9]. These characteristics are what led to the rise of prostacyclin analogs, such as iloprost, trepostinil, and epoprostenol, being used clinically in the treatment of pulmonary arterial hypertension [10–12]. For the FDA-approved prostacyclin analogs, iloprost can be administered through either the inhaled or intravenous routes, while epoprostenol is administered intravenously. Treprostinil can be given subcutaneously, intravenously, or orally [13,14]. While beraprost and cicaprost are also potent prostacyclin analogs, neither has been approved by the FDA [13].

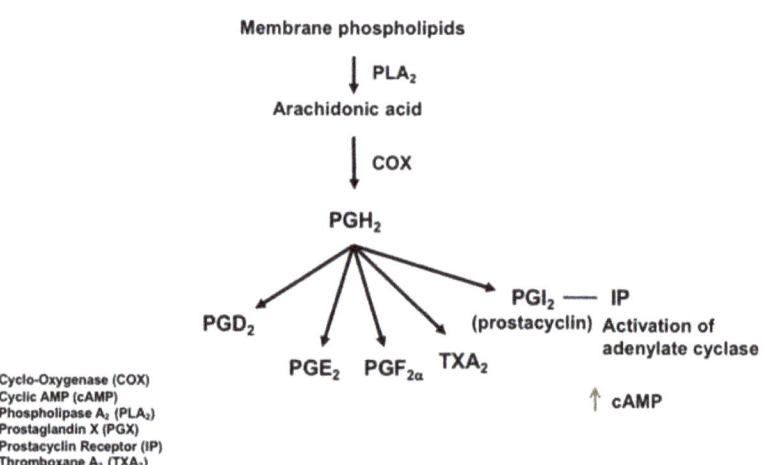

Pathway of Prostacyclin Production

Membrane phospholipids

↓ PLA_2

Arachidonic acid

↓ COX

PGH_2

PGD_2

PGE_2 $PGF_{2\alpha}$ TXA_2

PGI_2 —— IP
(prostacyclin) Activation of
adenylate cyclase

↑ cAMP

Cyclo-Oxygenase (COX)
Cyclic AMP (cAMP)
Phospholipase A_2 (PLA_2)
Prostaglandin X (PGX)
Prostacyclin Receptor (IP)
Thromboxane A_2 (TXA_2)

Figure 1. The pathway of prostacyclin production. The arrows show the downstream enzymatic pathways.

2. Prostacyclin Signaling and In Vivo Models That Suggest an Inability to Signal through the IP Receptor Augments Allergic Inflammation

The biological effects of prostacyclin are exerted by signaling through its primary receptor, IP, which is also known as PTGIR in humans. IP is a seven transmembrane spanning G protein-coupled receptor (GPCR) that, when activated, results in increased intracellular cyclic AMP (cAMP) [7,10]. The increase in cAMP levels that result from IP signaling activates protein kinase A (PKA), leading to the phosphorylation of other proteins leading to downstream vasodilatory effects [10]. In addition to prostacyclin signaling through IP, a peroxisome proliferator-activated nuclear receptor (PPAR) may also be stimulated to act as a transcription factor [15]. PPARs exist in multiple isoforms, and while prostacyclin can signal through PPARδ in mice, PPARγ can be activated by prostacyclin analogs [15,16].

The prostacyclin-IP signaling pathway has been the focus of multiple studies using IP knock-out (KO) mice in order to gain a greater understanding of how prostacyclin regulates the allergic airway inflammatory response (Figure 2); however, as described above, IP is not the sole signaling pathway responsible for the effects of prostacyclin.

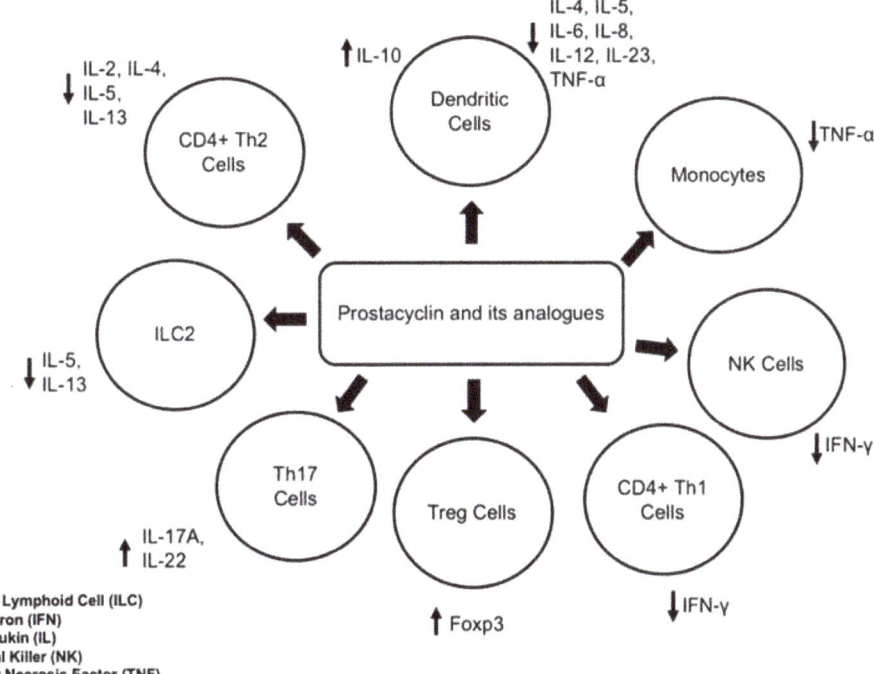

Figure 2. The effects of prostacyclin and its analogs on functions of leukocytes that are important in allergic inflammatory responses. The arrows show how prostacyclin and its analogues regulate specific cell types.

An important tool in understanding how endogenous prostacyclin signaling regulates allergic airway inflammation was the creation of the IP deficient, or knock-out (KO), mouse. Early studies first detailed the effects of the IP receptor signaling in allergic airway inflammation by sensitizing and airway-challenging IP KO mice with ovalbumin to elicit a pulmonary allergen-driven inflammatory response. These studies reported a multi-fold increase in the number of leukocytes in bronchoalveolar lavage fluid (BALF) in IP KO mice relative to their wild-type (WT) counterparts [17,18]. In addition, IP KO mice had a significant increase in the eosinophilic airway and lung inflammation compared to similarly ovalbumin-sensitized and -challenged WT mice. In the ovalbumin model, IP KO mice had more than five times the amount of IL-4 and IL-5 produced in bronchoalveolar lavage fluid (BALF) relative to WT mice [17]. Furthermore, there was also a three-fold increase in the amount of interferon (IFN)-γ produced by splenic CD4+ T cells within the IP KO mice when compared to WT mice [17]. The restraining effect of IP signaling on the production of IFN-γ has since been corroborated by a more recent study that also noted an increase in the level of IFN-γ production from Natural Killer (NK) cells in IP KO mice challenged with house dust mice allergen compared to WT mice [19].

3. Dendritic Cells

Myeloid dendritic cells (mDC) are monocyte-derived antigen-presenting cells that are vital for initiating and regulating the adaptive immune response [20]. More specifically, mDCs accumulate in airways that are challenged by allergens and are involved in inducing and maintaining inflammatory responses by activating naïve T cells in the secondary lymphoid organs, implicating mDCs in potentially having a crucial role in allergic inflammation [20].

In a study that determined the effects of prostacyclin on dendritic cell function, ovalbumin-sensitized and challenged mice treated with inhaled iloprost in vivo had decreased expression of IL-4, IL-5, and IL-13 in restimulated lymph node cells compared to mice treated with the iloprost vehicle [11]. Iloprost treatment significantly decreased the number of eosinophils and lymphocytes in the BAL compartment and reduced peribronchial inflammation and goblet cell hyperplasia compared to vehicle treatment [11]. In vitro, activated iloprost-treated mouse dendritic cells that expressed CC chemokine receptor 7 (CCR7) had decreased chemotactic responsiveness to CC chemokine ligand 19 (CCL19) compared to vehicle-treatment, perhaps explaining the effect of iloprost treatment on the reduction of dendritic cell migration to the lymph nodes in vivo [11].

Another group reported that iloprost dose-dependently decreased TNF-α, IL-6, and IL-8 secretion by human mDCs compared to vehicle treatment [21]. A second group reported that, compared to vehicle treatment, iloprost decreased IL-6, IL-12, IL-23, and TNF-α, while it increased IL-10 in bone marrow dendritic cells (BMDCs) that were stimulated with ovalbumin and then intratracheally adoptively transferred into mice that were subsequently ovalbumin challenged through the airway [9]. Further, mouse CD4+ T cells that expressed a T cell receptor specific for an ovalbumin peptide had reduced production of IL-4, IL-5, and IL-13 when these cells were stimulated with DCs that had been cultured with ovalbumin BMDCs in the presence of iloprost compared to vehicle-treated BMDCs [11]. These results show promise for the use of prostacyclin analogs in attenuating adaptive allergic inflammatory responses.

The results of experiments detailing the effect of prostacyclin in downregulating proinflammatory cytokine production by mouse DCs are similar to those in which human DCs have been studied. Iloprost and treprostinil suppressed TNF-α expression by mDCs activated by the toll-like receptor (TLR) agonist, poly I:C. TNF-α is an important proinflammatory cytokine that recruits immune cells, regulates chemokine production, releases histamine, upregulates adhesion molecules, and is potentially involved in airway remodeling in dendritic cells [13,20]. Compared to vehicle treatment, iloprost-treated human mDCs also decreased the production of IFN-γ by CD4+ helper T cells, while iloprost enhanced the production of the immunosuppressive cytokine IL-10 [20]. These effects were seemingly modulated through the IP and PGE$_2$ (EP) receptors but not PPARs [20]. Furthermore, the modulatory effects of treprostinil and iloprost in this study in which the cAMP pathway was activated were not completely IP-specific [20]. For instance, iloprost increased intracellular Ca2+ levels through EP1 receptor signaling and partly increased IL-10 levels while decreasing TNF-α via the EP1-Ca2+ pathway. In these studies, iloprost's suppressive effects on TNF-α in human mDCs were a result of MAPK-p38-ATF2 pathway signaling [20]. Thus, some prostacyclin analogs, particularly at higher concentrations, may have IP-independent effects by activating EP receptors. Additionally, the study also examined the in vitro effects of prostacyclin analogs on epigenetic regulation. Epigenetic regulation, observed by the activity of histone acetyltransferase and deacetylase, in this instance, regulates inflammatory gene expression [20]. In patients with asthma, there is an overexpression in inflammatory genes due to a decrease in histone deacetylase activity and an increase in histone acetyltransferase activity, and these changes in acetylation through epigenetic regulation also regulate the proliferation and differentiation of T lymphocytes [20,22]. In mDCs that were activated by poly I:C, iloprost downregulated H3K4 trimethylation of the TNFA gene promoter region and inhibited poly I: C-induced translocation of methyltransferases [20].

3.1. Monocytes

In vitro studies also suggest that prostacyclin decreased cytokine secretion by human monocytes. Beraprost, iloprost, and treprostinil dose-dependently suppressed TNF-α expression, and iloprost was the most efficient of the three analogs based on the concentration needed to achieve a partial reduction in cytokine production [13]. These results provide a potential role for prostacyclin in helping to control the symptoms of asthma that may be due to increased TNF-α levels. The effects of prostacyclin in restraining cytokine production in monocytes may not be IP-dependent, as is the case in studies in which DCs were used. For example, in a study that analyzed the effects of prostacyclin analogs on both Th1 and Th2 cytokines in human monocytes, prostacyclin analogs suppressed Th1-related chemokine expression via PPAR-γ [23]. Additionally, the same study reported that iloprost and treprostinil suppressed IP-10, a Th1-related chemokine protein, via the IP-receptor-cAMP pathway [23]. Overall, these studies reflect the importance of better understanding the multiple pathways by which prostacyclin acts, as they can provide several avenues in which to study prostacyclin analog efficacy.

3.2. CD4+ Th2 Cells

Naïve CD4+ T cell differentiation into the Th2 subset is implicated as a key driver of allergen-induced inflammatory diseases such as asthma, and multiple studies reveal that prostacyclin inhibits Th2 inflammation [24]. For instance, IP KO mice sensitized and challenged with an extract of the ubiquitous aeroallergen *Alternaria* had significantly greater numbers of IL-5+ and IL-13+ CD4+ T cells compared to WT mice, further solidifying that endogenous IP signaling is a critical restraining influence on CD4+ Th2 cell differentiation [24]. While IL-4 is recognized as an important cytokine in differentiating CD4+ T cells down the Th2 pathway, IL-33 also has this effect. Cicaprost dose-dependently decreased IL-33-induced production of IL-4, IL-5, and IL-13 by CD4+ cells from WT mice but not in IP KO CD4+ T cells [24]. Cicaprost's inability to suppress Th2 cytokine production in CD4+ Th2 cells from the IP KO mice confirmed the specificity of its effect on the prostacyclin-IP signaling pathway. Additionally, cicaprost decreased the IL-33-induced CD4+ Th2 cell production of IL-2 [24]. Prostacyclin reducing IL-2 could explain the decreased activation of the Th2 cells and their reduction in IL-5 and IL-13 production.

Signal Transducer and Activator of Transcription (STAT) 6 is a transcription factor that is activated by IL-4 and IL-13 and is critical for Th2 cell differentiation [25]. Indomethacin is a COX inhibitor that increases allergic proinflammatory cytokine responses in a STAT6-independent fashion [25]. Indomethacin administration likely resulted in increased allergic inflammation as a result of its decreasing prostacyclin production [25]. This was confirmed by a study using WT, STAT6 KO, IP KO, and IP-STAT6 double knock-out (DKO) mice. In this in vivo study in which ovalbumin was used to sensitize and challenge mice, IP KO mice had greater allergic lung inflammation compared to WT mice. STAT6 KO mice had undetectable levels of Th2 cytokines, while IP-STAT6 DKO mice also had significantly increased IL-5, IL-13, IL-1α, and IL-β protein expression compared to STAT6 KO mice [25]. This revealed that endogenous IP signaling inhibits a STAT6-independent pathway that can drive allergic inflammation [25].

3.3. Innate Allergic Inflammation and Group 2 Innate Lymphoid Cells (ILC2s)

ILC2s are tissue-resident cells that do not express T-cell, B-cell, or monocytic markers; however, they are able to produce Th2 cytokines, namely IL-5 and IL-13, at a markedly higher level than CD4+ Th2 cells [3]. ILC2s are instrumental in amplifying allergic inflammation in the lung [2].

In order to determine the effect of endogenous IP signaling on ILC2 function, mice were challenged with 4 consecutive days of *Alternaria* extract (Alt Ex) to elicit inflammation by innate immunity that precedes significant contribution from the adaptive immune response. In Alt Ex-challenged IP KO mice, there was an increase in lung IL-5 and IL-13 expression, as well as heightened airway eosinophilia and mucus compared to Alt Ex-challenged WT mice [2]. This revealed that endogenous IP signaling restrains ILC2-induced inflammation. In addition to these in vivo findings, in vitro data revealed that cicaprost inhibited IL-5 and IL-13 protein expression by IL-33-stimulated mouse ILC2s [2]. Likewise, in human ILC2s, cicaprost dose-dependently decreased IL-33-induced IL-5 and IL-13 production [2]. Others have reported similar findings. In a study examining mice stimulated with intranasal IL-33, the iloprost-treated group had lower mRNA expression levels of IL-5 and IL-13 alongside a reduction in the proliferation of ILC2s relative to mice treated with the vehicle for iloprost, demonstrating the attenuating effects of prostacyclin analogs on ILC2 type 2 cytokine production [26]. These findings were supported by another study that reported that iloprost directly suppressed ILC2 cytokine production following IL-33 activation [27].

3.4. Th17 Cells

Th17 cells are a subset of CD4+ helper T cells that produce the cytokines IL-17A, IL-17F, IL-21, and IL-22. The differentiation of naïve CD4+ T cells into Th17 cells requires the expression of TGF-β and IL-6 in mice, or TGF-β, IL-1 β, and IL-21 in humans [28]. When IL-17A and IL-17F are produced from Th17 cells, they act in a proinflammatory role and can induce other proinflammatory cytokines, such as IL-8, from the airway epithelium, resulting in neutrophil recruitment. IL-17A and IL-17F also can elicit smooth muscle contraction and airway mucus metaplasia. Both cytokines are increased in the airways of patients with severe asthma [28].

Eicosanoids clearly regulate the production of Th17 cytokines. COX-2 KO mice had significantly reduced numbers of Th17 cells in the lungs, BALF, and spleen following ovalbumin-sensitization and challenge compared to WT mice [28]. Further, IL-17A and IL-6 levels in the blood and BALF were markedly reduced in COX-2 KO mice relative to WT mice following the allergen challenge [28]. These investigators also examined the roles of several different prostaglandins in Th17 differentiation and demonstrated that prostacyclin increased Th17 differentiation in cells that express COX-2 and partially restored Th17 differentiation in mice that were deficient for COX-2 [28]. This finding was corroborated by another group that reported that when iloprost and cicaprost administration in the presence of IL-23 promoted Th17 differentiation and survival in vitro [29]. When prostacyclin analogs were administered in vitro to naïve CD4+ T cells from WT mice, they stimulated greater production of both IL-17A and IL-22 compared to vehicle treatment, indicating that the analogs supported Th17 differentiation and revealing another facet in prostacyclin's role in allergic inflammation [29].

γδ T cells have a first-line immunoprotective role against pathogens and environmental irritants in mucosal tissues [30]. A subset of γδ T cells, γδ-17 cells, produce IL-17. IP KO mice challenged by ovalbumin had a significant reduction in the amount of γδ-17 cells compared to WT mice, and iloprost augmented IL-17 production by γδ T cells, reflecting that both prostacyclin analogs and prostacyclin signaling play a key role in γδ T cell development and effector function [30].

3.5. Treg Cells

Regulatory T cells (Tregs) are critical for immune tolerance in that they suppress inflammation, promote tolerance, and inhibit the development of autoimmune disorders [9,31]. Development of Tregs is promoted by the transcription factor Forkhead box p3 (Foxp3) [31]. Regulatory T cells are crucial for suppressing type 2 inflammation and do so through expressing GATA-binding protein 3 (GATA3) and interferon regulatory factor 4 (IRF4) in order to inhibit Th2 cells [31]. Tregs that express the inhibitory receptor immunoglobulin-like transcript 3 (ILT3) are unable to suppress the Th2 response [31].

In vivo studies reveal that prostacyclin signaling promotes immune tolerance and Treg stability. In the ovalbumin sensitization and challenge model, immune tolerance can be induced by exposing WT mice to aerosolized ovalbumin prior to sensitization. IP KO mice did not develop tolerance in this protocol, suggesting that IP signaling was critical for tolerance induction [32]. Interestingly, in this study, a surprising finding was that there were more, not fewer, Treg in the lungs of IP KO mice. This result suggested that Treg in IP KO mice may be less functional than those in WT mice [32]. A follow-up study confirmed that IP signaling was critical for Treg effector function. Treg from IP KO mice had decreased Foxp3 expression compared to WT Treg, and Foxp3 expression is correlated with Treg suppressive function [31]. In an in vivo adoptive transfer model, Treg from IP KO mice was significantly less able to suppress allergic inflammation compared to WT Treg [31]. Lung IP KO Tregs isolated from mice had a significantly greater ILT3, revealing that prostacyclin signaling attenuated ILT3 expression on Tregs. Further, in vitro studies showed that cicaprost promoted Foxp3 expression in both mouse and human T cells polarized down the Treg pathway. Another group reported that in the ovalbumin-induced asthma model, iloprost promoted regulatory T cell differentiation from naïve T cells [9]. Thus, prostacyclin signaling is critical for optimal Treg function.

3.6. NK Cells

Natural Killer (NK) cells are cells of the innate immune system that serve to target and eliminate tumors and cells infected by viruses [19]. There have been conflicting reports on how exactly NK cells modulate allergic lung inflammation, where some have reported that NK cells play an inhibitory role, and others report that NK cells promote allergen-induced inflammation [19]. One study reported the role of prostacyclin signaling in NK cell function in allergic airway inflammation and found that IP KO mice had reduced allergic lung inflammation induced by house dust mites and decreased Th2 cytokine production [19]. While this finding is in contrast to data previously mentioned in this review, in this model, IP KO mice had a greater number of pulmonary NK cells than WT mice. Depleting NK cells restored allergic inflammation in the IP KO mice to levels seen in WT mice, and transferring NK cells into airways suppressed allergic inflammation [19]. Thus, this leads to the speculation that IP signaling promotes NK cell function to regulate allergies.

4. In Vivo Models that Support the Use of Prostacyclin in Reducing Airway Remodeling and Asthmatic Symptoms

The synthetic prostacyclin analog ONO-1301 reduced allergic inflammation, airway hyperresponsiveness, and remodeling in mice in the ovalbumin model [33]. Mice administered ONO-1301 had decreased goblet-cell metaplasia, reduced airway smooth muscle hypertrophy, and inhibited submucosal collagen deposition [33]. These results support the possibility that prostacyclin may be a potential therapeutic approach to reduce airway remodeling [18,34].

The relationship between cough reflex sensitivity and airway inflammation was investigated by observing the effect of the prostacyclin analog beraprost on asthmatic patients. Unfortunately, beraprost decreased the cough threshold and thus enhanced cough reflex sensitivity in the subjects with asthma [35]. Contrary to these findings, a more recent study examined the role of prostacyclin in the cough response by triggering bronchoconstriction via methacholine chloride (MCh) inhalation in guinea pigs [36]. In animals that were administered a high dose of prostacyclin, the number of coughs induced by bronchoconstriction was significantly decreased, and when an IP antagonist was incorporated, the number of coughs increased [36]. Thus, while there are conflicting reports on the exact effects of prostacyclin on the cough response, there is potential for prostacyclin analogs to reduce a nearly ubiquitous symptom of asthma and allergic inflammation.

5. Concluding Remarks

The landscape of asthma treatment has changed drastically over the last decade with the FDA approval of biologics that target specific molecules that contribute to allergic inflammation. Antibodies against IgE, IL-5, the IL-4 receptor α, and TSLP are all clinically efficacious. However, there remain patients who have uncontrolled asthma despite adequate trials of biological therapies, and this may be where prostacyclin may be useful. Future steps towards potentially utilizing prostacyclin analogs for allergic inflammation, particularly asthma, would require clinical trials. A study that examined the feasibility of administering inhaled iloprost in human patients with mild asthma found that this prostacyclin analog was safe [37]. While there are still aspects to learn about the mechanism for how prostacyclin signaling reduces allergic inflammatory responses, the published data in this review support further research into repurposing prostacyclin as a possible treatment for allergic inflammation and asthma.

Author Contributions: K.P. wrote all drafts of the manuscript and R.S.P.J. edited the manuscript drafts. All authors have read and agreed to the published version of the manuscript.

Funding: This project was supported by NIH/NIAID 5RO1 AI124456, 5RO1 AI145265, 5R21 AI145397, 2U19 AI095227, and U.S. Department of Veterans Affairs 5I01BX004299.

Institutional Review Board Statement: Not applicable.

Informed Consent Statement: Not applicable.

Data Availability Statement: Not applicable.

Conflicts of Interest: The authors declare no conflict of interest.

References

1. Kubo, M. Innate and adaptive type 2 immunity in lung allergic inflammation. *Immunol. Rev.* **2017**, *278*, 162–172. [CrossRef] [PubMed]
2. Zhou, W.; Toki, S.; Zhang, J.; Goleniewksa, K.; Newcomb, D.C.; Cephus, J.Y.; Dulek, D.E.; Bloodworth, M.H.; Stier, M.T.; Polosuhkin, V.; et al. Prostaglandin I2 Signaling and Inhibition of Group 2 Innate Lymphoid Cell Responses. *Am. J. Respir. Crit. Care Med.* **2016**, *193*, 31–42. [CrossRef] [PubMed]
3. Doherty, T.A.; Khorram, N.; Lund, S.; Mehta, A.K.; Croft, M.; Broide, D.H. Lung type 2 innate lymphoid cells express cysteinyl leukotriene receptor 1, which regulates TH2 cytokine production. *J. Allergy Clin. Immunol.* **2013**, *132*, 205–213. [CrossRef] [PubMed]
4. Wolterink, R.G.J.K.; KleinJan, A.; van Nimwegen, M.; Bergen, I.; de Bruijn, M.; Levani, Y.; Hendriks, R.W. Pulmonary innate lymphoid cells are major producers of IL-5 and IL-13 in murine models of allergic asthma. *Eur. J. Immunol.* **2012**, *42*, 1106–1116. [CrossRef]
5. Barnes, P.J. Pathophysiology of allergic inflammation. *Immunol. Rev.* **2011**, *242*, 31–50. [CrossRef] [PubMed]
6. Nørregaard, R.; Kwon, T.-H.; Frøkiær, J. Physiology and pathophysiology of cyclooxygenase-2 and prostaglandin E2 in the kidney. *Kidney Res. Clin. Pract.* **2015**, *34*, 194–200. [CrossRef]
7. Ricciotti, E.; FitzGerald, G.A. Prostaglandins and inflammation. *Arterioscler. Thromb. Vasc. Biol.* **2011**, *31*, 986–1000. [CrossRef]
8. Moncada, S.; Gryglewski, R.; Bunting, S.; Vane, J.R. An enzyme isolated from arteries transforms prostaglandin endoperoxides to an unstable substance that inhibits platelet aggregation. *Nature* **1976**, *263*, 663–665. [CrossRef]
9. Wong, T.-H.; Gau, R.-J.; Chen, Y.-F.; Shen, H.-H.; Lin, C.T.-Y.; Chen, S.-L.; Suen, J.-L. Dendritic cells treated with a prostaglandin I2 analog, iloprost, promote antigen-specific regulatory T cell differentiation in mice. *Int. Immunopharmacol.* **2019**, *79*, 106106. [CrossRef]
10. Dorris, S.L.; Peebles, R.S. PGI2 as a Regulator of Inflammatory Diseases. *Mediat. Inflamm.* **2012**, *2012*, 926968. [CrossRef]
11. Idzko, M.; Hammad, H.; Van Nimwegen, M.; Kool, M.; Vos, N.; Hoogsteden, H.C.; Lambrecht, B.N. Inhaled iloprost suppresses the cardinal features of asthma via inhibition of airway dendritic cell function. *J. Clin. Investig.* **2007**, *117*, 464–472. [CrossRef] [PubMed]
12. Mitchell, J.A.; Ahmetaj-Shala, B.; Kirkby, N.S.; Wright, W.R.; Mackenzie, L.S.; Reed, D.M.; Mohamed, N. Role of prostacyclin in pulmonary hypertension. *Glob. Cardiol. Sci. Pract.* **2014**, *2014*, 382–393. [CrossRef] [PubMed]
13. Wang, W.-L.; Kuo, C.-H.; Chu, Y.-T.; Huang, C.-H.; Lam, K.-P.; Huang, S.-K.; Jong, Y.-J.; Kuo, Y.-T.; Hung, C.-H. Prostaglandin I2 analogues suppress TNF-α expression in human monocytes via mitogen-activated protein kinase pathway. *Agents Actions* **2011**, *60*, 655–663. [CrossRef] [PubMed]
14. Kingman, M.S.; Tankersley, M.A.; Lombardi, S.; Spence, S.; Torres, F.; Chin, K.S. Prostacyclin administration errors in pulmonary arterial hypertension patients admitted to hospitals in the United States: A national survey. *J. Hear. Lung Transplant.* **2010**, *29*, 841–846. [CrossRef] [PubMed]
15. Mohite, A.; Chillar, A.; So, S.-P.; Cervantes, V.; Ruan, K.-H. Novel Mechanism of the Vascular Protector Prostacyclin: Regulating MicroRNA Expression. *Biochemistry* **2011**, *50*, 1691–1699. [CrossRef]
16. Lim, H.; Gupta, R.A.; Ma, W.-G.; Paria, B.C.; Moller, D.E.; Morrow, J.D.; Dubois, R.N.; Trzaskos, J.M.; Dey, S.K. Cyclo-oxygenase-2-derived prostacyclin mediates embryo implantation in the mouse via PPARdelta. *Genes Dev.* **1999**, *13*, 1561–1574. [CrossRef]
17. Takahashi, Y.; Tokuoka, S.; Masuda, T.; Hirano, Y.; Nagao, M.; Tanaka, H.; Inagaki, N.; Narumiya, S.; Nagai, H. Augmentation of allergic inflammation in prostanoid IP receptor deficient mice. *J. Cereb. Blood Flow Metab.* **2002**, *137*, 315–322. [CrossRef]

18. Nagao, K.; Tanaka, H.; Komai, M.; Masuda, T.; Narumiya, S.; Nagai, H. Role of Prostaglandin I2 in Airway Remodeling Induced by Repeated Allergen Challenge in Mice. *Am. J. Respir. Cell Mol. Biol.* **2003**, *29*, 314–320. [CrossRef]

19. Simons, B.; Ferrini, M.E.; Carvalho, S.; Bassett, D.J.P.; Jaffar, Z.; Roberts, K. PGI2 Controls Pulmonary NK Cells That Prevent Airway Sensitization to House Dust Mite Allergen. *J. Immunol.* **2016**, *198*, 461–471. [CrossRef]

20. Kuo, C.-H.; Lin, C.-H.; Yang, S.-N.; Huang, M.-Y.; Chen, H.-L.; Kuo, P.-L.; Hsu, Y.-L.; Huang, S.-K.; Jong, Y.-J.; Wei, W.-J.; et al. Effect of Prostaglandin I2 Analogs on Cytokine Expression in Human Myeloid Dendritic Cells via Epigenetic Regulation. *Mol. Med.* **2011**, *18*, 433–444. [CrossRef]

21. Muller, T.; Dürk, T.; Blumenthal, B.; Herouy, Y.; Sorichter, S.; Grimm, M.; Panther, E.; Cicko, S.; Norgauer, J.; Idzko, M. Iloprost has potent anti-inflammatory properties on human monocyte-derived dendritic cells. *Clin. Exp. Allergy* **2010**, *40*, 1214–1221. [CrossRef] [PubMed]

22. Henning, A.; Roychoudhuri, R.; Restifo, N.P. Epigenetic control of CD8+ T cell differentiation. *Nat. Rev. Immunol.* **2018**, *18*, 340–356. [CrossRef] [PubMed]

23. Kuo, C.-H.; Ko, Y.-C.; Yang, S.-N.; Chu, Y.-T.; Wang, W.-L.; Huang, S.-K.; Chen, H.-N.; Wei, W.-J.; Jong, Y.-J.; Hung, C.-H. Effects of PGI2 analogues on Th1- and Th2-related chemokines in monocytes via epigenetic regulation. *Klin. Wochenschr.* **2010**, *89*, 29–41. [CrossRef]

24. Zhou, W.; Zhang, J.; Toki, S.; Goleniewska, K.; Johnson, M.O.; Bloodworth, M.H.; Newcomb, D.C.; Peebles, R.S. The PGI2 Analog Cicaprost Inhibits IL-33–Induced Th2 Responses, IL-2 Production, and CD25 Expression in Mouse CD4+ T Cells. *J. Immunol.* **2018**, *201*, 1936–1945. [CrossRef]

25. Zhou, W.; Zhang, J.; Goleniewska, K.; Dulek, D.E.; Toki, S.; Newcomb, D.C.; Cephus, J.Y.; Collins, R.D.; Wu, P.; Boothby, M.R.; et al. Prostaglandin I2 Suppresses Proinflammatory Chemokine Expression, CD4 T Cell Activation, and STAT6-Independent Allergic Lung Inflammation. *J. Immunol.* **2016**, *197*, 1577–1586. [CrossRef] [PubMed]

26. Liu, J.; Jiang, X.; Li, L.; Liu, H.; Zhang, X.; Liu, K.; Yang, C. Iloprost inhibits acute allergic nasal inflammation by GATA3 -ILC2 pathway in mice. *Respir. Physiol. Neurobiol.* **2019**, *276*, 103364. [CrossRef] [PubMed]

27. Ikutani, M.; Tsuneyama, K.; Kawaguchi, M.; Fukuoka, J.; Kudo, F.; Nakae, S.; Arita, M.; Nagai, Y.; Takaki, S.; Takatsu, K. Prolonged activation of IL-5-producing ILC2 causes pulmonary arterial hypertrophy. *JCI Insight* **2017**, *2*, e90721. [CrossRef] [PubMed]

28. Li, H.; Bradbury, J.A.; Dackor, R.T.; Edin, M.L.; Graves, J.P.; DeGraff, L.M.; Wang, P.M.; Bortner, C.D.; Maruoka, S.; Lih, F.B.; et al. Cyclooxygenase-2 Regulates Th17 Cell Differentiation during Allergic Lung Inflammation. *Am. J. Respir. Crit. Care Med.* **2011**, *184*, 37–49. [CrossRef]

29. Zhou, W.; Dowell, D.R.; Huckabee, M.M.; Newcomb, D.C.; Boswell, M.G.; Goleniewska, K.; Lotz, M.T.; Toki, S.; Yin, H.; Yao, S.; et al. Prostaglandin I2 Signaling Drives Th17 Differentiation and Exacerbates Experimental Autoimmune Encephalomyelitis. *PLoS ONE* **2012**, *7*, e33518. [CrossRef]

30. Jaffar, Z.; Ferrini, M.E.; Shaw, P.K.; FitzGerald, G.A.; Roberts, K. Prostaglandin I2Promotes the Development of IL-17–Producing γδ T Cells That Associate with the Epithelium during Allergic Lung Inflammation. *J. Immunol.* **2011**, *187*, 5380–5391. [CrossRef]

31. Norlander, A.E.; Bloodworth, M.H.; Toki, S.; Zhang, J.; Zhou, W.; Boyd, K.; Polosukhin, V.V.; Cephus, J.-Y.; Ceneviva, Z.J.; Gandhi, V.D.; et al. Prostaglandin I2 signaling licenses Treg suppressive function and prevents pathogenic reprogramming. *J. Clin. Investig.* **2021**, *131*, e140690. [CrossRef] [PubMed]

32. Zhou, W.; Goleniewska, K.; Zhang, J.; Dulek, D.; Toki, S.; Lotz, M.T.; Newcomb, D.C.; Boswell, M.G.; Polosukhin, V.V.; Milne, G.; et al. Cyclooxygenase inhibition abrogates aeroallergen-induced immune tolerance by suppressing prostaglandin I2 receptor signaling. *J. Allergy Clin. Immunol.* **2014**, *134*, 698–705.e5. [CrossRef]

33. Yamabayashi, C.; Koya, T.; Kagamu, H.; Kawakami, H.; Kimura, Y.; Furukawa, T.; Sakagami, T.; Hasegawa, T.; Sakai, Y.; Matsumoto, K.; et al. A Novel Prostacyclin Agonist Protects against Airway Hyperresponsiveness and Remodeling in Mice. *Am. J. Respir. Cell Mol. Biol.* **2012**, *47*, 170–177. [CrossRef] [PubMed]

34. Hayashi, M.; Koya, T.; Kawakami, H.; Sakagami, T.; Hasegawa, T.; Kagamu, H.; Takada, T.; Sakai, Y.; Suzuki, E.; Gelfand, E.W.; et al. A prostacyclin agonist with thromboxane inhibitory activity for airway allergic inflammation in mice. *Clin. Exp. Allergy* **2010**, *40*, 317–326. [CrossRef]

35. Ishiura, Y.; Fujimura, M.; Nobata, K.; Oribe, Y.; Abo, M.; Myou, S. Prostaglandin I2 enhances cough reflex sensitivity to capsaicin in the asthmatic airway. *Cough* **2007**, *3*, 2. [CrossRef] [PubMed]

36. Sakai, T.; Hara, J.; Yamamura, K.; Okazaki, A.; Ohkura, N.; Sone, T.; Kimura, H.; Abo, M.; Yoshimura, K.; Fujimura, M.; et al. Role of prostaglandin I2 in the bronchoconstriction-triggered cough response in guinea pigs. *Exp. Lung Res.* **2018**, *44*, 455–463. [CrossRef]

37. Majeski, E.; Hoskins, A.; Dworski, R.; Sheller, J.R. Iloprost Inhalation in Mild Asthma. *J. Asthma* **2012**, *49*, 961–965. [CrossRef]

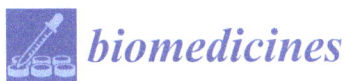 *biomedicines*

Review

The Potential Role of Serum and Exhaled Breath Condensate miRNAs in Diagnosis and Predicting Exacerbations in Pediatric Asthma

Natalia Kierbiedź-Guzik [1],* and Barbara Sozańska [2]

[1] 14th Paediatric Ward—Pulmonology and Allergology, J. Gromkowski Provincial Specialist Hospital, ul. Koszarowa 5, 51-149 Wrocław, Poland

[2] 1st Department and Clinic of Paediatrics, Allergology and Cardiology Wrocław Medical University, ul. Chałubińskiego 2a, 50-368 Wrocław, Poland

* Correspondence: natalia.kierbiedz@gmail.com

Abstract: Asthma is the most common chronic disease of the respiratory system in children and the number of new cases is constantly increasing. It is characterized by dyspnea, wheezing, tightness in the chest, or coughing. Due to diagnostic difficulties, disease monitoring, and the selection of safe and effective drugs, it has been shown that among the youngest patients, miRNAs fulfilling the above roles can be successfully used in common clinical practice. These biomolecules, by regulating the expression of the body's genes, influence various biological processes underlying the pathogenesis of asthma, such as the inflammatory process, remodeling, and intensification of airway obstruction. They can be detected in blood serum and in exhaled breath condensate (EBC). Among children, common factors responsible for the onset or exacerbation of asthma, such as infections, allergens, air pollution, or tobacco smoke present in the home environment, cause a change the concentration of miRNAs in the body. This is related to their significant impact on the modulation of the disease process. In the following paper, we review the latest knowledge on miRNAs and their use, especially as diagnostic markers in assessing asthma exacerbation, with particular emphasis on the pediatric population.

Keywords: miRNA; asthma; children; serum; exhaled breath condensate; diagnosis; exacerbation; biomarkers; factors

Citation: Kierbiedź-Guzik, N.; Sozańska, B. The Potential Role of Serum and Exhaled Breath Condensate miRNAs in Diagnosis and Predicting Exacerbations in Pediatric Asthma. *Biomedicines* **2023**, *11*, 763. https://doi.org/10.3390/biomedicines11030763

Academic Editor: Stanislawa Bazan-Socha

Received: 28 January 2023
Revised: 23 February 2023
Accepted: 27 February 2023
Published: 2 March 2023

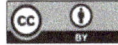

Copyright: © 2023 by the authors. Licensee MDPI, Basel, Switzerland. This article is an open access article distributed under the terms and conditions of the Creative Commons Attribution (CC BY) license (https://creativecommons.org/licenses/by/4.0/).

1. Introduction

Modern medicine is constantly developing, and new, minimally invasive methods are sought to facilitate accurate diagnosis and control the course of the disease. Undoubtedly, a breakthrough event was the recognition of microRNA molecules (miRNAs) which are involved in many biological processes in cells. These biomolecules can be found in blood serum, tissues, and exhaled breath condensate (EBC). They were discovered more than 30 years ago, but only recently have they become a special object of interest among scientists [1–3]. By changing their concentration in the blood serum and knowing the target site of action, they may serve as an extremely useful diagnostic and therapeutic tool allowing us to monitor the course of the disease and detect its exacerbations. Based on a large number of studies, it has been shown that they play a key role in the pathogenesis of allergic diseases (including asthma) by affecting the change in gene expression and modulation of inflammatory processes [4]. Thanks to their minimal invasiveness and the ease of obtaining them, miRNAs are becoming an extremely useful tool in the hands of physicians, especially among the pediatric population. The correct diagnosis of early childhood asthma among this group is often a major clinical problem [5]. Spirometry, i.e., a functional test of the respiratory system, is the gold standard for diagnosing asthma but it requires the cooperation of the patient which is only possible when the child is five to six years old. Due to the still small amount of data on the use of miRNAs among the pediatric population, there is a further need for research to assess their clinical utility in a group of young patients at high risk of an adverse course of the disease.

MiRNAs are small, non-coding RNA molecules, which usually consist of 18–25 nucleotides responsible for regulating gene expression at the translation level and affecting messenger RNA (mRNA) [1]. By binding to the 3′-UTR region, mRNAs lead to the inhibition of translation or degradation in this molecule. These biomarkers act by inhibiting the production of relevant proteins; therefore, it is assumed that the pro-inflammatory effects are probably due to indirect mechanisms [3,6,7]. Approximately 50% of the human genome is regulated by these molecules at the translation stage, which is why they have a significant impact on ensuring homeostasis in the body and coordination of the cell cycle, differentiation, apoptosis, and other physiological functions of cells [8]. Through detailed characterization of the miRNA profile in a given disease entity and correlation of this profile with the appropriate genes, a deeper understanding of the pathophysiological processes will be possible [1,4]. These biomolecules are characterized by high stability and tissue specificity, which emphasizes their additional advantages as new diagnostic markers [8]. MiRNAs have also been shown to be a promising target for potential therapeutic intervention [6,7]. We can divide them into intracellular and extracellular molecules. Thanks to the so-called exosomes, they are transported and transferred between different tissues and cells within the body [3]. Extensively conducted studies have shown a difference in the expression of miRNAs between asthmatics and healthy people. In some of them, the detailed molecular mechanism responsible for the biological processes taking place in cells has already been identified, but most of them are still undiscovered [3,6,7].

Asthma is a chronic inflammatory disease of the bronchial tree characterized by recurrent symptoms, such as cough, shortness of breath, wheezing, and chest tightness, that change in intensity over time. It is the most common chronic disease of the lower respiratory tract in children, usually diagnosed before the age of five (one to two years 34%, less than one year 32%). This may suggest over-diagnosis, because children often cough and wheeze with colds and chest infections, but this is not necessarily asthma [9]. In older children, lung function tests can be used to aid the diagnosis [10]. MiRNA in asthma, through indirect mechanisms, is responsible for the severity of inflammation, hyperresponsiveness, and remodeling of the airways, as well as resistance to standard therapy with inhaled steroids [6]. Moreover, allergens, infections, and air pollution may cause intensification and exacerbation of asthma (especially among children), change the concentration of miRNAs in the serum, and modulate the course of the disease process. The following publication, based on a literature review, aims to introduce miRNAs as new diagnostic markers that allow us to monitor the course of the disease, as well as to recognize and predict its exacerbation, with particular emphasis on the pediatric population [5]. This potential role of miRNAs in pediatric asthma we presented in Figure 1.

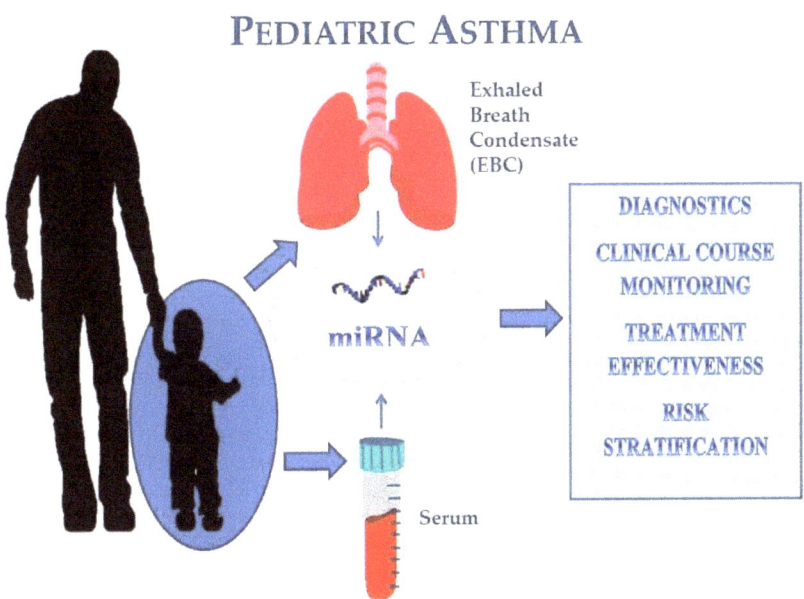

Figure 1. Serum and exhaled breath condensate-isolated miRNA and its potential role in asthma diagnostics and management in the pediatric population.

2. The Diagnostic Role of miRNAs

Due to diagnostic difficulties, delays in initiating appropriate treatment and the need to deal with complications of untreated diseases, asthma is a resource-consuming condition in the healthcare sector. Finding and implementing into clinical practice non-invasive, fast, and sensitive diagnostic methods that can undoubtedly be based on miRNA molecules would largely solve this growing problem. Research has been conducted on these biomolecules that could play a role in this process. Increased expression of miRNA-221 and miRNA-485-3p has been shown in the pediatric asthma population. The first molecule is associated with increased adhesion and migration of mast cells and cytokine production after the body comes into contact with the antigen. In addition, these biomolecules reduce the concentration of the Spred-2 protein (Sprouty-related EVH1 domain-containing 2), contributing to increased cell proliferation and the eosinophilic inflammatory response in the airways through IL-5 [7,11]. MiRNA-21 levels are higher in children with confirmed asthma and positively correlated with disease severity and serum and sputum eosinophilia in these patients. This molecule acts on the Smad-7 gene and inhibits the production of a protein that is an inhibitor of the TGFβ1/Smad pathway. The consequence of this is the excessive synthesis of collagen, α-smooth muscle actin, proliferation and differentiation of fibroblasts, and deposition of the extracellular matrix. This results in remodeling, fibrosis of the airways, and increased airway obstruction [12]. In a study conducted by M. Atashbasteh et al. among patients with severe asthma, increased expression of miRNA-125 was demonstrated, as well as decreased expression of miR-124, miR-130a, and miR-133b. The level of the first of these was correlated with the concentration of CRP and IgE in the serum. These molecules are involved in the pathway of phosphorylation of sphingosine to sphingosine-1 phosphate (S1P) by sphingosine kinase type 1 (SphK1). The effect of S1P on cells is possible by affecting receptors, e.g., S1PR and S2PR. The former is present in large amounts on the surface of lymphocytes and is involved in the process of their maturation (in particular, release from lymphatic organs). In addition to affecting the immune system cell population, S1P also participates in the activation of molecules that regulate inflammation, proliferation, and cell death: NF-kB (nuclear factor kappa B) and STAT3 (signal transducer and activator of transcription 3). For this reason, the significant role of this pathway in the development of autoimmune diseases is emphasized. The increased concentration of this compound in the airways of patients with asthma is responsible for the increased hyperreactivity of the smooth muscle cells of the bronchial tree and the increased inflammatory process. MiRNA-124 is associated with sphingosine kinase 1 (SphK1), which is responsible for the formation of S1P, miRNA-130a with an effect on the S1PR2 receptor (it was proven that the reduction in its expression is associated with an increase in the concentration of inflammatory mediators, including TNF-α and increased expression of inflammatory genes). MiRNA-133b, on the other hand, plays a significant role in controlling the level of sphingosine-1-phosphate receptor protein [13].

An increased blood concentration of some miRNAs in the pediatric population suffering from asthma, e.g., miRNA-3162-3p, miRNA-1260a, miRNA-let-7c-5p, and miRNA-494, has become the subject of further research interest in understanding their role in the pathogenesis of allergic diseases. Particular attention was paid to the miRNA-3162-3p increase in serum in a study of an allergic asthma model conducted in albumin-sensitized mice. Its relationship with β-catenin, which is responsible for the reconstruction of the respiratory tract, and its inhibitory effect on the expression of the gene encoding this protein was proven. The experimental use of antagomir (anti-miRNA) resulted in a reduction in airway hyperreactivity, inflammation, and an increase in B-catenin levels. Thus, signaling involving this molecule seems to be crucial in models of asthma provoked by allergens [14,15].

In childhood the model of allergic asthma dominates, with an increased Th2 cell response and eosinophilic inflammation of the airways. Eosinophils play a key role in the development and maintenance of the inflammatory process. It was shown that by their effect on smooth muscle cells (ASMC) in laboratory conditions, they promote proliferation and hypertrophy. This only occurs in the environment of eosinophilic cells obtained from the blood of sick people. These processes include, for example, TGF-β1 and WNT-5 genes [16]. Eosinophils are also a source of miRNAs which can be transferred between the cells of the body through exosomes, becoming a potential regulator of gene expression [17].

In a study evaluating differences in the expression of miRNAs in eosinophils in patients with the allergic march and healthy subjects, 18 biomarkers were isolated that were associated with the expression of genes involved in cellular regulation, immune response, angiogenesis, and smooth muscle cell proliferation. This highlights the role of miRNAs, which may play a role in the atopic march and the occurrence of many allergic diseases in one patient. Attention was paid to miRNA-590, which was then also shown to be down-expressed in previous studies. Its target is the CITED-2 gene, which is responsible for the regulation of the TGF-beta pathway and the proliferation of airway smooth muscle cells [18,19]. Another study demonstrated a higher concentration of miRNA-144-3p in severe disease and its positive correlation with blood eosinophilia. This biomolecule affects genes responsible for the inflammatory process and remodeling of the airways, e.g., GATA3, STAT6, SOCS5, RHOA, NR3C1, and PTEN, which makes it a potential diagnostic marker for severe asthma [20]. In non-allergic asthma, miRNA-629-3p, miRNA-223-3p, and miRNA-142-3p were significantly elevated in patients with severe symptoms and associated with increased inflammation mediated by neutrophils. In particular, the miRNA-629-3p molecule was responsible for the increased production of IL-8, which stimulates the migration of neutrophils, monocytes, and T cells and the adhesion of neutrophils to the endothelium [21]. Individual miRNAs also affect the expression of interleukins. Involvement in inflammatory processes, e.g., miRNA-1248 (increased concentration in asthmatics) stimulates the synthesis of IL-5, responsible for survival, growth, differentiation, and recruitment of eosinophils. MiRNA-181b-5p, on the other hand, showing reduced expression in people with asthma, is characterized by targeting the SPP1 molecule, i.e., phosphoprotein 1, otherwise known as osteopontin. It is a component of the extracellular matrix that is involved in the migration of eosinophils to the respiratory tract and the intensification of IL-13-induced expression of IL-1 and CCL 11 (eosinophil chemotactic protein) in bronchial epithelial cells [7,22]. MiR-146a and miR-106b, in turn, are upregulated in pediatric asthma patients and lead to increased production of IL-5 and IL-13, which stimulate inflammatory cell recruitment, epithelial cell hyperplasia, smooth muscle hyperplasia, goblet cell metaplasia, and extracellular matrix deposition in the respiratory tract [23].

3. Asthma Exacerbation and miRNAs

MiRNA molecules perform various functions in the body. In addition to the diagnostic role described above, they can be used to predict exacerbation of the disease with greater accuracy. The risk of exacerbation of the disease increases with the lack of use of inhaled corticosteroids, lack of adequate disease control, spirometric indices indicating deepening of obstruction, signs of eosinophilic inflammation, or exposure to allergens or irritants. In a group of children diagnosed with asthma and using anti-inflammatory treatment (inhaled steroids) for a period of 12 months, 12 miRNA molecules associated with exacerbations during observation were isolated. In addition, each doubling of the concentration of these molecules was associated with an increase in the risk of exacerbations by 25–67%, respectively. MiRNA-146b-5p, miRNA-206, and miRNA-720 were identified, which, in combination with clinical symptoms, enabled a better prediction of exacerbation of the disease in patients with asthma using inhaled corticosteroids, compared to a model based only on a single component. Involvement of these miRNAs in pathways involved in the pathogenesis of asthma was discovered, e.g., NF-kβ and GSK3 (glycogen synthase kinase-3)/AKT, which are responsible for remodeling the airways and deepening the inflammatory process [2].

MiRNAs are biomolecules that also play a key role in other obstructive respiratory diseases, including chronic obstructive pulmonary disease (COPD). Researchers compared circulating serum miRNAs associated with exacerbation of the disease in the pediatric population diagnosed with asthma and adults diagnosed with COPD. A total of 20 miRNA molecules were associated with worsening of symptoms in children and 5 of them (451b; 7-5p; 532-3p; 296-5p, and 766-3p) in the adult population with severe chronic obstructive pulmonary disease. Participation of these molecules in the signaling pathways MAPK (mitogen activated protein kinases) and PI3K-Akt, which are responsible for the increased response of both eosinophils and neutrophils, the production of immunoglobulin IgE, and the activation of tumor necrosis factor alpha (TNF-a), was proven. This leads to excessive production of interleukins, cytokines, and intensification of inflammation [24]. In addition, the MAPK pathway is activated by tobacco smoke, indicating its important role in the pathogenesis of COPD and neutrophilic asthma. Thanks to the analysis of the concentrations of appropriate miRNAs, it is also possible to identify the pathomechanism that may lead to exacerbation of symptoms among children with asthma who are exposed to tobacco smoke in the home environment. This is undoubtedly a factor that stimulates an increased immune response and affects the disease symptom severity. However, anti-inflammatory molecules have been identified that are also related to the concentration of the relevant miRNAs. One of them is annexin (ANXA1), also known as lipocortin I. It is a protein with a significant content in the secretions of the respiratory tract. It was shown that an increase in ANXA1 concentration was associated with the decreased concentration of miRNA-196-a2. It is also interesting that in subjects with a moderate disease severity, the level of ANXA 1 was higher than in those with severe asthma. In addition, miRNA-196-2a is responsible for the production of key interleukins involved in the pathogenesis of asthma, IL-5 and IL-13, whose role is described above [25–27]. Many factors can exacerbate the course of asthma, such as tobacco smoke, infections (mainly viral), allergens, irritants (e.g., aerosols or household cleaners, paint fumes, other occupational exposures), physical exertion, air pollution, medications, and foods. Respiratory infections caused by viruses, including RSV, influenza, and rhinoviruses, are of particular importance among the group of the youngest patients. When these pathogens infect human bronchial epithelial cells (HBECs), it was demonstrated that the NF-κB pathway and interferon signaling are activated to stimulate cellular responses, reduce viral replication, and avoid tissue damage. It was suspected that the HBEC cells of asthmatics impair the above-described processes and, consequently, exacerbate symptoms. Understanding miRNAs targeting the NF-κB and interferon pathway will uncover modulators of cellular responses and prevent the development of adverse events [28]. MiRNA-146a and miRNA-146b (miRNA-146a/b) are anti-inflammatory molecules more heavily produced in response to rhinovirus (RV) infection, targeting the NF-κB pathway specifically. In experimental animal models of allergic asthma, deprivation of HBEC cells of these miRNAs led to an increased inflammatory process involving Th1, Th17 lymphocytes with a reduced participation of Th2 lymphocytes. These molecules are therefore responsible for alleviating RV-induced allergic airway inflammation and represent a potential future therapeutic target [29]. Influenza virus is another important infectious agent responsible for exacerbating asthma symptoms. After infection of bronchial epithelial cells with H1N1 influenza virus in the laboratory, miRNA-22 growth was demonstrated only in a sample obtained from healthy individuals. The molecule blocks the CD147 receptor which is a transmembrane glycoprotein involved in the invasion of viral and bacterial infections. This molecule also participates in the remodeling of the respiratory tract through the increased synthesis of matrix metalloproteinases (MMPs). Therefore, asthma patients with low levels of miRNA-22 due to the inability to block CD147 lose one of the important defense barriers against viral infection, becoming more susceptible to infection. In the era of the COVID-19 pandemic, it was shown that the CD147 receptor is also responsible for the penetration of the SARS-CoV-2 virus into the cell. This proves the role of miRNA-22 in the defense process against a wider spectrum of viral infections than just influenza [30].

Unfortunately, not only infectious factors play a leading role in the pathogenesis of asthma in children, but also increasing air pollution and high concentrations of harmful substances in the environment. After measuring the content of PM 2.5 particles in the composition of the air at home, a significant correlation was shown between their concentration and the incidence of asthma. Moreover, greater exposure resulted in an increase in serum concentrations of miRNA-155, which is responsible for the enhancement of the type 2 immune response [31]. The relationship of this biomolecule was also confirmed with exposure to tobacco smoke, which is a special type of air pollution due to its local occurrence and relative ease of elimination from inhaled air compared to other factors. MiRNA-155-5p, miRNA-21-3p, and miRNA-18a-5 are a set of molecules that are overexpressed in the blood of mice exposed to cigarette smoke in utero, in which asthma was later induced with albumin. Additionally, their concentrations were positively correlated with proasthmatic Th2 cytokine levels in bronchoalveolar lavage fluid (BALF) samples [32]. Another aspect that was emphasized was the seasonal variability of miRNAs and its impact on the severity of the allergic process and asthma symptoms in the pediatric population, especially in the spring. It is at this time of the year patients are at risk of exacerbating asthmatic symptoms, especially those with hay fever. Of the 26 miRNAs studied, which were associated with a specific season and with the allergen causing the symptoms of this period, two miRNAs-328-3p and let-7d-3p were isolated. A decrease in the concentration of let-7d-3p was observed in spring and among those allergic to mulberry (spring blooming), while it increased after the allergen immunotherapy process (performed in patients allergic to wasp venom). The protective role of this molecule was proven, which is most likely achieved by reducing the concentration of IL-13. Its protective effect in relation to asthmatic patients is also supported by its abundant presence in the lung tissue. The role of miRNA-328-3p is more complex. It was observed that its concentration decreases in autumn. On the other hand, an increase was noted in patients with a concomitant allergy to aspergillus, which resulted in an exacerbation of symptoms. MiRNA-328-3p was shown to be involved in wound healing of the bronchial epithelium, but also facilitates the spread of bacterial infection in the lungs [33].

MiRNAs may participate in the process of airway remodeling, leading to airway obstruction and affecting airway function parameters. MiRNAs involved in a number of pathophysiological processes affect smooth muscle cells, the epithelium, and goblet cells and intensify the inflammatory process, causing narrowing of the bronchial lumen [34].

The relationship between 22 miRNAs and lung function parameters in the pediatric population was demonstrated. An example may be the following molecules: miRNA-186-5p, which participate in the release of acetylcholine and modulation of airway tone through the cholinergic pathway [35,36]; miRNA-203, which is associated with an increase in IgE concentration and intensifies the inflammatory process in the airways, leading to their obstruction [35,37]; and miRNA-26, which is released by bronchial smooth muscles after their physical stretching, causing cell hypertrophy. Over the course of many years of observation, it has also been proven that miRNA-145-5p is associated with an early decrease in FEV1 in children with asthma, leading to the development of COPD. It is also responsible for the increased proliferation of airway smooth muscle cells [38].

The results of the studies on miRNAs in pediatric asthma are summarized in Table 1.

Table 1. The relevance of miRNA in asthma based on studies conducted in the pediatric population.

Study	Population	miRNA	Gene	Biological Function
F. Liu et al. [11]	N = 12 (study with control group) Age: 4–6 years SAMPLE: serum	↑ miRNA-221 ↑ miRNA-485-3p	SPRED2	Decreased Spred-2 protein. Increased cell proliferation and eosinophilic inflammatory response in the airways through IL-5.
Y. Kang et al. [12]	N = 103 (study with control group) STUDY GROUP: ASTHMA Age: 9.3 ± 0.4 years CONTROL GROUP Age 9.6 ± 0.4 years SAMPLE: serum	↑ miRNA-21	Smad7	Decreased Smad7 protein. TGFβ1/Smad pathway. Excessive synthesis of collagen, α-smooth muscle actin, proliferation and differentiation of fibroblasts. Increased airway obstruction.
Y. Wang et al. [14]	N = 54 (study with control group) SAMPLE: serum	↑ miRNA-3162-3p ↑ miRNA-1260a, ↑ miRNA-let-7c-5p ↑ miRNA-494	CTNNB1	Decreased β-catenin. Intensification of airway hyperreactivity and inflammation.
H. Elnady et al. [23]	N = 50 (study with control group) STUDY GROUP: ASTHMA Age: 10.6 ± 0.7 years CONTROL GROUP Age: 11.0 ± 0.8 years SAMPLE: serum	↑ miRNA-146a ↑ miRNA-106b	-	Increased IL-5, IL-13. Stimulate inflammatory cell recruitment, epithelial cell and smooth muscle hyperplasia, goblet cell metaplasia, and extracellular matrix deposition in the respiratory tract.
L. He et al. [18]	N = 170 (study with control group) SAMPLE: serum	↑ miRNA-144-3p	GATA3, STAT6, SOCS5, RHOA, NR3C1 i PTEN	Increased eosinophilia, inflammatory process, and remodeling of the airways.
A. T. Kho et al. [2]	N = 153 (study with control group) STUDY GROUP: ASTHMA EXACERBATION Age: 8.9 ± 2.2 years CONTROL GROUP: NO EXACERBATION Age: 8.9 ± 2.0 years SAMPLE: serum	↑ miRNA-146b-5p ↑ miRNA-206 ↑ miRNA-720	-	Upregulation GSK3 by AKT and downregulation NF-kB pathway. Remodeling the airways and deepening the inflammatory process.

Table 1. *Cont.*

Study	Population	miRNA	Gene	Biological Function
A. Tiwari et al. [24]	N = 351 (study with control group) STUDY GROUP: ASTHMA EXACERBATION Age: 9.0 ± 1.9 years CONTROL GROUP: NO EXACERBATION Age: 9.4 ± 1.8 years SAMPLE: serum	↓ miRNA-451b ↓ miRNA-7-5p ↑ miRNA-532-3p ↑ miRNA-296-5p ↑ miRNA-766-3p)	Many genes involved in the production of more than 20 proteins.	Upregulation MAPK, PI3K-Akt (i.a). Increased eosinophils, neutrophils, IgE immunoglobulin, and the activation of tumor necrosis factor alpha (TNF-a). Excessive production of interleukins and cytokines and intensification of inflammation.
A. A. Ibrahim et al. [25]	N = 100 (study with control group) STUDY GROUP: MILD, MODERATE, SEVERE ASTHMA Age: 8.9 ± 1.3 years CONTROL GROUP Age: 8.2 ± 1.4 years SAMPLE: serum	↑ miRNA-196-2a	ANXA1	Downregukation Annexin (anti-inflammatory factor). Concentration: moderate asthma > severe asthma. Increased inflammatory reaction.
Q. Liu et al. [31]	N = 360 (study with control group) STUDY GROUP: ASTHMA Age: 10.8 ± 3.1 years CONTROL GROUP Age 10.1 ± 2.7 years SAMPLE: serum	↑ miRNA-155	-	Responsible for the enhancement of the type 2 immune response.
A. T. Kho et al. [35]	N = 360 (study without control group) Age: 8.8 ± 2.1 years SAMPLE: serum	↑ miRNA-186-5p ↑ miRNA-203 ↑ miRNA-26	≈50	Activation of cholinergic pathway, intensifies the inflammatory process in the airways leading to their obstruction. Hypertrophy of smooth muscles.
A. Tiwari et al. [33]	N = 398 (study without control group) Age: 5–12 years SAMPLE: serum	↑ let-7d-3p ↑ miRNA-328-3p	-	Decreased serum level of IL-13. Exacerbation of symptoms in patients allergic to aspergilus.
F. C. Mendes et al. [39]	N = 186 (study with control group) STUDY GROUP: ASTHMA Age: 8.7 ± 0.8 years CONTROL GROUP Age: 8.7 ± 0.8 years SAMPLE: exhaled breath condensate	↑ miRNA -155 ↑ miR-126-3p ↑ miR-133a-3p ↑ miR-145-5p, ↑ miRNA-423-3p	E.G RUNX3	GATA-3-upregulation of Th1/Th2 balance. Downregulation of GATA-3. Promotes a lymphocyte Th2 response. Increase in the levels of the IL-13 inflammatory response.
F. C. Mendes et al. [40]	N = 150 (study with control group) Age: 7–12 years SAMPLE: exhaled breath condensate	↑ miR-133a-3p	-	Upregulation of production of IL-13.

Abbreviations: SPRED2—Sprouty-related EVH1 domain-containing 2; Smad—suppressor of mother against decapentaplegic; TGFβ1—transforming growth factor β1; CTNNB1—catenin beta gene; IL—interleukin; GATA3—GATA binding protein three gene; STAT6—signal transducer and activator of transcription six gene; SOCS5—suppressor of cytokine signaling protein five gene; RHOA—Ras homolog family member A gene; NR3C1—nuclear receptor subfamily three group C member 1 gene; PTEN—phosphatase and tensin homolog gene; GSK3—glycogen synthase kinase-3; AKT—protein kinase *B*; NF-kB—nuclear factor kappa-light-chain-enhancer of activated B cells; MAPK—mitogen-activated protein kinases, PI3K—the phosphatidylinositol 3-kinase; Ige—immunoglobulin E; GATA3—GATA binding protein three; Th1—Type 1 T helper; Th2—Type 2 T helper.

4. Exhaled Breath Condensate

Examination of the exhaled breath condensate (EBC) is a new, non-invasive method that allows us to assess the inflammatory process within the respiratory tract and may be successfully used in children. The material is gathered by calm breathing for 10–15 min, and then cooling and accumulating the air exhaled into the capacitor. Thanks to the obtained condensate, it is possible to measure inflammatory markers in the collected material, as well as miRNA. In this way, a potentially useful, non-invasive technique was obtained for diagnosing and controlling the course of the disease and assessing the effectiveness of asthma treatment. The presence of miRNAs in EBC was confirmed for the first time in 2013. The difference in the expression of 11 miRNAs between asthmatics and healthy people was proven, as well as the greater stability of miRNA molecules in EBC compared to the material obtained from blood serum due to the difference in the number of miRNAs enclosed in exosomes [41,42].

It was found that the concentration of miRNA contained in EBC is related to the functional parameters of the respiratory tract. In the first study conducted among the pediatric population with diagnosed asthma in which the exhaled breath condensate was analyzed, the influence of a number of miRNAs (e.g., miRNA-155, miR-126-3p, miR-133a-3p, miR-145-5p, 3p) on lung function parameters and reversibility of airway obstruction was proven [39]. In subsequent studies, the relationship between miRNA-570-3p in EBC and spirometry results was also found through an inverse relationship between the expression of this molecule and FEV1 values. A similar relationship was obtained after examining miRNA-1248. With regard to the intensity of the inflammatory process, it was found that miRNA-570-3p affects the diverse expression of many cytokines, chemokines, and the HuR protein (it binds RNA and regulates post-transcriptional processes). Thus, this biomolecule becomes a potential regulator of inflammation in asthma [43]. In addition, attention was paid to miRNA-423, the relationship of which was proven with obesity. Obesity is known to be one of the factors predisposing a higher risk of developing asthma. Since asthma and obesity are characterized by chronic inflammation, it is likely that miRNAs may be misregulated in these diseases by modulating the immune cells found in EBCs. Interestingly, an unobvious relationship between the increase in the amount of fatty acids in the food consumed and the increase in the level of miRNA-133a-3p in the EBC affecting the inflammatory response in the condensate of exhaled air among children diagnosed with asthma was also noted [40].

The limitation of our work is the fact that some studies have been based on relatively small pediatric populations or studies with no control group. To present the trends and potential perspectives for future studies, we have presented studies conducted on adult populations or animal models in case of a lack of data on children.

5. Conclusions

In modern medicine we strive for an individual approach to each patient. This strategy is mainly based on clinical phenotyping, where biomarkers play an important role. Additionally, in childhood diseases, especially in asthma, problems with diagnostics and assessment of treatment efficacy often occur due to a lack of cooperation with young patient. Thus, many molecules, metabolites, and proteins remain the subject of research to find a simple, useful biomarker that may solve the abovementioned problems. The potential relevance of molecules, such as (in blood) eosinophil cationic protein, periostin, lipoxins, chitinases, YKL-40, (in exhaled breath) fractional exhaled nitric oxide, volatile organic compounds, evaluation of exhaled breath temperature, (in urine) bromotyrosine, metabolites of eicosanoids, eosinophil-derived neurotoxin in diagnostics and management of asthma were evaluated. Unfortunately, these biomarkers presented several limitations, e.g., particles detected in the urine do not directly reflect the inflammatory process in the respiratory tract and the concentration of some molecules changes during the growth of children or in the course of other diseases [44–46]. These facts make them useless in clinical practice. Therefore, understanding the importance of new, promising biomarkers

Biomedicines 2023, 11, 763

(miRNAs) and their role in metabolic pathways in childhood asthma seems to be crucial. Based on the considerations presented in this manuscript, it can be seen that miRNAs, in combination with disease symptoms, lung function tests, and allergy tests, seem to be a useful tool in the construction of predictive models, allowing for the identification of high-risk groups for the adverse course of the disease and increasing the probability of making an accurate diagnosis in an ambiguous case. In order for miRNAs to be introduced into common clinical practice, the methods of their detection should be characterized by high sensitivity and specificity. Based on many studies, it has been shown that they indeed have such potential; however, a lack of data prevents their successful implementation in clinical practice. Therefore, there is a need to conduct new analyses and search for solutions using miRNA molecules in the population of pediatric patients diagnosed or suspected of having bronchial asthma.

Author Contributions: N.K.-G. and B.S. conceived of the review and drafted the manuscript. The review was performed under the supervision of B.S. All authors have read and agreed to the published version of the manuscript.

Funding: This research received no external funding.

Institutional Review Board Statement: Not applicable.

Informed Consent Statement: Not applicable.

Data Availability Statement: No new data were created or analyzed in this study. Data sharing is not applicable to this article.

Conflicts of Interest: The authors declare no conflict of interest.

References

1. Gutierrez, M.J.; Gomez, J.L.; Perez, G.F.; Pancham, K.; Val, S.; Pillai, D.K.; Giri, M.; Ferrante, S.; Freishtat, R.; Rose, M.C.; et al. Airway Secretory MicroRNAome Changes during Rhinovirus Infection in Early Childhood. *PLoS ONE* **2016**, *11*, e0162244. [CrossRef] [PubMed]
2. Kho, A.T.; McGeachie, M.J.; Moore, K.G.; Sylvia, J.M.; Weiss, S.T.; Tantisira, K.G. Circulating MicroRNAs and Prediction of Asthma Exacerbation in Childhood Asthma. *Respir. Res.* **2018**, *19*, 128. [CrossRef] [PubMed]
3. Sharma, R.; Tiwari, A.; McGeachie, M.J. Recent MiRNA Research in Asthma. *Curr. Allergy Asthma Rep.* **2022**, *22*, 231–258. [CrossRef] [PubMed]
4. Taka, S.; Tzani-Tzanopoulou, P.; Wanstall, H.; Papadopoulos, N.G. MicroRNAs in Asthma and Respiratory Infections: Identifying Common Pathways. *Allergy Asthma Immunol. Res.* **2020**, *12*, 4. [CrossRef] [PubMed]
5. Weidner, J.; Bartel, S.; Kılıç, A.; Zissler, U.M.; Renz, H.; Schwarze, J.; Schmidt-Weber, C.B.; Maes, T.; Rebane, A.; Krauss-Etschmann, S.; et al. Spotlight on MicroRNAs in Allergy and Asthma. *Allergy* **2021**, *76*, 1661–1678. [CrossRef]
6. Lizzo, J.M.; Cortes, S. *Pediatric Asthma*; Mayo Clinic Press: Rochester, MN, USA, 2022.
7. Pattarayan, D.; Thimmulappa, R.K.; Ravikumar, V.; Rajasekaran, S. Diagnostic Potential of Extracellular MicroRNA in Respiratory Diseases. *Clin. Rev. Allergy Immunol.* **2018**, *54*, 480–492. [CrossRef]
8. Catalanotto, C.; Cogoni, C.; Zardo, G. MicroRNA in Control of Gene Expression: An Overview of Nuclear Functions. *Int. J. Mol. Sci.* **2016**, *17*, 1712. [CrossRef]
9. Ibrahim, A.A.; Elia Adil, N.; Ahmed, M.S.E. Diagnosis of Asthma in Childhood Age. *Arch. Asthma Allergy Immunol.* **2018**, *2*, 8–12. [CrossRef]
10. Yang, C.L.; Gaffin, J.M.; Radhakrishnan, D. Question 3: Can We Diagnose Asthma in Children under the Age of 5 years? *Paediatr. Respir. Rev.* **2019**, *29*, 25–30. [CrossRef]
11. Liu, F.; Qin, H.-B.; Xu, B.; Zhou, H.; Zhao, D.-Y. Profiling of MiRNAs in Pediatric Asthma: Upregulation of MiRNA-221 and MiRNA-485-3p. *Mol. Med. Rep.* **2012**, *6*, 1178–1182. [CrossRef]
12. Kang, Y.; Bai, M.; Deng, L.; Fan, L.; Wang, X. MiRNA-21 Regulates Bronchial Epithelial Cell Proliferation by Activating Tgfβ1/Smad Signaling Pathway and Its Correlation with Asthma Severity in Children. *Iran. J. Public Health* **2021**, *50*, 1973–1982. [CrossRef] [PubMed]
13. Atashbasteh, M.; Mortaz, E.; Mahdaviani, S.A.; Jamaati, H.; Allameh, A. Expression Levels of Plasma Exosomal MiR-124, MiR-125b, MiR-133b, MiR-130a and MiR-125b-1-3p in Severe Asthma Patients and Normal Individuals with Emphasis on Inflammatory Factors. *Allergy Asthma Clin. Immunol.* **2021**, *17*, 51. [CrossRef] [PubMed]
14. Fang, C.; Lu, W.; Li, C.; Peng, X.; Wang, Y.; Huang, X.; Yao, Z.; Cai, N.; Huang, Y.; Zhang, X.; et al. MiR-3162-3p Is a Novel MicroRNA That Exacerbates Asthma by Regulating β-Catenin. *PLoS ONE* **2016**, *11*, e0149257. [CrossRef] [PubMed]

15. Wang, Y.; Yang, L.; Li, P.; Huang, H.; Liu, T.; He, H.; Lin, Z.; Jiang, Y.; Ren, N.; Wu, B.; et al. Circulating MicroRNA Signatures Associated with Childhood Asthma. *Clin. Lab.* **2015**, *61*, 467–474. [CrossRef] [PubMed]
16. Januskevicius, A.; Vaitkiene, S.; Gosens, R.; Janulaityte, I.; Hoppenot, D.; Sakalauskas, R.; Malakauskas, K. Eosinophils Enhance WNT-5a and TGF-B1 Genes Expression in Airway Smooth Muscle Cells and Promote Their Proliferation by Increased Extracellular Matrix Proteins Production in Asthma. *BMC Pulm. Med.* **2016**, *16*, 94. [CrossRef]
17. Cañas, J.A.; Sastre, B.; Rodrigo-Muñoz, J.M.; del Pozo, V. Exosomes: A New Approach to Asthma Pathology. *Clin. Chim. Acta* **2019**, *495*, 139–147. [CrossRef]
18. He, L.; Liu, J.; Wang, X.; Wang, Y.; Zhu, J.; Kang, X. Identifying a Novel Serum MicroRNA Biomarker Panel for the Diagnosis of Childhood Asthma. *Exp. Biol. Med.* **2022**, *247*, 1732–1740. [CrossRef] [PubMed]
19. Bélanger, É.; Madore, A.-M.; Boucher-Lafleur, A.-M.; Simon, M.-M.; Kwan, T.; Pastinen, T.; Laprise, C. Eosinophil MicroRNAs Play a Regulatory Role in Allergic Diseases Included in the Atopic March. *Int. J. Mol. Sci.* **2020**, *21*, 9011. [CrossRef]
20. Rodrigo-Muñoz, J.M.; Gil-Martínez, M.; Lorente-Sorolla, C.; García-Latorre, R.; Valverde-Monge, M.; Quirce, S.; Sastre, J.; del Pozo, V. MiR-144-3p Is a Biomarker Related to Severe Corticosteroid-Dependent Asthma. *Front. Immunol.* **2022**, *13*, 858722. [CrossRef]
21. Maes, T.; Cobos, F.A.; Schleich, F.; Sorbello, V.; Henket, M.; de Preter, K.; Bracke, K.R.; Conickx, G.; Mesnil, C.; Vandesompele, J.; et al. Asthma Inflammatory Phenotypes Show Differential MicroRNA Expression in Sputum. *J. Allergy Clin. Immunol.* **2016**, *137*, 1433–1446. [CrossRef]
22. Huo, X.; Zhang, K.; Yi, L.; Mo, Y.; Liang, Y.; Zhao, J.; Zhang, Z.; Xu, Y.; Zhen, G. Decreased Epithelial and Plasma MiR-181b-5p Expression Associates with Airway Eosinophilic Inflammation in Asthma. *Clin. Exp. Allergy* **2016**, *46*, 1281–1290. [CrossRef] [PubMed]
23. Elnady, H.G.; Sherif, L.S.; Kholoussi, N.M.; Ali Azzam, M.; Foda, A.R.; Helwa, I.; Sabry, R.N.; Eissa, E.; Fahmy, R.F. Aberrant Expression of Immune-Related MicroRNAs in Pediatric Patients with Asthma. *Int. J. Mol. Cell Med.* **2020**, *9*, 246–255. [CrossRef] [PubMed]
24. Tiwari, A.; Hobbs, B.D.; Li, J.; Kho, A.T.; Amr, S.; Celedón, J.C.; Weiss, S.T.; Hersh, C.P.; Tantisira, K.G.; McGeachie, M.J. Blood MiRNAs Are Linked to Frequent Asthma Exacerbations in Childhood Asthma and Adult COPD. *Noncoding RNA* **2022**, *8*, 27. [CrossRef] [PubMed]
25. Ibrahim, A.A.; Ramadan, A.; Wahby, A.A.; Draz, I.H.; El Baroudy, N.R.; Abdel Hamid, T.A. Evaluation of MiR-196a2 Expression and Annexin A1 Level in Children with Bronchial AsthmaEvaluation of MiR-196a2 Expression and Annexin A1 Level in Children. *Allergol. Immunopathol.* **2020**, *48*, 458–464. [CrossRef] [PubMed]
26. Lee, S.-H.; Lee, P.-H.; Kim, B.-G.; Seo, H.-J.; Baek, A.-R.; Park, J.-S.; Lee, J.-H.; Park, S.-W.; Kim, D.-J.; Park, C.-S.; et al. Annexin A1 in Plasma from Patients with Bronchial Asthma: Its Association with Lung Function. *BMC Pulm. Med.* **2018**, *18*, 1. [CrossRef] [PubMed]
27. Hussein, M.H.; Toraih, E.A.; Aly, N.M.; Riad, E.; Fawzy, M.S. A Passenger Strand Variant in MiR-196a2 Contributes to Asthma Severity in Children and Adolescents: A Preliminary Study. *Biochem. Cell Biol.* **2016**, *94*, 347–357. [CrossRef] [PubMed]
28. Jartti, T.; Gern, J.E. Role of Viral Infections in the Development and Exacerbation of Asthma in Children. *J. Allergy Clin. Immunol.* **2017**, *140*, 895–906. [CrossRef] [PubMed]
29. Laanesoo, A.; Urgard, E.; Periyasamy, K.; Laan, M.; Bochkov, Y.A.; Aab, A.; Magilnick, N.; Pooga, M.; Gern, J.E.; Johnston, S.L.; et al. Dual Role of the MiR-146 Family in Rhinovirus-induced Airway Inflammation and Allergic Asthma Exacerbation. *Clin. Transl. Med.* **2021**, *11*, e427. [CrossRef]
30. Moheimani, F.; Koops, J.; Williams, T.; Reid, A.T.; Hansbro, P.M.; Wark, P.A.; Knight, D.A. Influenza A Virus Infection Dysregulates the Expression of MicroRNA-22 and Its Targets; CD147 and HDAC4, in Epithelium of Asthmatics. *Respir. Res.* **2018**, *19*, 145. [CrossRef]
31. Liu, Q.; Wang, W.; Jing, W. Indoor Air Pollution Aggravates Asthma in Chinese Children and Induces the Changes in Serum Level of MiR-155. *Int. J. Environ. Health Res.* **2019**, *29*, 22–30. [CrossRef]
32. Xiao, R.; Noël, A.; Perveen, Z.; Penn, A.L. In Utero Exposure to Second-Hand Smoke Activates pro-Asthmatic and Oncogenic MiRNAs in Adult Asthmatic Mice. *Environ. Mol. Mutagen.* **2016**, *57*, 190–199. [CrossRef]
33. Tiwari, A.; Wang, A.L.; Li, J.; Lutz, S.M.; Kho, A.T.; Weiss, S.T.; Tantisira, K.G.; McGeachie, M.J. Seasonal Variation in MiR-328-3p and Let-7d-3p Are Associated With Seasonal Allergies and Asthma Symptoms in Children. *Allergy Asthma Immunol. Res.* **2021**, *13*, 576. [CrossRef]
34. Liang, J.; Liu, X.-H.; Chen, X.-M.; Song, X.-L.; Li, W.; Huang, Y. Emerging Roles of Non-Coding RNAs in Childhood Asthma. *Front. Pharm.* **2022**, *13*, 856104. [CrossRef] [PubMed]
35. Kho, A.T.; Sharma, S.; Davis, J.S.; Spina, J.; Howard, D.; McEnroy, K.; Moore, K.; Sylvia, J.; Qiu, W.; Weiss, S.T.; et al. Circulating MicroRNAs: Association with Lung Function in Asthma. *PLoS ONE* **2016**, *11*, e0157998. [CrossRef] [PubMed]
36. Nadorp, B.; Soreq, H. Predicted Overlapping MicroRNA Regulators of Acetylcholine Packaging and Degradation in Neuroinflammation-Related Disorders. *Front. Mol. Neurosci.* **2014**, *7*, 9. [CrossRef]
37. Lv, Y.; Qi, R.; Xu, J.; Di, Z.; Zheng, H.; Huo, W.; Zhang, L.; Chen, H.; Gao, X. Profiling of Serum and Urinary MicroRNAs in Children with Atopic Dermatitis. *PLoS ONE* **2014**, *9*, e115448. [CrossRef]

38. Tiwari, A.; Li, J.; Kho, A.T.; Sun, M.; Lu, Q.; Weiss, S.T.; Tantisira, K.G.; McGeachie, M.J. COPD-Associated MiR-145-5p Is Downregulated in Early-Decline FEV1 Trajectories in Childhood Asthma. *J. Allergy Clin. Immunol.* **2021**, *147*, 2181–2190. [CrossRef] [PubMed]

39. Mendes, F.C.; Paciência, I.; Ferreira, A.C.; Martins, C.; Rufo, J.C.; Silva, D.; Cunha, P.; Farraia, M.; Moreira, P.; Delgado, L.; et al. Development and Validation of Exhaled Breath Condensate MicroRNAs to Identify and Endotype Asthma in Children. *PLoS ONE* **2019**, *14*, e0224983. [CrossRef]

40. Mendes, F.C.; Paciência, I.; Cavaleiro Rufo, J.; Silva, D.; Delgado, L.; Moreira, A.; Moreira, P. Dietary Acid Load Modulation of Asthma-Related MiRNAs in the Exhaled Breath Condensate of Children. *Nutrients* **2022**, *14*, 1147. [CrossRef]

41. Szymczak, I.; Wieczfinska, J.; Pawliczak, R. Molecular Background of MiRNA Role in Asthma and COPD: An Updated Insight. *Biomed Res. Int.* **2016**, *2016*, 7802521. [CrossRef]

42. Sinha, A.; Yadav, A.K.; Chakraborty, S.; Kabra, S.K.; Lodha, R.; Kumar, M.; Kulshreshtha, A.; Sethi, T.; Pandey, R.; Malik, G.; et al. Exosome-Enclosed MicroRNAs in Exhaled Breath Hold Potential for Biomarker Discovery in Patients with Pulmonary Diseases. *J. Allergy Clin. Immunol.* **2013**, *132*, 219–222.e7. [CrossRef] [PubMed]

43. Roff, A.N.; Craig, T.J.; August, A.; Stellato, C.; Ishmael, F.T. MicroRNA-570-3p Regulates HuR and Cytokine Expression in Airway Epithelial Cells. *Am. J. Clin. Exp. Immunol.* **2014**, *3*, 68–83. [PubMed]

44. Tiotiu, A. Biomarkers in Asthma: State of the Art. *Asthma Res. Pract.* **2018**, *4*, 10. [CrossRef] [PubMed]

45. Pite, H.; Morais-Almeida, M.; Mensinga, T.; Diamant, Z. Non-Invasive Biomarkers in Asthma: Promises and Pitfalls. In *Asthma—From Childhood Asthma to ACOS Phenotypes*; InTech: London, UK, 2016.

46. James, A.; Hedlin, G. Biomarkers for the Phenotyping and Monitoring of Asthma in Children. *Curr. Treat Options Allergy* **2016**, *3*, 439–452. [CrossRef] [PubMed]

Disclaimer/Publisher's Note: The statements, opinions and data contained in all publications are solely those of the individual author(s) and contributor(s) and not of MDPI and/or the editor(s). MDPI and/or the editor(s) disclaim responsibility for any injury to people or property resulting from any ideas, methods, instructions or products referred to in the content.

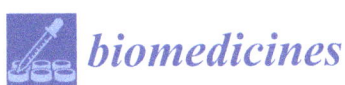

Article

Side-Directed Release of Differential Extracellular Vesicle-associated microRNA Profiles from Bronchial Epithelial Cells of Healthy and Asthmatic Subjects

Viktoria E. M. Schindler [1,†], Fahd Alhamdan [1,†], Christian Preußer [2,3], Lukas Hintz [1], Bilal Alashkar Alhamwe [2,4], Andrea Nist [5], Thorsten Stiewe [5], Elke Pogge von Strandmann [2,3], Daniel P. Potaczek [1], Clemens Thölken [6,†] and Holger Garn [1,*,†]

[1] Translational Inflammation Research Division & Core Facility for Single Cell Multiomics, Philipps University of Marburg–Medical Faculty, Member of the German Center for Lung Research (DZL) and the Universities of Giessen and Marburg Lung Center, 35043 Marburg, Germany; schindlerviktoria@t-online.de (V.E.M.S.); alhamdaf@staff.uni-marburg.de (F.A.); hintz@staff.uni-marburg.de (L.H.); potaczek@staff.uni-marburg.de (D.P.P.)

[2] Institute for Tumor Immunology, Philipps University of Marburg–Medical Faculty, 35043 Marburg, Germany; preusserc@staff.uni-marburg.de (C.P.); bilal.alashkaralhamwe@staff.uni-marburg.de (B.A.A.); elke.poggevonstrandmann@uni-marburg.de (E.P.v.S.)

[3] Core Facility Extracellular Vesicles, Philipps University of Marburg–Medical Faculty, 35043 Marburg, Germany

[4] College of Pharmacy, International University for Science and Technology (IUST), Daraa 15, Syria

[5] Institute of Molecular Oncology & Genomics Core Facility, Philipps University of Marburg–Medical Faculty, Member of the German Center for Lung Research (DZL) and the Universities of Giessen and Marburg Lung Center, 35043 Marburg, Germany; andrea.nist@imt.uni-marburg.de (A.N.); stiewe@uni-marburg.de (T.S.)

[6] Institute of Medical Bioinformatics and Biostatistics, Philipps University of Marburg–Medical Faculty, 35043 Marburg, Germany; thoelken@uni-marburg.de

* Correspondence: garn@staff.uni-marburg.de; Tel.: +49-6421-2866040

† These authors contributed equally to this work.

Citation: Schindler, V.E.M.; Alhamdan, F.; Preußer, C.; Hintz, L.; Alashkar Alhamwe, B.; Nist, A.; Stiewe, T.; Pogge von Strandmann, E.; Potaczek, D.P.; Thölken, C.; et al. Side-Directed Release of Differential Extracellular Vesicle-associated microRNA Profiles from Bronchial Epithelial Cells of Healthy and Asthmatic Subjects. *Biomedicines* **2022**, *10*, 622. https://doi.org/10.3390/biomedicines10030622

Academic Editors: Berislav Bošnjak and Stanislawa Bazan-Socha

Received: 16 February 2022
Accepted: 27 February 2022
Published: 7 March 2022

Publisher's Note: MDPI stays neutral with regard to jurisdictional claims in published maps and institutional affiliations.

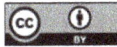

Copyright: © 2022 by the authors. Licensee MDPI, Basel, Switzerland. This article is an open access article distributed under the terms and conditions of the Creative Commons Attribution (CC BY) license (https://creativecommons.org/licenses/by/4.0/).

Abstract: Extracellular vesicles (EVs) are released by virtually all cells and may serve as intercellular communication structures by transmitting molecules such as proteins, lipids, and nucleic acids between cells. MicroRNAs (miRNAs) are an abundant class of vesicular RNA playing a pivotal role in regulating intracellular processes. In this work, we aimed to characterize vesicular miRNA profiles released in a side-directed manner by bronchial epithelial cells from healthy and asthmatic subjects using an air−liquid interface cell culture model. EVs were isolated from a culture medium collected from either the basolateral or apical cell side of the epithelial cell cultures and characterized by nano-flow cytometry (NanoFCM) and bead-based flow cytometry. EV-associated RNA profiles were assessed by small RNA sequencing and subsequent bioinformatic analyses. Furthermore, miRNA-associated functions and targets were predicted and miRNA network analyses were performed. EVs were released at higher numbers to the apical cell side of the epithelial cells and were considerably smaller in the apical compared to the basolateral compartment. EVs from both compartments showed a differential tetraspanins surface marker expression. Furthermore, 236 miRNAs were differentially expressed depending on the EV secretion side, regardless of the disease phenotype. On the apical cell side, 32 miRNAs were significantly altered in asthmatic versus healthy conditions, while on the basolateral cell side, 23 differentially expressed miRNAs could be detected. Downstream KEGG pathway analysis predicted mTOR and MAPK signaling pathways as potential downstream targets of apically secreted miRNAs. In contrast, miRNAs specifically detected at the basolateral side were associated with processes of T and B cell receptor signaling. The study proves a compartmentalized packaging of EVs by bronchial epithelial cells supposedly associated with site-specific functions of cargo miRNAs, which are considerably affected by disease conditions such as asthma.

Biomedicines **2022**, *10*, 622

Keywords: bronchial epithelial cells; extracellular vesicles; miRNAs; airway epithelium; asthma; cellular compartmentalization

1. Introduction

Asthma is a common non-communicable inflammatory disease of the airways, affecting more than 339 million people worldwide, and is a major cause of morbidity around the globe [1,2]. Disease pathogenesis in asthma involves the interaction of many different cell types within the respiratory tract, including CD4+ T-cells, granulocytes, dendritic cells, macrophages, myeloid-derived regulatory cells, natural killer cells, smooth muscle cells, and airway epithelial cells [3]. These various types of cells communicate via many different signaling mechanisms, such as soluble factors, including cytokines and chemokines. In the past decade, a new mechanism of intercellular communication by extracellular vesicles (EVs) was discovered [4]. They have been found in all body fluids, including in blood [5], urine [6], and bronchoalveolar lavage fluid (BALF) [7]. All EVs are composed of a lipid bilayer containing transmembrane proteins and can be classified into exosomes, microvesicles, and apoptotic bodies depending on size, structural components, and generation process [8]. While exosomes are approximately 30–150 nm in diameter and are derived from the exocytosis of multivesicular bodies, microvesicles are shed at the cell surface and are 50–1000 nm in size [9,10]. EVs express membrane proteins, which frequently have been used as surface markers to identify specific EV subsets such as exosomes, or to trace the cell of origin. Universally expressed exosomal proteins such as the tetraspanins CD9, CD63, and CD81 are therefore commonly used as exosomal markers to distinguish exosomes from other EV subsets [11], although conflicting data describe the expression on both exosomes and microvesicles [12].

EVs function as intercellular communicators transporting diverse lipids, proteins, and nucleic acids, such as DNA and certain types of RNA including messenger RNA (mRNA) and small RNAs, such as microRNAs (miRNAs), small interfering RNAs (siRNAs), transfer RNAs (tRNAs), and PIWI-associated RNAs (piRNAs) [13]. Small RNAs are less than 200 nucleotides long and are not translated into proteins, but rather regulate biological processes by interfering with mRNA translation. MiRNAs are defined as short non-coding single-stranded RNAs with a length of approximately 22 nucleotides. They target mRNA, inducing mRNA degradation or inhibiting protein translation, and thereby regulate gene expression [14]. Vesicular miRNAs are protected from degradation by RNA-degrading enzymes (RNAses) in body fluids due to the protective shell provided by the vesicles lipid bilayer, and therefore can be shuttled between cells [15].

The airway epithelium is known to account for a variety of abnormal responses in asthma, such as epithelial mucus metaplasia [16,17]. Increasing evidence further suggests an active role of lung epithelial cells in the initiation and perpetuation of local immune mechanisms not only by the secretion of cytokines, but also as a major producer of EVs [18–21]. Many studies have described a potential proinflammatory role of EVs in allergy and asthma, but with few studies specifically addressing the role of EVs derived from airway epithelial cells. Vesicles secreted by lung epithelial cells have been shown to prime immune cells toward proinflammatory features [22]. Furthermore, a differential expression of extracellular miRNAs in asthmatic patients compared to non-asthmatics with a downstream regulatory impact on inflammation has been described [23,24]. However, to the best of our knowledge, so far, no study has explicitly distinguished between vesicular miRNA profiles on the apical and basolateral cell side of airway epithelial cells.

The purpose of this study was to investigate vesicle characteristics and vesicular miRNA profiles associated with EVs derived from the airway epithelial cells of healthy and asthmatic subjects depending on the cell side of secretion. Therefore, an air−liquid-interface cell culture model of airway epithelial cells was used for sample collection. We then performed small RNA sequencing and conducted extensive bioinformatic analyses to identify vesicular miRNA signatures. Furthermore, miRNA associated roles, functions, and targets were predicted by associated target genes, and miRNA network analysis was conducted to reveal closely related functional clusters within the identified set.

2. Materials and Methods

2.1. Cell Culture

MucilAir™ primary human bronchial epithelial cells were purchased from Epithelix (Epithelix, Sárl, Geneve, Switzerland) and cultured using air−liquid interface conditions. Cultures were established from three different healthy non-smoking donors (two males and one female, aged 15, 41, and 71 years, respectively) and three different asthmatic non-smoking donors (two males and one female, aged 36, 50, and 55 years, respectively). MucilAir™ cell culture medium (Epithelix) was exchanged and the cells were washed carefully with a medium from the apical side to remove residual mucus on a regular basis, according to the manufacturer's instructions. The cell culture medium was continuously collected over one month from the basolateral and apical cell sides. While basal samples were directly retrieved from the bottom chamber of the culture system, for collection of the apical samples, the cells were incubated with 200 µL apically applied cell culture medium for 30 min at 37 °C, and afterwards they were washed by carefully pipetting up and down. All samples were stored at −80 °C until further use. The general experimental downstream workflow is shown in Figure 1.

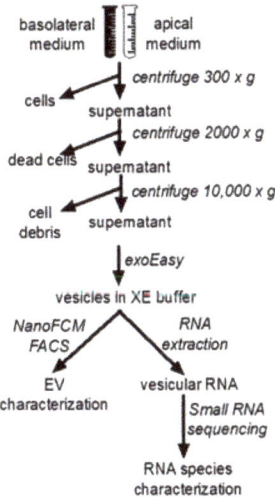

Figure 1. Schematic overview of EV preparation steps.

2.2. EV Isolation

After thawing at room temperature, conditioned medium samples were sequentially centrifuged at 4 °C to remove cell debris and large vesicles (10 min at 500× g, 20 min at 2000× g and 30 min at 10,000× g). Next, the samples were passed through a 0.22 µm filter (Millex-GS Syringe filter unit, Merck KGaA, Darmstadt, Germany) and the EVs were isolated using the exoEasy kit (Qiagen GmbH, Hilden, Germany) from 4 mL of basolaterally and 600 µL of apically collected conditioned medium, according to the manufacturer's protocol [25].

2.3. NanoFCM Analysis

For the Flow Nano Analyzer (NanoFCM Co. Ltd., Nottingham, UK) analysis, the system was calibrated using 200 nm polystyrene beads (NanoFCM Co. Ltd., Nottingham, UK) with a defined concentration of 5.7×10^8 particles/mL, which were also used as a reference for the particle concentration. In addition, monodisperse silica beads (NanoFCM Co. Ltd., Nottingham, UK) of four different sizes were used as reference standards to calibrate the size of the EVs. Freshly filtered (0.22 μm) PBS was analyzed as a background signal, which was subtracted from the other measurements. EV samples were diluted with filtered PBS resulting in a particle count in an optimum range of 2500–12,000 events, and sample data were collected for 1 min with a sample pressure of 0.4 kPa. Particle concentration and size distribution were calculated using the NanoFCM software NF Profession v1.08) (NanoFCM Co. Ltd., Nottingham, UK). Median and interquartile range (IQR) were calculated using R software v4.1.0 (R Foundation, Vienna, Austria).

2.4. Total Protein Quantification

The EV sample protein concentration measurement was performed on NanoDrop™ (Thermo Fisher Scientific, Waltham, MA, USA) at 280 nm, with an estimated percent extinction coefficient of 10. The analysis was performed in triplicate on non-diluted EV isolates.

2.5. Bead-Based Flow Cytometry

EVs were detected by bead-based flow cytometry as previously described by Benedikter et al., with some adaptations [26]. Briefly, 4 μm aldehyde/sulphate latex beads at 3.5×10^8/mL (Thermo Fisher Scientific, Waltham, MA, USA) were incubated with 0.125 mg/mL of an equal mixture of three monoclonal antibodies (anti-human CD9 (clone M-L13), anti-human CD63 (clone H5C6), anti-human CD81 (clone JS-81); all antibodies were purchased from BD Biosciences, Franklin Lakes, NJ, USA) overnight in an MES buffer (Sigma Aldrich, St. Louis, MO, USA) on a shaker at 6500 rpm. The coated beads were stored in PBS containing 0.1% (m/v) glycine and 0.1% (m/v) sodium azide at 4 °C until use. Before use, the beads were washed with PBS containing 2% (w/v) bovine serum albumin (BSA). Then, 1×10^6 beads in 1 μL were incubated overnight with 100 μL of isolated EVs suspended in PBS at a concentration of 1.6×10^7 particles/mL based on NanoFCM measurements. Detection was performed as described previously, with either one or a mixture of the following phycoerythrin (PE)-labelled antibodies: anti-human CD9, anti-human CD63, and anti-human CD81 (same clones as above) [26]. Stained beads were suspended in 150 μL PBS and were analyzed using a BD FACSCanto II and FACS Diva v8.0.1 analysis software (BD Biosciences, Franklin Lakes, NJ, USA). To quantify the EV surface marker expression, relative fluorescence units (RFU) were calculated by multiplying the percentage of PE-positive beads with the median fluorescent intensity (MFI) of the positive bead population, as described by Benedikter et al. [26].

2.6. Statistical Analysis of Numerical Data

Data were analyzed using GraphPad Prism v7 (GraphPad Software Inc., San Diego, CA, USA) using Student's unpaired t-test for concentration and size distribution, and the Whitney−Mann U-test for FACS analysis with p-values * < 0.05, ** < 0.01, *** < 0.001, and **** < 0.0001. Data are presented as mean $\pm$ SEM.

2.7. Vesicular RNA Extraction

RNA extraction was performed from 200 μL of EV solution using the miRNeasy kit (Qiagen GmbH, Hilden, Germany), according to the manufacturer's instructions. The RNA concentration was assessed using the Qubit™ microRNA Assay Kit (Thermo Fisher Scientific, Waltham, MA, USA). RNA size distribution and yield were analyzed using the Agilent 2100 Bioanalyzer with the Small RNA analysis kit (Agilent Technologies, Santa Clara, CA, USA).

2.8. Small RNA Sequencing

Small RNA libraries were constructed using NEBNext Small RNA Library Prep Set for Illumina (New England Biolabs, Ipswich, MA, USA), according to the manufacturer's protocol, with minor modifications for the low RNA input. Briefly, 3 ng of RNA was used for the library preparation. The 3′ SR Adapter, SR RT Primer, and 5′ SR Adapter were diluted 1:4, and the RNA was ligated with both adapters, and was reverse transcribed, barcoded, and amplified for 15 cycles. The generated libraries were cleaned up using AMPure XP Beads (Beckman Coulter, Brea, CA, USA) and quantified using the Qubit™ dsDNA HS Assay (Thermo Fisher Scientific, Waltham, MA, USA) and the Bioanalyzer High Sensitivity DNA Analysis kit (Agilent Technologies) prior to sequencing on a NextSeq550 platform (Illumina, San Diego, CA, USA) with High Output Kit v2.5 and 50 bases single-reads, according to the manufacturer's instructions.

2.9. Bioinformatic Analysis

The reads were first trimmed for the first three nucleotides (-u 3) and adapters overlapping at least five nucleotides with the read (-O 5) using cutadapt v2.9 [27]. Reads shorter than 15 nucleotides were discarded (-m 15). Trimmed reads were mapped using bwa-mem v0.7.17-r1188 in three steps, with the minimum score output (-T) and seed length (-k) set to 15 [28]. The reads were mapped successively against a custom list of transcripts containing ribosomal RNAs (rRNAs) from rFam 14.1, mature miRNAs from miRbase 22.1, ncRNAs from ENSEMBL release 97, piRNAs from piRNA-DB v1.7.5, and cDNAs from ENSEMBL release 97 as the references. In this order, unmapped reads from each step were mapped against the next reference to assure unique attribution per RNA type. The reads were counted per transcript with Samtools v1.10 [29], and 374 miRNAs with more than 10 reads across all samples were analyzed using R package DESeq2 v1.28.1 for the differential gene expression [30]. Differences were classified as significant with a threshold of absolute value of fold change (FC) > 2 and FDR < 0.05. Principal component analysis was conducted and visualized using R package pcaExplorer v2.14.2 based on variance stabilized transformed read counts of miRNAs [31]. Heatmaps were generated using R package pheatmap v1.0.12 with default clustering parameters. KEGG (Kyoto Encyclopedia of Genes and Genomes) pathway analyses were performed using DIANA-miRPath v3.0 with a FDR threshold < 0.05 and other default settings [32]. miRNAs function, family, disease, and regulatory proteins were analyzed using TAM 2.0 by masking cancer-related terms and keeping the other default settings [33]. Network analysis was conducted by miRTargetLink Human with strong evidence, and the resulting genes were uploaded on STRING v11.0 for the Reactome pathways [34].

3. Results

3.1. EVs Secreted by Airway Epithelial Cells Are Mainly Released at the Apical Cell Surface

To confirm that the isolated particles were indeed EVs, and to compare numbers and composition of apically versus basolaterally released EVs, NanoFCM analysis and bead-based flow cytometry with staining for characteristic tetraspanin surface markers of EVs were performed. Particle concentrations and size profiles showed significant differences in NanoFCM analysis, depending on their isolation side. Generally, epithelial cells secreted significantly larger quantities of particles at the apical cell surface compared to the basolateral side. NanoFCM analysis showed higher particle concentrations in apically obtained EV samples (Figure 2A). This finding was further confirmed by the results of protein concentration analyses, as depicted in Figure 2B. Furthermore, the size of particles retrieved from the apical cell side wash corresponded to the typical size range of exosomes with a mean median size of 75 nm (62–95 nm). Contrarily, particles isolated from the basolateral side were considerably larger in size with a mean median size of 169 nm (140–192 nm), consistent in size with microvesicles rather than with exosomes (Figure 2C,D). No differences in concentration or size range were observed between particles from healthy and asthmatic subjects.

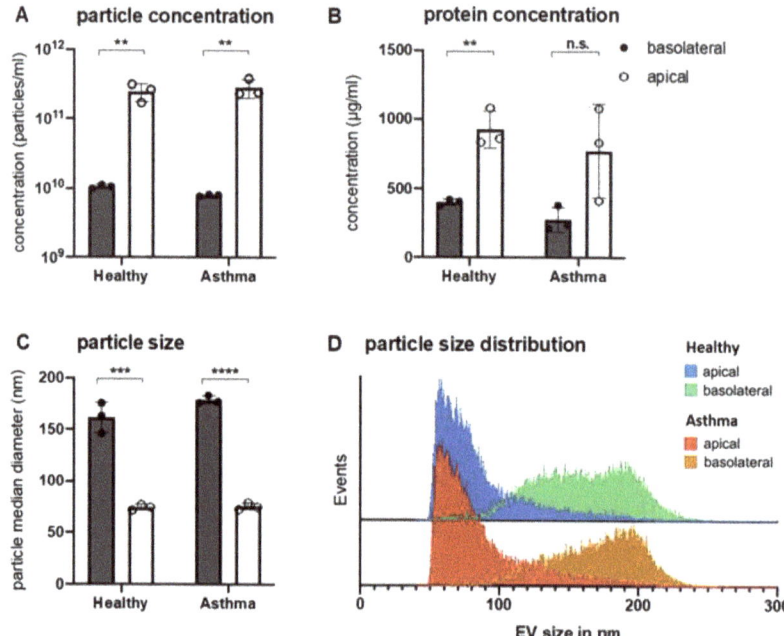

Figure 2. EV characteristics in apically and basolaterally secreted vesicles. (**A**), Particle concentration after EV isolation analyzed by NanoFCM. (**B**), Protein concentration in EV isolates measured by NanoDrop Protein A280. (**C**), Median particle diameter and (**D**) size distribution of EVs isolated from the apical or basolateral side of bronchial epithelial cell cultures from healthy and asthmatic subjects analyzed by NanoFCM. Bars represent mean ± SD; dots indicate individual samples. ** $p < 0.01$, *** $p < 0.001$, **** $p < 0.0001$. EV—extracellular vesicle; n.s.—not significant.

3.2. Differential Surface Marker Expression Profiles between Apically and Basolaterally Released EVs

Bead-based flow cytometry using cocktails of antibodies directed towards the EV-identifying tetraspanin surface markers CD9, CD63, and CD81 for bead binding and detection did not reveal any significant differences between apical and basolateral EVs. However, when examining the expression of singular surface proteins, vesicles secreted to the basolateral side showed a higher expression of CD9 and CD81 compared to apically secreted vesicles, while for CD63, such a difference could not be observed (Figure 3A,B). When further looking at the subgroups, namely EVs from asthmatic and healthy subjects, these differences in marker expression depending on secretion side were similarly represented. However, CD9 expression by apical compared to basolateral EVs seemed to differ to a greater extent in the EVs of healthy subjects. When comparing the surface marker expression of EVs from healthy and asthmatic subjects, subtle distinctions in the expression of CD9 were observed on the basolateral side, but not for the other tetraspanins. No differences could be found in these groups for vesicles from the apical cell side (Figure 3C). This differential representation of selective marker proteins on EVs was generally suggestive for compositional differences, depending on the cell side of secretion.

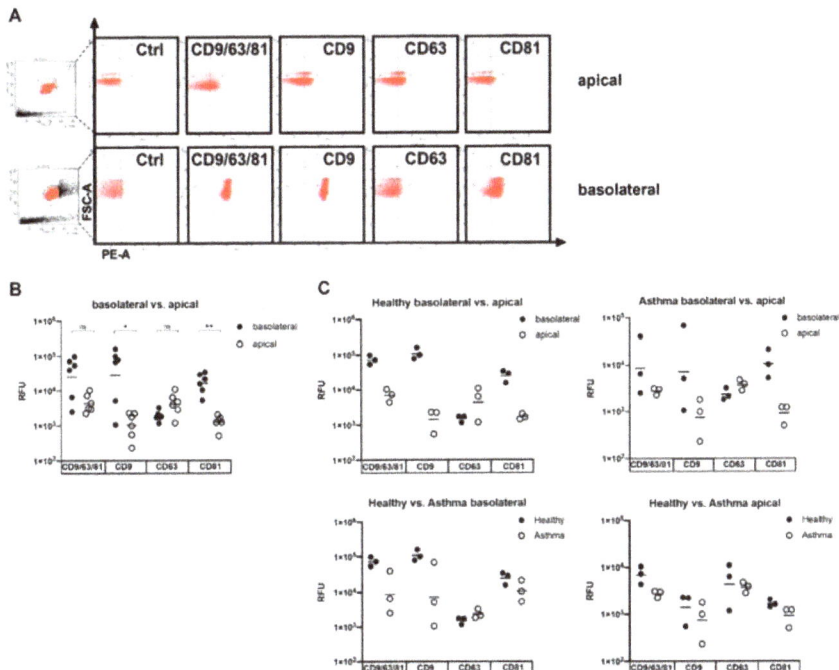

Figure 3. Bead-based flow cytometry analysis of tetraspanins surface marker expression on EVs released by airway epithelial cells. Vesicles were captured using beads coated with a mixture of CD9-, CD63-, and CD81-specific antibodies. Specific secondary antibodies coupled with either CD9, CD63, or CD81, or a combination of all three, were used for detection. (**A**) The results of one representative experiment demonstrating tetraspanin expression on EVs isolated from apical and basolateral cell culture medium are shown. (**B**) Tetraspanin expression in EVs isolated from basolateral versus apical cell culture medium regardless of disease expression. (**C**) Comparison of the surface marker expression of apical and basolateral EVs in healthy and asthmatic subjects. n = 3 in each group, * $p < 0.05$, ** $p < 0.01$. EV—extracellular vesicle; ns—not significant; RFU—relative fluorescent units.

3.3. Apically and Basolaterally Released EVs Show Distinct RNA Cargo Composition

Small RNAs were isolated from EVs retrieved from the apical and basolateral compartments of airway epithelial air−liquid interface cultures from healthy and asthmatic subjects (each n = 3), and were further analyzed by small RNA sequencing. All libraries exhibited a minimum of 7.5 million uniquely mapped reads and were thus comparable in efficiency. RNA composition was determined by counting the percentages of reads mapped to different species of RNA, such as rRNAs, long-non-coding RNAs (lncRNAs), miRNAs, mRNAs, and piRNAs. Our analysis showed a significant difference in the composition of RNA subtypes between apical and basolateral EV populations. Apical EVs contained comparable proportions of miRNAs (37.3%) and lncRNAs (33.3%) as te most prominent fractions, while basolateral EVs contained miRNAs only at a percentage of 2.3% and were rather dominated by a high percentage of lncRNAs (50.5%; Supplementary Figure S1).

Further focusing on miRNAs composition, apical and basolateral vesicles could be clearly separated from each other as two distinct populations in a principal component analysis. Moreover, in each of these populations, two clearly different clusters representing either the healthy or the asthmatic condition were clearly distinguishable (Figure 4). When looking at differences in miRNAs composition between apical and basolateral EVs in all 12 samples, we found 236 significantly differentially expressed miRNAs between the two subgroups, of which 151 miRNAs were more and 85 miRNAs less abundant in the apical compared to the basolateral EVs (Figure 5A,B). More frequent miRNAs in the apical population were assigned to different miRNA families (groups of miRNAs with a high sequence similarity deriving from distinct genomic loci) than those found at higher levels in the basolateral EVs (Figure 5C,D). In apically secreted EVs, all family members of the miR-30 (6/6) and the miR-941 (5/5) family were present, pointing to a significant association of these miRNAs to processes specifically important to the apical environment. Additionally, 10 out of 12 miRNAs from the let-7, 6 out of 8 of the miR-10, and 5 out of 8 of the miR-17 families were present. On the basolateral side, the most represented miRNA family was the miR-320 family with 7 out of 8 members, followed by the miR-181 (4/6), the miR-550 (3/5), the let-7 (3/12), and the miR-154 (3/19) families.

We then investigated whether these differentially distributed EV miRNAs could be linked to specific biological effects by evaluating the KEGG pathways and biological functions predicted to be affected by them, according to the two databases, DIANA-miRPath v3.0 and TAM 2.0. As shown in Figure 6, the significantly associated KEGG pathways of the preferentially apically secreted miRNAs included, among others, the mTOR and MAPK signaling pathways. Interestingly, miRNAs on the basolateral side were associated with processes of T and B cell receptor signaling, along with others (Figure 6A). Thus, associated KEGG pathways deviated in apically and basolaterally secreted EVs, suggesting different downstream functions for EVs depending on the site of action that are linked to diverse potential biological functions, as shown in Figure 6B. Significantly enriched target regulatory proteins can be found in Figure 6C. The results showed very distinct differences in miRNA composition as well as in downstream targeted proteins and pathways of vesicular RNA, depending on their cell side of secretion.

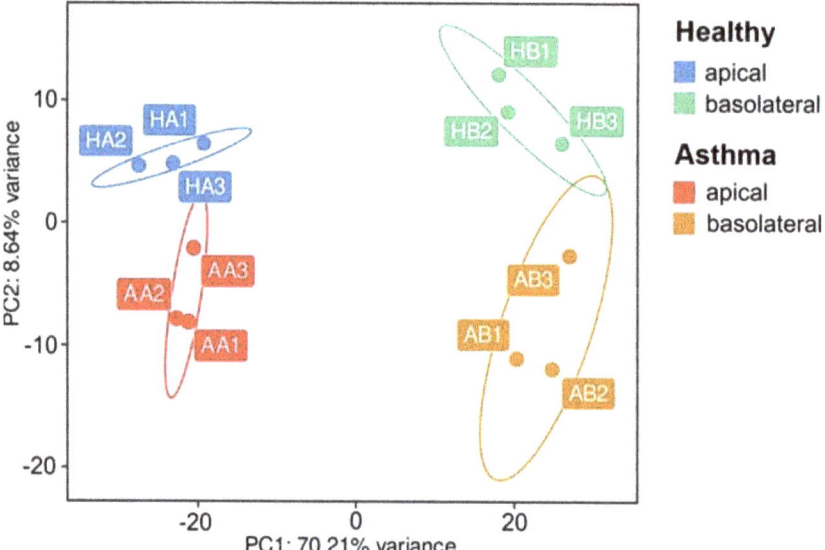

Figure 4. PCA plot depicting the clustering of 12 EV samples according to their miRNA cargo depending on disease condition and cellular side of EV release. PCA—principal component analysis; EV—extracellular vesicle.

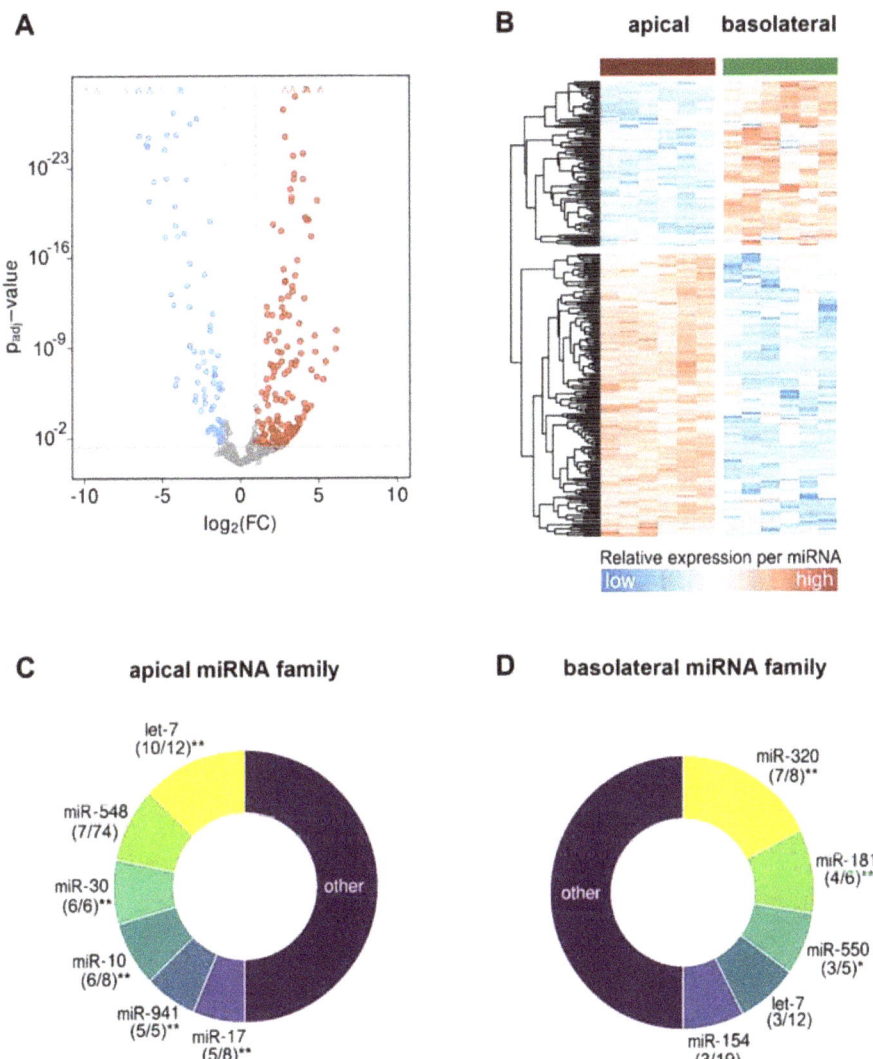

Figure 5. Differential expression analysis of vesicular miRNAs in apical versus basolateral compartments of bronchial epithelial cell cultures. (**A,B**) Volcano plot and heat map showing the differentially expressed miRNAs within EVs secreted to the apical versus basolateral compartment at $p_{adj} < 0.05$ and FC $\geq$ 2, and (**C,D**) donut charts showing the distribution of the mainly represented miRNA families in both compartments. Digits in brackets depict the number of enriched miRNA family members out of the total number of miRNAs belonging to the respective family, * $p < 0.05$, ** $p < 0.01$, miRNA—microRNA; EV—extracellular vesicle; FC—fold change.

A   **Enriched KEGG pathways: apical vs. basolateral**

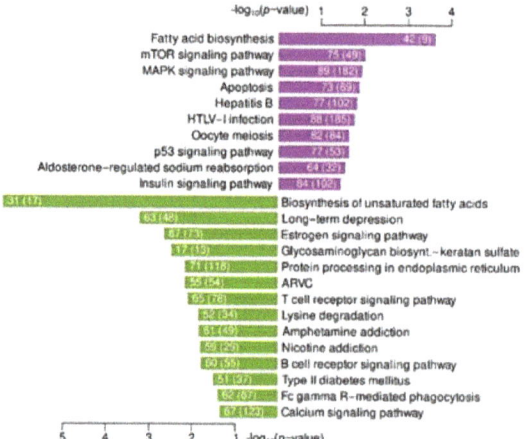

B   **Enriched biological functions: apical vs. basolateral**

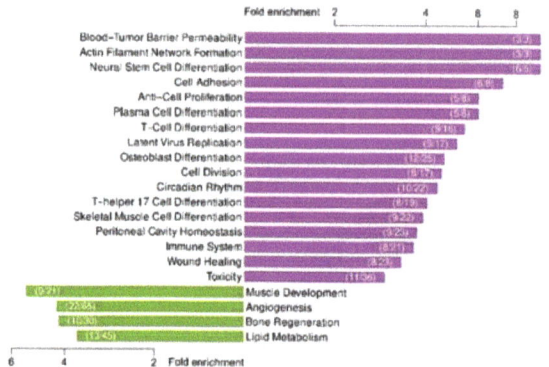

C   **Enriched target proteins: apical vs. basolateral**

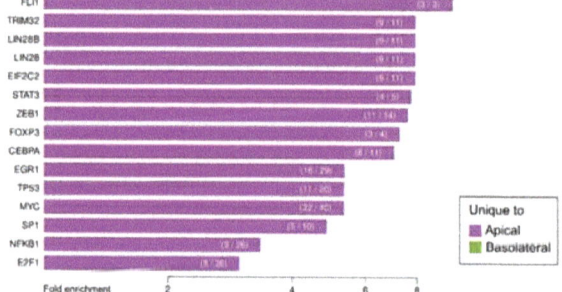

Figure 6. Functional analysis of miRNAs differentially expressed in EVs released by bronchial epithelial cells to the apical versus basolateral compartments. (**A**) KEGG pathway and (**B**) biological functions analyses of differentially expressed miRNAs in both compartments and (**C**) target proteins potentially regulated by the differentially expressed miRNAs. EV—extracellular vesicle.

3.4. Small RNA Cargo Is Altered in Vesicles from Asthmatic Subjects

We additionally checked whether EVs derived from epithelial cells of healthy and asthmatic subjects differed in their miRNA expression profiles regardless of the secretion side, and found overall 12 miRNAs differentially represented in the two groups, with 6 being up- and 6 down-regulated in the vesicles of asthmatics (Supplementary Figure S2). A more complex picture was obtained when additionally taking the EV secretion side into account (Figure 7A). In apical EVs, 32 miRNAs showed a significant difference in abundances in the two groups, 29 of which were up- and 3 of which were down-regulated in the vesicles of asthmatics (Figure 6A, left). On the basolateral side, 23 miRNAs with a divergent expression profile were detected, 9 being significantly upregulated and 14 being downregulated in asthmatics (Figure 7A, right), with 5 out of 12 being family members of the let-7 family and with 3 out of 8 being members of the miR-10 family (Figure 6C). Specifically, the miR-9 family showed significant differences between the healthy and the asthmatic phenotype origin in both EV secretion compartments (Figure 7B,C). The KEGG pathway terms and biological functions associated with differentially abundant miRNAs in apical and basolateral EVs from asthmatic versus healthy subject's bronchial epithelial cell cultures are shown in Supplementary Figure S3A,B, respectively. Enriched associated diseases included a variety of inflammatory conditions, among them asthma, especially when the analysis was based on the signals from the basolateral side (Supplementary Figure S3C). Significantly enriched target regulatory proteins in asthmatic subjects were HIF1A and NFKB1 (Supplementary Figure S3D). The target genes of the EV-derived miRNAs differentially expressed between both conditions are shown in Supplementary Figure S4A,B, associated with some of the most significant pathways.

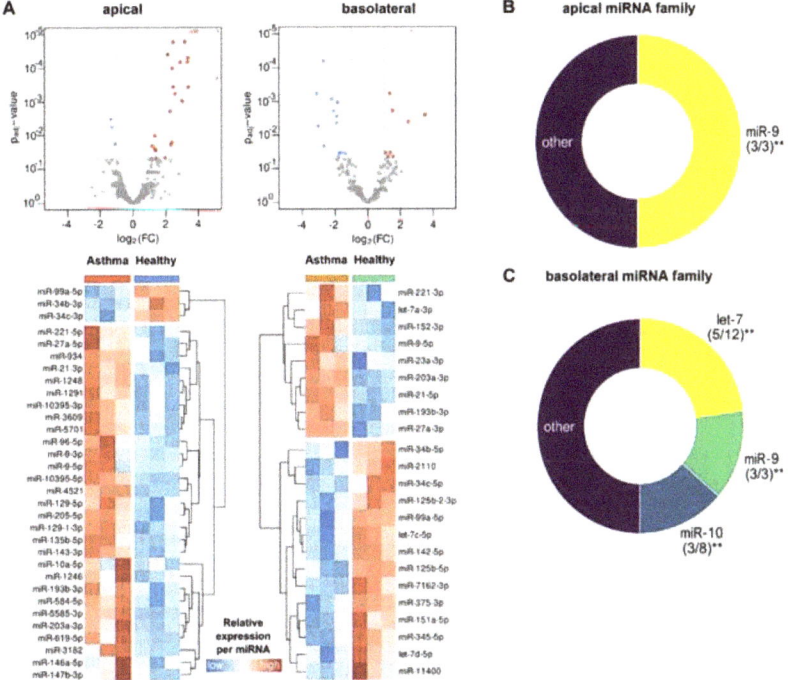

Figure 7. Differential miRNA expression analysis per disease condition (asthma versus healthy) and

compartment (apical and basolateral). (**A**) Volcano plot and heat map of differentially expressed miRNAs of asthma versus healthy comparison in EVs from the apical (left) and basolateral (right) cell culture compartments at $p_{adj} < 0.05$ and FC $\geq$ 2, and (**B**,**C**) donut charts showing the distribution of the mainly represented miRNA families in the asthma versus healthy comparison in both compartments. Digits in brackets depict the number of enriched miRNA family members out of total number of miRNAs belonging to the respective family, ** $p < 0.01$. miRNA—microRNA; EV—extracellular vesicle; FC—fold change.

4. Discussion

In the past decade, the role of EVs as communication structures between neighboring or remote cells has been increasingly recognized. The presence of EV-associated RNAs has been attested by next-generation sequencing in numerous body fluids, including blood plasma and sputum [35]. Specific miRNA signatures hold the potential for being used as fingerprints, helping to identify phenotypes or states of diseases and gain more insights into their underlying pathological mechanisms. Plenty of studies have analyzed miRNA profiles in patients with asthma compared to subjects not affected by this disease, some with a specific focus on the role of airway epithelial cells in EV-related miRNA generation [36]. However, to date, no investigations have explicitly distinguished between EV RNA profiles in polarized airway epithelial cells depending on their direction of secretion. Hence, no distinction has been made between their supposed location of action being either the outer epithelial environment, e.g., sputum, or compartments within the body, such as lung interstitium, tissue, or even blood plasma.

According to the results of the NanoFCM particle characterization, EV populations isolated from the apical cell side were mainly composed of vesicles with diameters matching the size range of the exosomes. Contrarily, on the basolateral cell side, median vesicle diameters were noticeably larger, consistent rather with the size of the microvesicles than with the exosomes [37,38]. FACS analysis for exosomal marker proteins revealed the presence of exosomes in both apical and basolateral samples, although apical EVs seemed to express exosomal marker proteins to a greater extent than the basolateral vesicles.

In our study, we were able to observe distinct differences in EV-associated miRNA patterns secreted by bronchial epithelial cells from healthy and asthmatic subjects, depending on the side of EV secretion. Interestingly, secretion patterns of EV miRNAs varied more distinctly based on the side of secretion than the pathophysiological condition. This knowledge might be essential for future investigations into potential biomarkers analyzed in different compartments such as sputum and plasma. Bartel et al. recently published a PCR-based study comparing the expression of specific miRNAs in EVs secreted by normal human bronchial epithelial cells to the basolateral and apical cell side. Interestingly, there were some notable overlaps in miRNAs, including miR-34b and miR-21 preferentially identified on the apical side, while other differentially expressed miRNAs in this study could not be observed in our analysis [39]. Notably, serum levels of miR-21 have been previously reported to be an efficient biomarker for asthma patients [40]. Further, treatment with a miR-21-specific antagomir was demonstrated to reduce airway hyperresponsiveness and restore steroid sensitivity in mice with ovalbumin-induced allergic airway inflammation [41]. The differentially expressed miR-10 on the apical side was found to regulate the proliferation of airway smooth muscle cells by suppressing the phosphoinositide 3-kinase (PI3K) pathway [42]. Moreover, MAPK and mTOR signaling pathways were enriched as potential targets for differentially expressed miRNAs on the apical side. Activation of the mTOR pathway has been shown to lead to tight junction susceptibility and epithelial–mesenchymal transition (EMT), which can in turn play an essential role in airway remolding in asthma pathogenesis [43,44]. Accordingly, inhibition of MAPK signaling pathway led to a significant reduction in the allergic inflammation of the airways [45]. In contrast, miR-221, which was downregulated on the basolateral side, was shown to play a unique role in controlling the differentiation of Th17 and regulatory T (Treg) cells through targeting SOCS-1 (suppressor of cytokine signaling 1) [46]. Likewise, T and B cell receptor signaling pathways have been associated with miRNAs dominantly secreted to the basolateral side. These pathways have been intensively investigated as key regulators of the antigen recognition in the adaptive immune response and have been utilized as key therapy targets in asthmatic patients [47,48]. Taken together, our observations strongly indicate a compartmentalized packaging and side-specific release of EVs by bronchial epithelial cells, pointing to site-specific functions of these structures at least partially mediated by their miRNA cargo.

While differences in miRNA profiles from apical versus basolateral sides were more pronounced, a number of significant alterations in the levels of certain EV-associated miRNAs (or their families) were also observed between cells of an asthmatic or healthy origin, either at one or at both sides. For example, EV miRNAs belonging to the miR-9 family were upregulated in both apical and basolateral vesicles of asthmatic patients. Increased levels of miR-9 have already been linked to steroid-resistant and neutrophilic, but not eosinophilic asthma [49]. Interestingly, Bazzoni et al. observed a miR-9-dependent inhibition of NFκB1 transcription in human neutrophils and monocytes exposed to proinflammatory signals, suggesting that the rapid induction of miR-9 operates as a feedback control of NFκB1-dependent cellular response [50]. Accordingly, NFκB1 was found among the predicted targets of miRNAs, specifically present in asthmatic samples in our investigation. Several independent studies further identified enhanced NFκB-pathway activation in asthmatic tissue [51].

Interestingly enough, miR-34b and miR-34c were downregulated when associated with EVs released by epithelial cells from asthmatic subjects at both compartments, even though they were generated from opposite DNA strands, dependent on the compartment. The levels of miR-34b/c have been found to be significantly lowered in murine mouse models of ovalbumin-induced allergic airway inflammation and have been suggested to play a regulatory role in the activation of the Nrf2-/ARE pathway [52]. Disruption of Nrf2-expression augmented airway inflammation and hyperresponsiveness [53–55]. Moreover, in a clinical study by Solberg et al., treatment with corticosteroids resulted in increased levels of miR-34b/c in BALF of patients suffering from asthma, while the administration of IL-13 was able to repress its expression in an air–liquid interface bronchial epithelial cell culture model [56]. This suggests a protective role of miR-34b/c against allergic and asthmatic cellular responses, and hints toward a diagnostic potential of the miR-34 family.

Generally, miRNA of the let-7 family showed a higher expression in apical compared to basolateral EVs. However, in basolateral EVs, the let-7 family was the miRNA subgroup with the largest divergence between asthmatic and healthy subjects, with 5 out of 12 total family members showing significant alterations, while on the apical side, no differences in expression were found. In contrast to this finding, Levänen et al. described significant variations in 16 miRNA, including the let-7 and miR-200 families and miR-99 (as seen in our study) in BALF [24]. Interestingly, while let-7c and let-7d were downregulated, let-7a showed an upregulation in EVs released by cells from asthmatics. miRNAs of the let-7 family are among the most intensely studied miRNAs, with two studies proposing the exosome-mediated transfer of let-7 miRNAs to various immune cells as a suppressive mechanism used by Treg cells (let-7d), and reporting the inhibition of Treg cell generation and function by these miRNAs (let-7i) [57,58].

There are some limitations to this study that should be mentioned. One limitation is the small sample size, yet the major goal of the study was a general overview of EV fingerprints in different cellular compartments, rather than assessing the function of singular EV miRNAs. For a more detailed analysis, further studies investigating the role of single miRNA are required to give the data a clinical significance. Another limitation is that there was no information available about the clinical details and/or the asthmatic phenotype of the patients whose cells were involved in the study. Lastly, as miRNAs can be secreted by almost every cell type, the overall in vivo situation can largely dissociate from in vitro observed conditions. Dissecting the contribution of individual cell types in the production of specific miRNA is, on the other hand, essential to understand their role in disease pathogenesis.

In summary, in this study, we provide a general overview of miRNA-composition in EVs secreted by airway epithelial cells. We were able to reveal distinctly differing miRNA expression profiles depending on the vesicle side of secretion and disease condition. This emphasizes the importance of taking the vesicle site of action into consideration for further research to which the data presented in this study provide a sound basis.

Supplementary Materials: The following supporting information can be downloaded at: https://www.mdpi.com/article/10.3390/biomedicines10030622/s1. Supplementary Figure S1: Comparison of EV total RNA composition between basolateral and apical compartments regardless of disease expression in percentage of reads mapped to indicated RNA species. EV—extracellular vesicle; rRNA—ribosomal RNA; mRNA—messenger RNA; lncRNAs—long-non-coding RNAs; piRNA—PIWI-associated RNAs; miRNA—microRNA. Supplementary Figure S2: Differential miRNA expression analysis per disease condition (asthma versus healthy) regardless of compartment (apical and basolateral). (A) Volcano plot and (B) heat map exhibiting the differently expressed miRNAs of the asthma versus healthy comparison at $p_{adj} < 0.05$ and FC $\geq$ 2. miRNA—microRNA; FC—fold change. Supplementary Figure S3: Functional analysis of the differentially expressed miRNAs in the asthma versus healthy comparison in each apical and basolateral compartment. (A) KEGG pathway and (B) biological function analyses of differentially expressed vesicular miRNAs of asthma versus healthy in each apical and basolateral compartment, (C) enriched diseases, and (D) target proteins potentially regulated by the differentially expressed miRNAs. miRNA—microRNA. Supplementary Figure S4: mRNA–miRNA network analysis involving differentially regulated miRNAs of the asthma versus healthy comparison in (A) the apical and (B) the basolateral compartments associated with biological pathways of potential target genes. miRNA—microRNA.

Author Contributions: H.G., D.P.P., V.E.M.S. and F.A.—designed the experiments. V.E.M.S.—isolated the material and performed EV and RNA isolation. F.A.—prepared the material for sequencing. A.N. and T.S.—implemented sequencing analysis. C.P., B.A.A. and E.P.v.S.—implemented NanoFCM analysis. V.E.M.S. and L.H.—performed FACS analysis. C.T. and F.A.—performed the bioinformatics analysis. V.E.M.S., H.G. and F.A.—drafted the manuscript. All authors have read and agreed to the published version of the manuscript.

Funding: This research was funded by the German Center for Lung Research (DZL); the German Academic Exchange Service (DAAD; F.A., personal reference number: 91726294); the HessenFonds, World University Service (WUS; F.A.); the Hessen State Ministry for Higher Education, Research and the Arts (HMWK; F.A.); and the German Research Foundation (DFG; E.P.v.S., B.A.A. and T.S., Grant 512416910386–GRK 2573/1).

Institutional Review Board Statement: Not applicable.

Informed Consent Statement: Not applicable.

Data Availability Statement: The data presented in this study and underlying raw data are available on reasonable request from the corresponding author.

Acknowledgments: We would like to thank our funding institutions.

Conflicts of Interest: Authors declared no conflict of interest.

References

1. GBD 2016 Disease and Injury Incidence and Prevalence Collaborators; Vos, T.; Abajobir, A.A.; Abate, K.H.; Abbafati, C.; Abbas, K.M.; Abd-Allah, F.; Abdulkader, R.S.; Abdulle, A.M.; Abebo, T.A.; et al. Global, regional, and national incidence, prevalence, and years lived with disability for 328 diseases and injuries for 195 countries, 1990–2016: A systematic analysis for the Global Burden of Disease Study 2016. *Lancet* **2017**, *390*, 1211–1259. [CrossRef]
2. WHO. SGlobal Health Estimates: Life Expectancy and Leading Causes of Death and Disability. 2022. Available online: https://www.who.int/data/gho/data/themes/mortality-and-global-health-estimates (accessed on 7 January 2022).
3. Vieira Braga, F.A.; Kar, G.; Berg, M.; Carpaij, O.A.; Polanski, K.; Simon, L.M.; Brouwer, S.; Gomes, T.; Hesse, L.; Jiang, J.; et al. A cellular census of human lungs identifies novel cell states in health and in asthma. *Nat. Med.* **2019**, *25*, 1153–1163. [CrossRef] [PubMed]

4. Mathivanan, S.; Ji, H.; Simpson, R.J. Exosomes: Extracellular organelles important in intercellular communication. *J. Proteom.* **2010**, *73*, 1907–1920. [CrossRef] [PubMed]
5. Caby, M.P.; Lankar, D.; Vincendeau-Scherrer, C.; Raposo, G.; Bonnerot, C. Exosomal-like vesicles are present in human blood plasma. *Int. Immunol.* **2005**, *17*, 879–887. [CrossRef]
6. Pisitkun, T.; Shen, R.F.; Knepper, M.A. Identification and proteomic profiling of exosomes in human urine. *Proc. Natl. Acad. Sci. USA* **2004**, *101*, 13368–13373. [CrossRef]
7. Admyre, C.; Grunewald, J.; Thyberg, J.; Bripenäck, S.; Tornling, G.; Eklund, A.; Scheynius, A.; Gabrielsson, S. Exosomes with major histocompatibility complex class II and co-stimulatory molecules are present in human BAL fluid. *Eur. Respir. J.* **2003**, *22*, 578–583. [CrossRef]
8. György, B.; Szabó, T.G.; Pásztói, M.; Pál, Z.; Misják, P.; Aradi, B.; László, V.; Pállinger, É.; Pap, E.; Kittel, Á.; et al. Membrane vesicles, current state-of-the-art: Emerging role of extracellular vesicles. *Cell. Mol. Life Sci.* **2011**, *68*, 2667–2688. [CrossRef]
9. Cocucci, E.; Meldolesi, J. Ectosomes and exosomes: Shedding the confusion between extracellular vesicles. *Trends Cell Biol.* **2015**, *25*, 364–372. [CrossRef]
10. Heijnen, H.F.G.; Schiel, A.E.; Fijnheer, R.; Geuze, H.J.; Sixma, J.J. Activated Platelets Release Two Types of Membrane Vesicles: Microvesicles by Surface Shedding and Exosomes Derived from Exocytosis of Multivesicular Bodies and a-Granules. *Blood* **1999**, *94*, 3791–3799. [CrossRef]
11. Théry, C.; Ostrowski, M.; Segura, E. Membrane vesicles as conveyors of immune responses. *Nat. Rev. Immunol.* **2009**, *9*, 581–593. [CrossRef]
12. Mathieu, M.; Névo, N.; Jouve, M.; Valenzuela, J.I.; Maurin, M.; Verweij, F.J.; Palmulli, R.; Lankar, D.; Dingli, F.; Loew, D.; et al. Specificities of exosome versus small ectosome secretion revealed by live intracellular tracking of CD63 and CD9. *Nat. Commun.* **2021**, *12*, 4389. [CrossRef] [PubMed]
13. Großhans, H.; Filipowicz, W. The expanding world of small RNAs. *Nature* **2008**, *451*, 414–416. [CrossRef] [PubMed]
14. Bartel, D.P. MicroRNAs. *Cell* **2004**, *116*, 281–297. [CrossRef]
15. Valadi, H.; Ekström, K.; Bossios, A.; Sjöstrand, M.; Lee, J.J.; Lötvall, J.O. Exosome-mediated transfer of mRNAs and microRNAs is a novel mechanism of genetic exchange between cells. *Nat. Cell Biol.* **2007**, *9*, 654–659. [CrossRef]
16. Locksley, R.M. Asthma and Allergic Inflammation. *Cell* **2010**, *140*, 777–783. [CrossRef]
17. Potaczek, D.P.; Miethe, S.; Schindler, V.; Alhamdan, F.; Garn, H. Role of airway epithelial cells in the development of different asthma phenotypes. *Cell. Signal.* **2020**, *69*, 109523. [CrossRef]
18. Torregrosa Paredes, P.; Esser, J.; Admyre, C.; Nord, M.; Rahman, Q.K.; Lukic, A.; Rådmark, O.; Grönneberg, R.; Grunewald, J.; Eklund, A.; et al. Bronchoalveolar lavage fluid exosomes contribute to cytokine and leukotriene production in allergic asthma. *Allergy Eur. J. Allergy Clin. Immunol.* **2012**, *67*, 911–919. [CrossRef]
19. Wahlund, C.J.E.; Eklund, A.; Grunewald, J.; Gabrielsson, S. Pulmonary Extracellular Vesicles as Mediators of Local and Systemic Inflammation. *Front. Cell Dev. Biol.* **2017**, *5*, 39. [CrossRef]
20. Nagano, T.; Katsurada, M.; Dokuni, R.; Hazama, D.; Kiriu, T.; Umezawa, K.; Kobayashi, K.; Nishimura, Y. Crucial Role of Extracellular Vesicles in Bronchial Asthma. *Int. J. Mol. Sci.* **2019**, *20*, 2589. [CrossRef]
21. Alashkar Alhamwe, B.; Miethe, S.; Pogge von Strandmann, E.; Potaczek, D.P.; Garn, H. Epigenetic Regulation of Airway Epithelium Immune Functions in Asthma. *Front. Immunol.* **2020**, *11*, 1747. [CrossRef]
22. Kulshreshtha, A.; Ahmad, T.; Agrawal, A.; Ghosh, B. Proinflammatory role of epithelial cell-derived exosomes in allergic airway inflammation. *J. Allergy Clin. Immunol.* **2013**, *131*, 1194–1203. [CrossRef] [PubMed]
23. van den Berge, M.; Tasena, H. Role of microRNAs and exosomes in asthma. *Curr. Opin. Pulm. Med.* **2019**, *25*, 87–93. [CrossRef] [PubMed]
24. Levänen, B.; Bhakta, N.R.; Torregrosa Paredes, P.; Barbeau, R.; Hiltbrunner, S.; Pollack, J.L.; Sköld, C.M.; Svartengren, M.; Grunewald, J.; Gabrielsson, S.; et al. Altered microRNA profiles in bronchoalveolar lavage fluid exosomes in asthmatic patients. *J. Allergy Clin. Immunol.* **2013**, *131*, 894–903. [CrossRef] [PubMed]
25. Enderle, D.; Spiel, A.; Coticchia, C.M.; Berghoff, E.; Mueller, R.; Schlumpberger, M.; Sprenger-Haussels, M.; Shaffer, J.M.; Lader, E.; Skog, J.; et al. Characterization of RNA from exosomes and other extracellular vesicles isolated by a novel spin column-based method. *PLoS ONE* **2015**, *10*, e0136133. [CrossRef]
26. Benedikter, B.J.; Volgers, C.; van Eijck, P.H.; Wouters, E.F.M.; Savelkoul, P.H.M.; Reynaert, N.L.; Haenen, G.R.M.M.; Rohde, G.G.U.; Weseler, A.R.; Stassen, F.R.M. Cigarette smoke extract induced exosome release is mediated by depletion of exofacial thiols and can be inhibited by thiol-antioxidants. *Free Radic. Biol. Med.* **2017**, *108*, 334–344. [CrossRef]
27. Martin, M. Cutadapt removes adapter sequences from high-throughput sequencing reads. *EMBnet. J* **2011**, *17*, 10. [CrossRef]
28. Li, H. Aligning sequence reads, clone sequences and assembly contigs with BWA-MEM. *arXiv Preprint* **2013**, arXiv:1303.3997.
29. Li, H.; Handsaker, B.; Wysoker, A.; Fennell, T.; Ruan, J.; Homer, N.; Marth, G.; Abecasis, G.; Durbin, R. The Sequence Alignment/Map format and SAMtools. *Bioinformatics* **2009**, *25*, 2078–2079. [CrossRef]
30. Love, M.I.; Huber, W.; Anders, S. Moderated estimation of fold change and dispersion for RNA-seq data with DESeq2. *Genome Biol.* **2014**, *15*, 550. [CrossRef]
31. Marini, F.; Binder, H. PcaExplorer: An R/Bioconductor package for interacting with RNA-seq principal components. *BMC Bioinform.* **2019**, *20*, 331. [CrossRef]

32. Vlachos, I.S.; Zagganas, K.; Paraskevopoulou, M.D.; Georgakilas, G.; Karagkouni, D.; Vergoulis, T.; Dalamagas, T.; Hatzigeorgiou, A.G. DIANA-miRPath v3.0: Deciphering microRNA function with experimental support. *Nucleic Acids Res.* **2015**, *43*, W460–W466. [CrossRef] [PubMed]

33. Li, J.; Han, X.; Wan, Y.; Zhang, S.; Zhao, Y.; Fan, R.; Cui, Q.; Zhou, Y. TAM 2.0: Tool for MicroRNA set analysis. *Nucleic Acids Res.* **2018**, *46*, W180–W185. [CrossRef] [PubMed]

34. Hamberg, M.; Backes, C.; Fehlmann, T.; Hart, M.; Meder, B.; Meese, E.; Keller, A. MiRTargetLink—miRNAs, genes and interaction networks. *Int. J. Mol. Sci.* **2016**, *17*, 564. [CrossRef] [PubMed]

35. Turchinovich, A.; Drapkina, O.; Tonevitsky, A. Transcriptome of extracellular vesicles: State-of-the-art. *Front. Immunol.* **2019**, *10*, 202. [CrossRef]

36. Alashkar Alhamwe, B.; Potaczek, D.P.; Miethe, S.; Alhamdan, F.; Hintz, L.; Magomedov, A.; Garn, H. Extracellular Vesicles and Asthma—More Than Just a Co-Existence. *Int. J. Mol. Sci.* **2021**, *22*, 4984. [CrossRef]

37. Mohan, A.; Agarwal, S.; Clauss, M.; Britt, N.S.; Dhillon, N.K. Extracellular vesicles: Novel communicators in lung diseases. *Respir. Res.* **2020**, *21*, 1–21. [CrossRef]

38. Pastor, L.; Vera, E.; Marin, J.M.; Sanz-Rubio, D. Extracellular Vesicles from Airway Secretions: New Insights in Lung Diseases. *Int. J. Mol. Sci.* **2021**, *22*, 583. [CrossRef]

39. Bartel, S.; La Grutta, S.; Cilluffo, G.; Perconti, G.; Bongiovanni, A.; Giallongo, A.; Behrends, J.; Kruppa, J.; Hermann, S.; Chiang, D.; et al. Human airway epithelial extracellular vesicle miRNA signature is altered upon asthma development. *Allergy Eur. J. Allergy Clin. Immunol.* **2020**, *75*, 346–356. [CrossRef]

40. Sawant, D.; Yao, W.; Wright, Z.; Sawyers, C.; Tepper, R.; Gupta, S.; Kaplan, M.; Dent, A. Serum MicroRNA-21 as a Biomarker for Allergic Inflammatory Disease in Children. *MicroRNA* **2015**, *4*, 36–40. [CrossRef]

41. Kim, R.Y.; Horvat, J.C.; Pinkerton, J.W.; Starkey, M.R.; Essilfie, A.T.; Mayall, J.R.; Nair, P.M.; Hansbro, N.G.; Jones, B.; Haw, T.J.; et al. MicroRNA-21 drives severe, steroid-insensitive experimental asthma by amplifying phosphoinositide 3-kinase–mediated suppression of histone deacetylase 2. *J. Allergy Clin. Immunol.* **2017**, *139*, 519–532. [CrossRef]

42. Hu, R.; Pan, W.; Fedulov, A.V.; Jester, W.; Jones, M.R.; Weiss, S.T.; Panettieri, R.A.; Tantisira, K.; Lu, Q. MicroRNA-10a controls airway smooth muscle cell proliferation via direct targeting of the PI3 kinase pathway. *FASEB J.* **2014**, *28*, 2347–2357. [CrossRef] [PubMed]

43. Saito, M.; Mitani, A.; Ishimori, T.; Miyashita, N.; Isago, H.; Mikami, Y.; Noguchi, S.; Tarui, M.; Nagase, T. Active mTOR in lung epithelium promotes epithelial-mesenchymal transition and enhances lung fibrosis. *Am. J. Respir. Cell Mol. Biol.* **2020**, *62*, 699–708. [CrossRef] [PubMed]

44. Gong, J.H.; Cho, I.H.; Shin, D.; Han, S.Y.; Park, S.H.; Kang, Y.H. Inhibition of airway epithelial-to-mesenchymal transition and fibrosis by kaempferol in endotoxin-induced epithelial cells and ovalbumin-sensitized mice. *Lab. Investig.* **2014**, *94*, 297–308. [CrossRef] [PubMed]

45. Alam, R.; Gorska, M.M. Mitogen-activated protein kinase signalling and ERK1/2 bistability in asthma. *Clin. Exp. Allergy* **2011**, *41*, 149–159. [CrossRef]

46. Guan, Y.; Ma, Y.; Tang, Y.; Liu, X.; Zhao, Y.; An, L. MiRNA-221-5p suppressed the Th17/Treg ratio in asthma via RORγt/Foxp3 by targeting SOCS1. *Allergy Asthma Clin. Immunol.* **2021**, *17*, 123. [CrossRef]

47. Minervina, A.; Pogorelyy, M.; Mamedov, I. T-cell receptor and B-cell receptor repertoire profiling in adaptive immunity. *Transpl. Int.* **2019**, *32*, 1111–1123. [CrossRef]

48. Foth, S.; Völkel, S.; Bauersachs, D.; Zemlin, M.; Skevaki, C. T cell Repertoire during Ontogeny and Characteristics in Inflammatory Disorders in Adults and Childhood. *Front. Immunol.* **2021**, *11*, 3826. [CrossRef]

49. Li, J.J.; Tay, H.L.; Maltby, S.; Xiang, Y.; Eyers, F.; Hatchwell, L.; Zhou, H.; Toop, H.D.; Morris, J.C.; Nair, P.; et al. MicroRNA-9 regulates steroid-resistant airway hyperresponsiveness by reducing protein phosphatase 2A activity. *J. Allergy Clin. Immunol.* **2015**, *136*, 462–473. [CrossRef]

50. Bazzoni, F.; Rossato, M.; Fabbri, M.; Gaudiosi, D.; Mirolo, M.; Mori, L.; Tamassia, N.; Mantovani, A.; Cassatella, M.A.; Locati, M. Induction and regulatory function of miR-9 in human monocytes and neutrophils exposed to proinflammatory signals. *Proc. Natl. Acad. Sci. USA* **2009**, *106*, 5282–5287. [CrossRef]

51. Edwards, M.R.; Bartlett, N.W.; Clarke, D.; Birrell, M.; Belvisi, M.; Johnston, S.L. Targeting the NF-κB pathway in asthma and chronic obstructive pulmonary disease. *Pharmacol. Ther.* **2009**, *121*, 1–13. [CrossRef]

52. Ho, C.Y.; Lu, C.C.; Weng, C.J.; Yen, G.C. Protective Effects of Diallyl Sulfide on Ovalbumin-Induced Pulmonary Inflammation of Allergic Asthma Mice by MicroRNA-144, -34a, and -34b/c-Modulated Nrf2 Activation. *J. Agric. Food Chem.* **2016**, *64*, 151–160. [CrossRef] [PubMed]

53. Rangasamy, T.; Guo, J.; Mitzner, W.A.; Roman, J.; Singh, A.; Fryer, A.D.; Yamamoto, M.; Kensler, T.W.; Tuder, R.M.; Georas, S.N.; et al. Disruption of Nrf2 enhances susceptibility to severe airway inflammation and asthma in mice. *J. Exp. Med.* **2005**, *202*, 47–59. [CrossRef] [PubMed]

54. Wakabayashi, N.; Slocum, S.L.; Skoko, J.J.; Shin, S.; Kensler, T.W. When NRF2 Talks, Who's Listening? *Antioxid. Redox Signal.* **2010**, *13*, 1649–1663. [CrossRef] [PubMed]

55. Malhotra, D.; Portales-Casamar, E.; Singh, A.; Srivastava, S.; Arenillas, D.; Happel, C.; Shyr, C.; Wakabayashi, N.; Kensler, T.W.; Wasserman, W.W.; et al. Global mapping of binding sites for Nrf2 identifies novel targets in cell survival response through chip-seq profiling and network analysis. *Nucleic Acids Res.* **2010**, *38*, 5718–5734. [CrossRef] [PubMed]

56. Solberg, O.D.; Ostrin, E.J.; Love, M.I.; Peng, J.C.; Bhakta, N.R.; Hou, L.; Nguyen, C.; Solon, M.; Nguyen, C.; Barczak, A.J.; et al. Airway epithelial miRNA expression is altered in asthma. *Am. J. Respir. Crit. Care Med.* **2012**, *186*, 965–974. [CrossRef] [PubMed]

57. Okoye, I.S.; Coomes, S.M.; Pelly, V.S.; Czieso, S.; Papayannopoulos, V.; Tolmachova, T.; Seabra, M.C.; Wilson, M.S. MicroRNA-Containing T-Regulatory-Cell-Derived Exosomes Suppress Pathogenic T Helper 1 Cells. *Immunity* **2014**, *41*, 89–103. [CrossRef]

58. Kimura, K.; Hohjoh, H.; Fukuoka, M.; Sato, W.; Oki, S.; Tomi, C.; Yamaguchi, H.; Kondo, T.; Takahashi, R.; Yamamura, T. Circulating exosomes suppress the induction of regulatory T cells via let-7i in multiple sclerosis. *Nat. Commun.* **2018**, *9*, 17. [CrossRef]

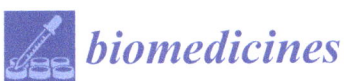

Article

Predictive Response to Immunotherapy Score: A Useful Tool for Identifying Eligible Patients for Allergen Immunotherapy

Ilaria Mormile [1], Francescopaolo Granata [2,*], Aikaterini Detoraki [2], Daniela Pacella [3], Francesca Della Casa [1], Felicia De Rosa [1], Antonio Romano [4], Amato de Paulis [1,5] and Francesca Wanda Rossi [1,5]

[1] Department of Translational Medical Sciences, University of Naples Federico II, 80131 Naples, Italy; ilariamormile@virgilio.it (I.M.); francesca.dellacasa4@gmail.com (F.D.C.); felicia.derosa@libero.it (F.D.R.); depaulis@unina.it (A.d.P.); francescawanda.rossi@unina.it (F.W.R.)
[2] Department of Internal Medicine, Clinical Immunology, Clinical Pathology, and Infectious Diseases, Azienda Ospedaliera Universitaria Federico II, 80131 Naples, Italy; caterina.detoraki@gmail.com
[3] Department of Public Health, University of Naples Federico II, 80131 Naples, Italy; daniela.pacella@unina.it
[4] Department of Neurosciences, Reproductive and Odontostomatological Sciences, Maxillofacial Surgery Unit, University of Naples Federico II, 80131 Naples, Italy; romano.antonio1972@gmail.com
[5] Center for Basic and Clinical Immunology Research (CISI), WAO Center of Excellence, University of Naples Federico II, 80131 Naples, Italy
* Correspondence: frapagra@hotmail.com; Tel.: +39-081-7462218

Citation: Mormile, I.; Granata, F.; Detoraki, A.; Pacella, D.; Della Casa, F.; De Rosa, F.; Romano, A.; de Paulis, A.; Rossi, F.W. Predictive Response to Immunotherapy Score: A Useful Tool for Identifying Eligible Patients for Allergen Immunotherapy. *Biomedicines* 2022, 10, 971. https://doi.org/10.3390/biomedicines10050971

Academic Editor: Stanisława Bazan-Socha

Received: 28 February 2022
Accepted: 20 April 2022
Published: 22 April 2022

Publisher's Note: MDPI stays neutral with regard to jurisdictional claims in published maps and institutional affiliations.

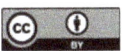

Copyright: © 2022 by the authors. Licensee MDPI, Basel, Switzerland. This article is an open access article distributed under the terms and conditions of the Creative Commons Attribution (CC BY) license (https://creativecommons.org/licenses/by/4.0/).

Abstract: A specific predictive tool of allergen immunotherapy (AIT) outcome has not been identified yet. This study aims to evaluate the efficacy of a disease score referred to as Predictive Response to Immunotherapy Score (PRIS) to predict the response to AIT and identify eligible patients. A total of 110 patients diagnosed with allergic rhinitis with or without concomitant asthma were enrolled in this study. Before beginning sublingual immunotherapy (SLIT), patients were evaluated by analyzing clinical and laboratory parameters. A specific rating was assigned to each parameter to be combined in a total score named PRIS. At baseline (T0) and follow-up [after 12 (T12) and 24 months (T24) of SLIT], a Visual Analogue Scale (VAS) was used to calculate a mean symptom score (MSS). Finally, the percentage variation between the MSS at T0 and at T12 [ΔMSS-12(%)] and T24 [ΔMSS-24 (%)] was measured. We observed a significant improvement of symptoms at T12 and T24 compared to T0 in all groups undergoing SLIT. PRIS was effective in predicting ΔMSS-24 (%) in patients treated with single-allergen SLIT. In addition, PRIS was effective in predicting ΔMSS-24 (%) in both patients with only rhinitis and with concomitant asthma. PRIS assessment can represent a useful tool to individuate potential responders before SLIT prescription.

Keywords: allergic rhinitis; allergen immunotherapy; bronchial asthma; component-resolved diagnosis; sublingual immunotherapy

1. Introduction

Allergic rhinitis and bronchial asthma are widespread diseases that can impact social life, school learning, and work productivity when poorly controlled by conventional therapy [1]. In addition, allergic rhinitis is considered one of the major risk factors for asthma, as up to 40% of patients with allergic rhinitis have or will go on to develop it [2]. Allergen immunotherapy (AIT) is the only disease-modifying treatment for allergic diseases, as it can prevent both the onset of new allergic sensitizations and disease progression [3]. AIT should be considered in those subjects with inadequate response or adverse effects to conventional medications such as antihistamines, topical intranasal antihistamines, and intranasal corticosteroid sprays [4–6]. Two routes of administration of AIT, subcutaneous (SCIT) or sublingual (SLIT), are currently used in clinical practice and have shown good efficacy in the treatment of allergic rhinitis and bronchial asthma [7]. International guidelines recommend that maintenance therapy for both SCIT and SLIT should be continued for at least three years [4,6,7]. Hence, AIT is a long-lasting and expensive treatment, especially if the patient is being treated for more than a few allergens. In addition, in clinical studies, it has been frequently observed that a percentage of patients undergoing AIT do not have significantly beneficial effects [8]. Indeed, the efficacy of AIT ranges between 60% and 90% [9].

Several studies have tried to identify some biomarkers able to predict AIT response through the years. For instance, the assessment of serum-specific IgE [10] and the specific and total IgE ratio has been proposed as a biomarker of AIT efficacy [11]. Other studies suggested a possible correlation between some subtypes of IgG (IgG1, sIgG4) and clinical outcomes [12,13]. Finally, changes in cytokine pattern (e.g., IL-4, IL-13, IL-10) have been associated with AIT response [9,14,15]. However, there is no consensus on the use of these markers in the clinical routine.

The diagnostic approach to allergic disease has significantly been improved by the Component-Resolved Diagnosis (CRD), which provides information about patients' sensitization at the molecular component level by integrating the Skin Prick Test (SPT) and the specific IgE assay with extractive allergen results. Indeed, CRD can increase awareness about the major allergen sensitization and help avoid the administration of AIT for irrelevant allergens, improving its clinical efficacy and cost effectiveness [16,17]. However, the studies which tried to establish a direct link between CRD and AIT outcomes have shown conflicting results.

This study aims to develop and validate a disease score, referred to as Predictive Response to Immunotherapy Score (PRIS), combining clinical features and laboratory results to predict the likelihood of clinical improvement during AIT and identify eligible patients.

2. Materials and Methods

2.1. Patients

Defining the primary outcome as the relationship between the total PRIS score and the ΔMSS, a minimum sample size of 85 patients achieves 80% power assuming a medium effect size (d = 0.3; [18]). A two-tailed test on Pearson's correlation was considered with a significance level α = 0.05. Therefore, 110 patients (68 males and 42 females) diagnosed with allergic rhinitis with or without concomitant asthma at the Division of Allergy and Clinical Immunology of the University of Naples Federico II, Naples, Italy, were enrolled in this prospective cohort single-center study. All the patients presented a history of symptoms related to allergen exposure (rhinitis and/or asthma), documented positive SPT for pollen and/or perennial allergens, and allergen-specific IgE test. Spirometry was used to diagnose asthma [19].

We included both monosensitized and polysensitized patients with uncontrolled allergies despite optimal pharmacotherapy. Patients under six years of age were excluded. We also excluded patients with asthma not adequately controlled by pharmacotherapy [20–22] as assessed by Asthma Control Test (ACT) [23–25]. Finally, we excluded patients with nasal polyposis diagnosed by nasal endoscopy.

Demographic and clinical data were collected from patient medical charts and diaries. Data were available for all 110 patients.

Rhinitis and asthma symptoms were singularly measured using a Visual Analogue Scale (VAS) at baseline (T0) and after 12 (T12) and 24 months (T24) of SLIT treatment. In particular, patients were asked to place a mark on a 10 cm line for rating the severity and frequency of each symptom [26,27]. The symptoms evaluated for allergic rhinitis were sneezing, nasal congestion, rhinorrhea, and nasal, throat, eyes, and ears itching, while chest tightness, breathlessness, wheezing, and coughing were assessed for bronchial asthma. The VAS was anchored at 0 with "no symptoms" and 10 with "very severe symptoms". The VAS also included the assessment of the frequency of symptoms (0 with "no symptoms in the last 30 days" and at 10 with "I have experienced symptoms every day in the past 30 days"). In addition, we instructed patients to record monthly in a diary their symptoms, the number of asthma exacerbations, and on-demand therapy [28–30]. When the patients were visited, they were asked to complete the VAS by checking their diaries. This helped patients take note of their clinical conditions both during and out of season. In particular, when the VAS was administrated for evaluating the asthma exacerbation, 0 corresponded to no exacerbation while 10 implied frequent exacerbations. All the patients enrolled were switched to the same on-demand therapy with second-generation oral antihistamines and intranasal corticosteroids. Patients with asthma were treated using inhaled corticosteroids (ICS) and long-acting β-agonists (LABAs) as the controller and the quick relief therapy. The patients were instructed to record monthly on the provided diary the use of on-demand therapy. Subsequently, when the patients were visited, their perception of on-demand therapy use was evaluated by the VAS (10 implied the highest medication use, while 0 corresponded to no medication use). The mark was then measured in millimeters for all the items explored to provide the VAS score and normalized to 100. For each patient, we assessed the mean symptom score (MSS) based on VAS results at T0 (MSS-0), T12 (MSS-12), and T24 (MSS-24). As efficacy index of SLIT, we calculated the percentage difference between the MSS-0 and MSS-12 [ΔMSS-12(%) = (MSS-0–MSS-12)/MSS-0*100], and between MSS-0 and MSS-24 [ΔMSS-24(%) = (MSS-0–MSS-24)/MSS-0*100]. Based on the ΔMSS-12(%) and ΔMSS-24(%) results, patients' SLIT outcome was stratified into quartiles (first quartile = ΔMSS ≥ 75% = very high symptom improvement; second quartile = 50% ≤ ΔMSS < 75% = high symptom improvement, third quartile = 25% ≤ ΔMSS < 50% = mild symptom improvement, fourth quartile = ΔMSS < 25% = low symptom improvement, Table 1).

Table 1. Classification of patients treated with sublingual immunotherapy (SLIT) based on ΔMSS. Patients were stratified based on ΔMSS to identify patients who had a better clinical response as compared to those with a poor response to SLIT. ΔMSS-12: evaluation after 12 months of SLIT treatment; ΔMSS-24: evaluation after 24 months of SLIT treatment.

	ΔMSS	ΔMSS-12 (N, %)	ΔMSS-24 (N, %)
Very high symptom improvement	ΔMSS ≥ 75%	39 (39.80%)	41 (41.84%)
High symptom improvement	50% ≤ ΔMSS < 75%	37 (37.76%)	41 (41.84%)
Mild symptom improvement	25% ≤ ΔMSS < 50%	10 (10.20%)	14 (14.29%)
Low symptom improvement	ΔMSS < 25%	12 (12.24%)	2 (2.04%)
	Total	98 (100.00%)	98 (100.00%)

All procedures performed in this study were in accordance with the ethical standards of the study center and with the 1964 Helsinki Declaration and its later amendments or comparable ethical standards. All the subjects enrolled gave informed consent to participate in the study.

2.2. Predictive Response to Immunotherapy Score (PRIS)

We tried to develop a specific disease index for predicting SLIT efficacy so that patients could choose whether to undergo SLIT based on their chance of success. We identified eight parameters that might contribute to SLIT responsiveness. Each parameter was assigned a score range, and three to five groups were established (Table 2). The parameters were chosen based on clinical practice, literature review, and previous work evaluating AIT responsiveness and possible predictive factors. The parameters included age, clinical features, disease onset, number of allergen sensitizations, presence of symptoms following exposure to the allergen(s) to which the patient is sensitized, specific IgE/total IgE ratio, IgE level for CRD, and allergen dominance (Table 2).

Table 2. Predictive Response to Immunotherapy Score (PRIS).

Parameter	Group	Score	Score Range
Age (years)	0–12	15	3–15
	13–18	12	
	19–28	9	
	29–38	6	
	>38	3	
Clinical features	Rhinitis	9	3–9
	Rhinitis + Asthma	6	
	Rhinitis + Asthma + Other Allergies	3	
Disease onset (years)	3	9	3–9
	4–10	6	
	>10	3	
Number of allergen sensitizations [a]	1	16	4–16
	2–3	12	
	4–5	8	
	>5	4	
Presence of symptoms following exposure to allergen(s) to which the patient is sensitized	Symptoms when exposed to 1 allergen	12	3–12
	Symptoms when exposed to 2 allergens	9	
	Symptoms when exposed to 3 allergens	6	
	Symptoms when exposed to ≥4 allergens	3	
Specific IgE/total IgE (s/t) ratio	$s/t \geq 0.2$	12	4–12
	$0.2 > s/t \geq 0.05$	8	
	$s/t < 0.05$	4	
Component-Resolved Diagnosis for major allergens	High Positive (IgE ≥ 3.50 KUA/L)	12	0–12
	Positive (0.35 ≤ IgE < 3.50)	6	
	Negative (IgE < 0.35 KUA/L)	0	
Allergen dominance [b]	1	15	0–15
	2	10	
	3	5	
	>3	0	
Total			20–100

[a] Assessed with Skin Prick Test and/or specific IgE; ImmunoCAP 250, Phadia, Sweden. [b] The number of dominant allergens was assessed as described in the Methods Section 2.5 (Immunotherapy).

Total PRIS was calculated for each patient when he/she completed the diagnostic evaluation. Each patient was informed about his/her PRIS value and spontaneously decided to undergo SLIT treatment and be enrolled in this study. PRIS value could potentially range from 20 to 100. Therefore, PRIS stratification in quartiles would be as follows: first quartile = PRIS ≥ 80; second quartile = 80 > PRIS ≥ 60; third quartile = 60 > PRIS ≥ 40; fourth quartile = PRIS < 40. However, the PRIS values of patients enrolled in this study ranged from 41 to 93. Therefore, we had no patients in the fourth quartile.

2.3. Skin Prick Test

SPT was performed on the forearms of all enrolled subjects to confirm the diagnosis of a suspected type I allergy and identify the sensitization type. We used specific inhalant allergen extracts (Gramineae grass pollen (Gramineae mix/Phleum Pratense/Cynodon Dactilon), ambrosia, mugwort, wall pellitory (Parietaria Judaica/Parietaria Officinalis), olive pollen (Olea Europea), cypress pollen (Cupressaceae), birch, cat, dog, house dust mite (Dermatophagoides farina/Dermatophagoides pteronissinus), molds (Alternaria

Alternata/Aspergillus/Cladosporium), a histamine positive control, and normal saline as a negative control. The test was interpreted after 15–20 min of application, with a positive result defined as a wheal $\geq$3 mm diameter.

2.4. In Vitro Tests

Total IgE and specific IgE Assay (ImmunoCAP 250; Phadia, Sweden) were performed in patients with positive SPT to evaluate the major inhalant allergen. The level of awareness towards the main inhalant allergen was increased using the CRD. We evaluated IgE antibodies to Phl p1 (Timothy grass), Phl p5 (Timothy grass), Bet v1 and Bet v2 (Betula verrucose), Amb a1 (Ambrosia), Art v1 (Mugwort), Par j2 (Wall pellitory), Ole e1 (Olea europea), Cup a1 (Cupressus arizonica), Fel d1 (cat), Can f1 (dog), Der p1 (House dust mite), Der p2 (House dust mite), and Alt a1 (Alternaria alternata). IgE levels were considered positive at the level $\geq$0.35 kUA/l. Patients with IgE antibodies to Bet v2 were excluded to rule out profilin allergy [31–33].

2.5. Immunotherapy

SLIT was performed using allergen medicines currently authorized and marketed in Italy (Oralvac Plus®/Allergy Therapeutics; Sulgen®/Roxall-Aristegui; SlitONE Ultra®, Grazax®, Accarizax®/ALK Abellò; Lais®/Lofarma). The allergen(s) used for immunotherapy (dominant allergen(s)) had to be clinically relevant to the patient's clinical history, and it was identified according to the result of SPT and specific IgE assay. In detail, a difference of wheal diameter $\geq$5 mm compared to the other allergen tested at SPT and a difference of half a logarithm of the IgE level for a specific allergen compared to the other allergens was required to identify the dominant allergen(s). When applicable, the awareness of the major allergens was increased using CRD. Patients with one dominant allergen underwent a single-allergen SLIT; those with two dominant allergens underwent a two-allergen SLIT (Table 3). The evaluating physicians performed the first SLIT administration, then the patients were carefully instructed about the self-administration, and written instructions were provided to follow administration protocol.

Table 3. Allergen(s) used for sublingual immunotherapy (SLIT).

	Allergen(s)	Number of Patients N (%)
Single-allergen SLIT	Parietaria	38 (38.77%)
	House dust mite	18 (18.36%)
	Gramineae grass	18 (18.36%)
	Alternaria	1 (1.02%)
	Olive	1 (1.02%)
Two-allergen SLIT	Parietaria + Gramineae grass	27 (27.55%)
	Parietaria + mugwort	2 (2.04%)
	House dust mite + Parietaria	1 (1.02%)
	Gramineae grass + mugwort	1 (1.02%)
	Gramineae grass + olive	1 (1.02%)
	Olive + mugwort	1 (1.02%)
	Parietaria + olive	1 (1.02%)

2.6. Data Analysis

Data were summarized by descriptive analysis. Means and SD were calculated for continuous variables, while absolute values and frequency (percentage) were calculated for categorical variables. The assessment of the significance of the results obtained was performed with repeated-measures 1-way ANOVA with "MSS" (MSS-0, MSS-12, and MSS-24) as a within-subject factor. To test the predictive value of PRIS on ΔMSS-24(%) as well as of the PRIS parameters we used linear regression analysis. Analysis of dependent variable ΔMSS-24 was performed with independent 1-way ANOVA considering the stratification of patients according to the PRIS value as a between-subject independent variable (PRIS ≥ 80; 80 > PRIS ≥ 60; 60 > PRIS ≥ 40; PRIS < 40). The level of significance was set at α = 0.05.

3. Results

3.1. Demographic Data

A total of 110 patients, 68 males (61.8%) and 42 females (38.1%), were enrolled in this study. The cohort was White-Caucasian. The average age at enrollment was 24.87 ± 10.80 years (6–63). During AIT, 12 patients (10.9%) dropped and were excluded from the overall assessment which was performed only on the 98 patients who completed the 24-month immunotherapy. Therefore, the evaluation of a total of 98 patients who completed the 24-month SLIT treatment were included in the T12 and T24 evaluations. All patients enrolled were affected by allergic rhinitis (n = 98; 100%), and 49 out of 98 (50%) presented with concomitant allergic asthma.

3.2. Evaluation of Sublingual Immunotherapy Efficacy

Of the 98 total patients, 66 (67.34%) patients underwent SLIT for a single allergen and 32 (32.65%) underwent SLIT for two allergens (Table 3). Each patient received the maximum tolerated dose, per the manufacturers' recommendations. SLIT was well tolerated, and no discontinuation due to severe adverse drug effects was registered.

Patients experienced a significant improvement in symptoms at T12 (mean MSS-12 = 31.11 ± 16.88) and T24 (mean MSS-24 = 27.07 ± 15.01) compared to T0 (mean MSS-0 = 80.97 ± 8.24). Indeed, ANOVA conducted on MSS revealed a significant difference between MSS-0 and MSS-12 ($p < 0.001$) and MSS-0 and MSS-24 ($p < 0.001$) (Figure 1A). Although an additional symptom improvement was recorded at T24, no significant difference was observable between MSS-12 and MSS-24 ($p = 0.07$). Accordingly, after 12 or 24 months of SLIT, the clinical improvement assessed by ΔMSS-12(%) and ΔMSS-24(%) was 61.35% and 67.71%, respectively.

To evaluate whether the number of allergens administered may affect SLIT efficacy, we compared patients undergoing single-allergen SLIT (Mono SLIT) with patients undergoing two-allergen SLIT (MIX-SLIT). Both patient groups showed a significant improvement of symptoms at T12 (Mono SLIT-MSS-12 = 29.68 ± 17.59; MIX-SLIT-MSS-12 = 34.06 ± 15.15) and T24 (Mono SLIT-MSS-24 = 26.00 ± 14.91; MIX-SLIT-MSS-24 = 29.28 ± 12.05) as compared to T0 (Mono SLIT-MSS-0 = 81.55 ± 7.75; MIX-SLIT-MSS-0 = 79.75 ± 9.18) (Figure 1B). In addition, no significant difference was found when ANOVA was conducted by comparing ΔMSS-12(%) and ΔMSS-24(%) in patients treated with a single-allergen SLIT and patients treated with a two-allergen SLIT ($p = 0.11$ and $p = 0.07$, respectively). These results indicate that the efficacy is comparable when one or two allergens are used for SLIT.

Next, we compared SLIT efficacy between patients with only rhinitis and rhinitis associated with asthma. Figure 1C illustrates that both patient groups showed a significant improvement in symptoms at T12 (rhinitis-MSS-12 = 25.90 ± 13.95; rhinitis+asthma-MSS-12 = 36.33 ± 18.05) and T24 (rhinitis-MSS-24 = 22.61 ± 11.71; rhinitis+asthma-MSS-24 = 31.53 ± 14.90) as compared to T0 (rhinitis-MSS-0 = 78.33 ± 8.55; rhinitis+asthma-MSS-0 = 83.60 ± 7.07). When ANOVA was conducted on ΔMSS, values revealed that ΔMSS-12(%) and ΔMSS-24(%) were significantly higher in patients with only rhinitis compared to patients with rhinitis and concomitant asthma ($p < 0.05$) (Figure 1C). These results indicate that SLIT was effective in both patients with allergic rhinitis and concomitant asthma. However, they also suggest that patients affected only by rhinitis can experience a better response to SLIT compared to patients with associated asthma.

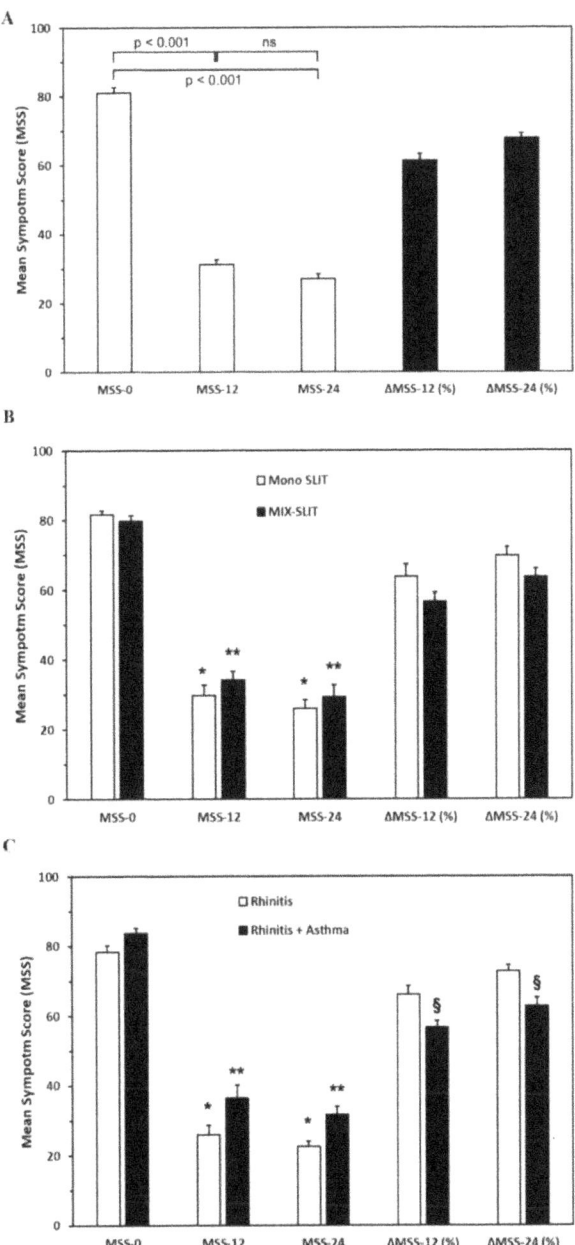

Figure 1. Sublingual immunotherapy (SLIT) efficacy assessment in the whole cohort (**A**), in patients treated with single-allergen (Mono SLIT) and two-allergen SLIT (MIX-SLIT) (**B**), and with allergic rhinitis and concomitant asthma (**C**). MSS-0: mean symptom score at T0; MSS-12: mean symptom score at T12; MSS-24: mean symptom score at T24; ΔMSS-12 (%): percentage difference between the MSS-0 and MSS-12; ΔMSS-24 (%): percentage difference between MSS-0 and MSS-24; ns: not significant; *,**: $p < 0.001$; §: $p < 0.05$.

3.3. Validation of the Predictive Response to Immunotherapy Score (PRIS)

Linear regression analysis was used to test the predictive value of PRIS on our efficacy index of SLIT [ΔMSS-24 (%)]. Figure 2 shows that overall PRIS significantly predicted ΔMSS-24 (%) ($R = 0.622$; $F (1,97) = 60.810$; $p < 0.001$).

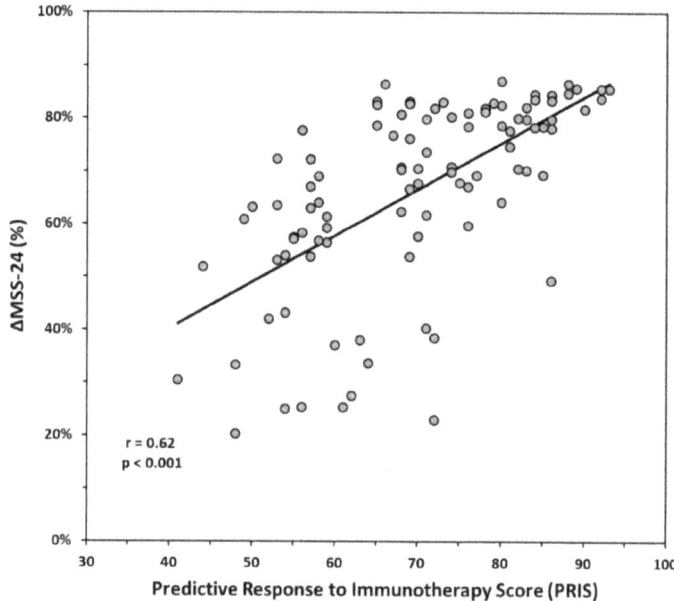

Figure 2. Correlation analysis revealed a significant direct correlation between the Predictive Response to Immunotherapy Score (PRIS) and ΔMSS-24 ($p < 0.001$).

In addition, regression analysis verified that PRIS significantly predicted ΔMSS-24 (%) in patients treated with a single-allergen SLIT (Mono-SLIT: $R = 0.708$; $F (1.65) = 64.453$; $p < 0.001$; Figure 3A) as well as in patients treated with a two-allergen SLIT (MIX-SLIT: $R = 0.599$; $F (1.31) = 16.833$; $p < 0.001$; Figure 3B), suggesting that PRIS has the same efficacy in predicting SLIT outcome when one or two allergens are used for SLIT.

Furthermore, regression analysis also showed that PRIS significantly predicted ΔMSS-24 (%) in both patients with only rhinitis ($R = 0.660$; $F (1.48) = 36.313$; $p < 0.001$; Figure 3C) and in patients with rhinitis associated with asthma ($R = 0.674$; $F (1.48) = 39.207$; $p < 0.001$; Figure 3D), suggesting that PRIS is as effective as in predicting SLIT outcome in both patients with rhinitis and with concomitant asthma. Together these results indicate that PRIS can be used to predict the efficacy of SLIT independent of the number of allergens used with SLIT and the patient's clinical condition.

Finally, in order to check that all parameters that compose the PRIS score contribute to the prediction of the outcome, linear regression analysis was also used to test the association of all individual PRIS components with ΔMSS-24 (%). As shown in Table 4, all PRIS parameters are significant predictors for our outcome, and the parameters' score categories (assumed in the model on an ordinal scale) adequately reflect the difference progression in comparison with the references.

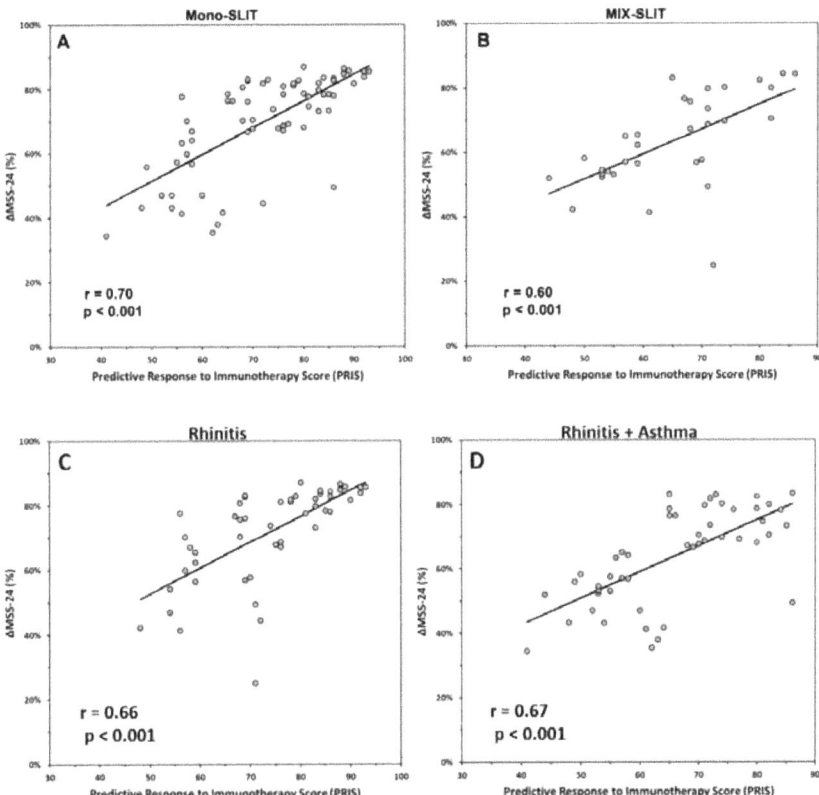

Figure 3. Correlation analysis revealed a significant direct correlation between the Predictive Response to Immunotherapy Score (PRIS) and ΔMSS-24 for both patients treated with single-allergen (**A**) and multiple-allergen (**B**) sublingual immunotherapy (SLIT) ($p < 0.001$), and between PRIS and ΔMSS-24 for both patients with only rhinitis (**C**) and with both asthma and rhinitis (**D**) ($p < 0.001$).

Table 4. Linear regression models using as predictors all PRIS parameters.

PRIS Parameter		N	Outcome ΔMSS-24(%)		
			Beta	95% CI	*p*-Value
Age (years)		98			<0.001
Group	*Score*				
>38	3		—	—	
29–38	6		0.01	−0.09, 0.10	
19–28	9		0.13	0.04, 0.22	
13–18	12		0.13	0.03, 0.23	
0–12	15		0.19	0.08, 0.30	
Clinical features		98			<0.001
Group	*Score*				
Rhinitis + Asthma + Other Allergies	3		—	—	
Rhinitis + Asthma	6		0.12	0.02, 0.22	
Rhinitis	9		0.19	0.09, 0.29	

Table 4. *Cont.*

PRIS Parameter		N	Outcome ΔMSS-24(%)		
			Beta	**95% CI**	**p-Value**
Disease onset (years)		98			0.006
Group	*Score*				
>10	3		—	—	
4–10	6		0.09	0.03, 0.16	
≤3	9		0.11	0.03, 0.18	
Number of allergen sensitizations		98			0.003
Group	*Score*				
>5	4		—	—	
4–5	8		−0.02	−0.12, 0.07	
2–3	12		0.05	−0.04, 0.15	
1	16		0.16	0.04, 0.29	
Symptoms when exposed to		98			<0.001
Group	*Score*				
3 allergens	6		—	—	
2 allergens	9		0.04	−0.04, 0.11	
1 allergen	12		0.15	0.07, 0.22	
Specific IgE/Total IgE (s/t) ratio		98			<0.001
Group	*Score*				
s/t < 0.05	4		—	—	
0.2 > s/t ≥ 0.05	8		0.05	−0.02, 0.13	
s/t ≥ 0.2	12		0.15	0.07, 0.22	
CRD for major allergens		98			<0.001
Group	*Score*				
Negative (IgE < 0.35 KUA/L)	0		—	—	
Positive (0.35 ≤ IgE < 3.50)	6		0.11	0.00, 0.21	
High Positive (IgE ≥ 3.50 KUA/L)	12		0.20	0.09, 0.31	
Allergen Dominance		98			0.002
Group	*Score*				
3	5		—	—	
2	10		0.02	−0.08, 0.12	
1	15		0.12	0.02, 0.22	

3.4. Stratification in Quartiles

We stratified patients into quartiles to gain insights into the relationship between immunotherapy efficacy and PRIS. Patients were first stratified in quartiles based on ΔMSS (%) to identify patients who had a better clinical response than those with a poor response to SLIT (Table 1). Overall, the vast majority of patients obtained a significant symptom improvement (very high or high) after 12-(72 out of 98 patients; 77.56%) and 24-month SLIT (82 out of 98 patients; 81.64%).

We then stratified patients in quartiles based on PRIS values (PRIS ≥ 80; 80 > PRIS ≥ 60; 60 > PRIS ≥ 40) to identify patients who had more chances to obtain a significant response to SLIT. ANOVA conducted on ΔMSS-24 (%) revealed a significant difference between the three groups (F (2.97) = 16.32; $p < 0.001$). Post hoc comparisons revealed a significant higher value of ΔMSS-24 (%) for PRIS $\geq$ 80 (mean $\pm$ SD 78.91 $\pm$ 8.16) than 80 > PRIS $\geq$ 60 (post hoc $p < 0.001$; mean $\pm$ SD 66.25 $\pm$ 18.31) and 60 > PRIS $\geq$ 40 (post hoc $p < 0.001$; mean $\pm$ SD 54.02 $\pm$ 15.16) (Figure 4). In addition, ΔMSS-24 (%) for 80 > PRIS $\geq$ 60 (mean $\pm$ SD 66.25 $\pm$ 18.31) was significantly higher than 60 > PRIS $\geq$ 40 (post hoc $p < 0.001$; mean $\pm$ SD 54.02 $\pm$ 15.16). These results indicate that patients with a higher PRIS value have more chances to obtain a higher ΔMSS-24 (%).

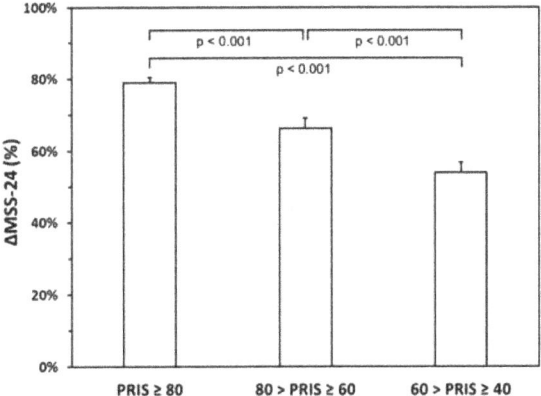

Figure 4. Stratification of patients in three groups according to the Predictive Response to Immunotherapy Score (PRIS) results and their ΔMSS-24. A significant difference was found between the three groups (F (2.97) = 16.32; $p < 0.001$).

Finally, we categorized patients by matching quartile stratification based on ΔMSS-24 (%) with quartile stratification based on PRIS. Figure 5 shows that most patients with a PRIS $\geq$ 80 experienced a very high improvement, whereas patients with 60 > PRIS $\geq$ 40 mostly experienced a high improvement. Patients with 80 > PRIS $\geq$ 60 were homogeneously distributed in ΔMSS-24 (%) quartiles. These data strongly suggest that PRIS can effectively predict the clinical response that patients may expect from SLIT.

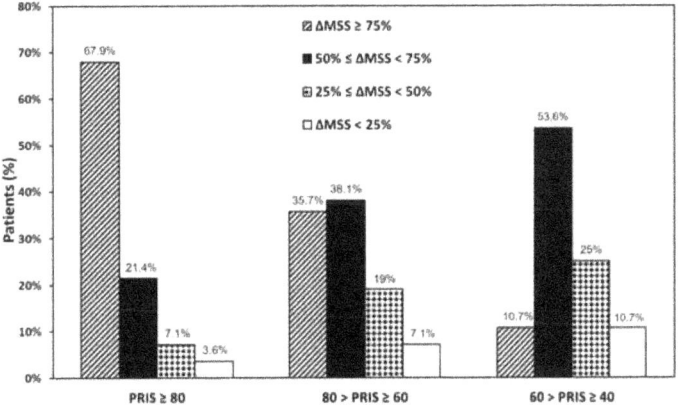

Figure 5. Stratification of patients in three groups according to the Predictive Response to Immunotherapy Score (PRIS) results and their ΔMSS-24. Most patients with a PRIS $\geq$ 80 experienced a very high improvement, whereas patients with 60 > PRIS $\geq$ 40 mostly experienced a high improvement. Patients with 80 > PRIS $\geq$ 60 were homogeneously distributed in ΔMSS-24 (%) quartiles.

4. Discussion

AIT is the only disease-modifying and potentially resolving treatment available for patients with IgE-mediated allergic diseases, and its efficacy has been proven with a high degree of evidence [34–36]. However, one of the major problems of AIT management in clinical practice is that current guidelines give no clear indication about the algorithm to be used for choosing patients eligible for this treatment [37–40]. This could be one of the reasons for the low patient compliance with AIT reported in many clinical studies [41–43]. The introduction of personalized medicine, envisioned as a patient-tailored diagnostic and therapeutic approach, is currently influencing all fields of medicine; therefore, dedicated tools for identifying patients eligible for AIT are strongly needed [13].

According to current guidelines, AIT is indicated in patients with allergic rhinitis, with or without co-existing asthma [37–40]. Identification of the allergen(s) driving symptoms is the first level of patient stratification to ensure that the correct allergen solution is used for AIT. However, this treatment is preferentially used in patients with few sensitizations or polysensitized patients with one to three dominant allergens in clinical practice. In addition, to take advantage of AIT long-term effects, younger patients with few allergic diseases and a recent onset of allergic rhinitis are preferred for AIT. Previous studies have tried to correlate AIT response with a single marker. For instance, changes in cytokine pattern, such as an increase in Th2-dependent cytokines IL-4 and IL-13, have been associated with AIT response [9]. In addition, IL-10 mRNA levels have been suggested to be predictive of clinical responses to AIT [14]. IL-10 producing regulatory B- and T-cells specific for allergens were reported to increase during AIT or following the natural allergen exposure [15]. However, no cytokine has been clearly established as a marker for AIT efficacy to be used in the clinical routine. In addition, the specific and total IgE ratio has been formerly proposed as a biomarker of AIT efficacy [11,44]. A study by Di Lorenzo et al. [11] analyzing 279 monosensitized patients treated with both SCIT and SLIT immunotherapy found that specific IgE/total IgE ratio >16.2 (i.e., specific IgE/total IgE ratio × 100) was associated with an effective response to AIT. On the contrary, a randomized, double-blind, placebo-controlled clinical trial by Fujimura et al. [44] reported that patients with specific IgE/total IgE ratio <0.19 achieved better AIT outcomes. Other authors have suggested considering allergen-specific IgE level rather than the specific IgE/total IgE ratio, describing higher specific IgE levels in AIT responders than in non-responder adults [45] and children with allergic rhinitis [46]. The same research group has proposed a cut-off value of allergen-specific IgE levels (>9.74 kUA/L) that could predict a successful response to AIT [10]. Nonetheless, these observations were based on a small number of studied patients, with a consistent discrepancy between the sample size of the responders and non-responders, which should be considered a limitation of these results [9]. We chose to use the specific IgE/total IgE ratio rather than allergen-specific IgE level, because we would need a normalized specificity index that could be easily stratified into categories. In addition, the linear regression analysis of PRIS parameters (Table 4) shows that the ratio was a significant PRIS predictor ($p < 0.001$). CRD can help to differentiate patients with genuine sensitization from those with cross-reactive sensitization to other allergen sources [1,17,47]. This could help avoid administering irrelevant allergens in AIT, improving its clinical efficacy and cost effectiveness [1,17,47]. A pilot study by di Coste et al. [1] including 36 children with allergic rhinoconjunctivitis monosensitized to grass pollen aimed to evaluate the correlation between the sensitization to different molecular Phleum pratense (Phl p) allergens and clinical efficacy of SLIT. The authors performed serum analysis of specific IgE to Phl p 1, 2, 4, 5, 6, 7, 11, and 12, and showed that SLIT was effective irrespective of the patients' baseline sensitization to either single or multiple grass pollen allergens [1]. However, a direct correlation between IgE sensitization for other major allergens detected at the molecular component level and AIT outcome has currently not been found. Finally, other potential biomarkers that have been suggested for the assessment of AIT efficacy are the assessment of IgG1 and IgG4 levels [12] or the basophil activation test [48,49], but they did not show real reliability, and there is no consensus in their usage in patients undergoing SLIT [50].

Indeed, numerous studies indicate IgG1 and IgG4 levels increase during SLIT, but they may reflect compliance instead of clinical efficacy [12,50].

To approach the heterogeneity of allergic patients, we developed a multi-parameter score, namely PRIS, potentially able to predict AIT effectiveness and identify eligible patients. PRIS includes clinical and laboratory parameters (Table 2) chosen based on clinical practice, literature review, and previous work evaluating AIT responsiveness and possible predictive factors [1,10–13,44,46,48,49,51–53]. We rated each PRIS parameter to reach a maximum of 100 points to mimic the odds of achieving a clinical improvement, thereby making it easy to be used by clinicians and intelligible by the patients. We included age, number of allergic diseases, and disease onset as clinical parameters. In addition, we tried to increase the awareness of the major allergen(s) responsible for clinical symptoms by including in the PRIS the evaluation of the occurrence of symptoms following the exposure to one or more allergens [51]. As diagnostic parameters, we started by evaluating the sensitization profiles of patients, and we included the number of sensitizations, CRD, and the specific/total IgE ratio. This last parameter was preferred to specific IgE level because we would need a normalized specificity index. Finally, we included the number of dominant allergens used to calculate PRIS and decide the allergen(s) to be used with SLIT.

To our knowledge, this study is the first time that a multi-parameter score has been effective in identifying patients eligible for SLIT in a real-life setting. Overall, PRIS strongly correlates with symptom improvement after 24 months of SLIT (Figure 2), and it was effective in patients undergoing single-allergen SLIT (Figure 3A) as well as in patients treated with a two-allergen SLIT (Figure 3B). Furthermore, PRIS was a good predictor in both patients with only rhinitis (Figure 3C) and patients with rhinitis associated with asthma (Figure 3D). Together, these results indicate that PRIS can be used to predict the efficacy of SLIT regardless of the patient's clinical condition, the product, and the number of allergens used for SLIT. Our observations suggest that PRIS also effectively predicts the degree of clinical response patients may expect from SLIT. Indeed, we observed that patients with a higher PRIS value have significantly more chances of achieving a higher symptom improvement (Figure 4). In addition, we reported that most patients with PRIS ≥ 80 experienced a very high improvement, whereas patients with 60 > PRIS ≥ 40 mostly experienced a high improvement (Figure 5). Further studies are needed to confirm these observations on a larger scale.

One of the surprising observations in our study was to find such high patient compliance to AIT. Indeed, we observed that only 10.9% of patients included in our study did not complete the 24-month follow-up. These data are dramatically lower than that reported by most studies (30–40%) [41–43]. We cannot exclude the possibility that the limited number of patients influenced compliance in our study. However, we believe that one of the reasons for the high patient compliance in our cohort is that the knowledge of their PRIS value conferred them a sort of awareness about the goal they could achieve with SLIT.

The clinical efficacy of AIT is measured using various scores as study endpoints. According to EAACI recommendations [37–40], we used a combined symptom and medication score (MSS) to permit the comparison of results with other studies. Our results confirmed that SLIT effectively improves symptoms of rhinitis and/or asthma after 12 months of SLIT treatment (Figure 1A). Although an additional symptom improvement was recorded after 24 months, no significant difference was observable between MSS-12 and MSS-24 (Figure 1A). Another interesting point of reflection is that up to a 30% improvement is achieved with placebo in AIT placebo-controlled studies [54]. This placebo effect is substantially less than >75% in nearly half of the patients in the present study (Table 1). However, as this study was open, there is no way to evaluate a contribution of the placebo effect on the perceived effects of the AIT. We also observed a significant response in both monosensitized and polysensitized patients (Figure 1B) and patients with or without allergic asthma (Figure 1C). In our cohort, a better efficacy was found in patients with only rhinitis than in patients with rhinitis associated with asthma (Figure 1C). However, further studies are needed to confirm this observation.

Our study is subject to some limitations. First, the sample size was small, but our encouraging results showed that a strong direct correlation between PRIS and SLIT outcome (Figures 2 and 3) could be a starting point for multi-center studies, which could validate PRIS on a larger scale. Second, we used different products for SLIT, and we cannot exclude the possibility that data on SLIT efficacy can be influenced by the product used. However, we avoided any product comparison because products for SLIT cannot be compared at present due to their heterogeneous composition [55,56]. From our perspective, combining several parameters routinely used in clinical practice to obtain a disease score rather than relying on a single parameter or a single product for SLIT may help better manage the within-subject variability.

In conclusion, AIT is very demanding for the patients since it is expensive and requires a long period to achieve a sustained response [7,37]. Therefore, a specific tool able to predict SLIT efficacy is worth being used in clinical practice to select eligible patients and improve patients' compliance to complete the course of treatment.

Author Contributions: Conceptualization, I.M. and F.G.; Data curation, I.M., F.G., A.D., D.P. and F.D.R.; Formal analysis, I.M., F.G., A.D., D.P., F.D.C., F.D.R. and A.R.; Investigation, I.M., A.D., D.P., F.D.C., F.D.R. and A.R.; Methodology, I.M., A.D., D.P., F.D.C., F.D.R. and A.R.; Project administration, F.G. and A.d.P.; Resources, F.G., A.D., A.d.P. and F.W.R.; Supervision, F.G., A.d.P. and F.W.R.; Validation, I.M., F.G., A.D., D.P., F.D.C., F.D.R., A.R., A.d.P. and F.W.R.; Visualization, I.M. and F.G.; Writing—original draft, I.M., F.G., F.D.C. and F.D.R.; Writing—review and editing, I.M., F.G., A.D., D.P., A.R., A.d.P. and F.W.R. All authors have read and agreed to the published version of the manuscript.

Funding: This research received no external funding.

Institutional Review Board Statement: The study was conducted in accordance with the Declaration of Helsinki and approved by the Ethics Committee of the University of Naples Federico II (protocol code 75/21).

Informed Consent Statement: This study was performed in accordance with the principles of the Helsinki Declaration. Informed consent was obtained from all subjects involved in the study.

Data Availability Statement: The data presented in this study are available on request from the corresponding author.

Conflicts of Interest: The authors declare no conflict of interest.

References

1. di Coste, A.; Occasi, F.; De Castro, G.; Zicari, A.M.; Galandrini, R.; Giuffrida, A.; Indinnimeo, L.; Duse, M. Predictivity of clinical efficacy of sublingual immunotherapy (SLIT) based on sensitisation pattern to molecular allergens in children with allergic rhinoconjunctivitis. *Allergol. Immunopathol.* **2017**, *45*, 452–456. [CrossRef] [PubMed]
2. Wheatley, L.M.; Togias, A. Clinical practice. Allergic rhinitis. *N. Engl. J. Med.* **2015**, *372*, 456–463. [CrossRef] [PubMed]
3. Dhami, S.; Kakourou, A.; Asamoah, F.; Agache, I.; Lau, S.; Jutel, M.; Muraro, A.; Roberts, G.; Akdis, C.A.; Bonini, M.; et al. Allergen immunotherapy for allergic asthma: A systematic review and meta-analysis. *Allergy* **2017**, *72*, 1825–1848. [CrossRef]
4. Penagos, M.; Eifan, A.O.; Durham, S.R.; Scadding, G.W. Duration of Allergen Immunotherapy for Long-Term Efficacy in Allergic Rhinoconjunctivitis. *Curr. Treat. Options Allergy* **2018**, *5*, 275–290. [CrossRef] [PubMed]
5. Cox, L.; Nelson, H.; Lockey, R.; Calabria, C.; Chacko, T.; Finegold, I.; Nelson, M.; Weber, R.; Bernstein, D.I.; Blessing-Moore, J.; et al. Allergen immunotherapy: A practice parameter third update. *J. Allergy Clin. Immunol.* **2011**, *127*, S1–S55. [CrossRef] [PubMed]
6. Muraro, A.; Roberts, G.; Halken, S.; Agache, I.; Angier, E.; Fernandez-Rivas, M.; Gerth van Wijk, R.; Jutel, M.; Lau, S.; Pajno, G.; et al. EAACI guidelines on allergen immunotherapy: Executive statement. *Allergy* **2018**, *73*, 739–743. [CrossRef]
7. Alvaro-Lozano, M.; Akdis, C.A.; Akdis, M.; Alviani, C.; Angier, E.; Arasi, S.; Arzt-Gradwohl, L.; Barber, D.; Bazire, R.; Cavkaytar, O.; et al. EAACI Allergen Immunotherapy User's Guide. *Pediatr Allergy Immunol* **2020**, *31*, 1–101. [CrossRef]
8. Sokolowska, M.; Boonpiyathad, T.; Escribese, M.M.; Barber, D. Allergen-specific immunotherapy: Power of adjuvants and novel predictive biomarkers. *Allergy* **2019**, *74*, 2061–2063. [CrossRef]
9. Ciprandi, G.; Tosca, M.A.; Silvestri, M. The practical role of serum allergen-specific IgE as potential biomarker for predicting responder to allergen immunotherapy. *Expert Rev. Clin. Immunol.* **2014**, *10*, 321–324. [CrossRef]
10. Ciprandi, G.; Silvestri, M. Serum specific IgE: A biomarker of response to allergen immunotherapy. *J. Investig. Allergol. Clin. Immunol.* **2014**, *24*, 35–39.

11. Di Lorenzo, G.; Mansueto, P.; Pacor, M.L.; Rizzo, M.; Castello, F.; Martinelli, N.; Ditta, V.; Lo Bianco, C.; Leto-Barone, M.S.; D'Alcamo, A.; et al. Evaluation of serum s-IgE/total IgE ratio in predicting clinical response to allergen-specific immunotherapy. *J. Allergy Clin. Immunol.* **2009**, *123*, 1103–1110. [CrossRef] [PubMed]
12. Shamji, M.H.; Kappen, J.H.; Akdis, M.; Jensen-Jarolim, E.; Knol, E.F.; Kleine-Tebbe, J.; Bohle, B.; Chaker, A.M.; Till, S.J.; Valenta, R.; et al. Biomarkers for monitoring clinical efficacy of allergen immunotherapy for allergic rhinoconjunctivitis and allergic asthma: An EAACI Position Paper. *Allergy* **2017**, *72*, 1156–1173. [CrossRef] [PubMed]
13. Incorvaia, C.; Ridolo, E.; Bagnasco, D.; Scurati, S.; Canonica, G.W. Personalized medicine and allergen immunotherapy: The beginning of a new era? *Clin. Mol. Allergy* **2021**, *19*, 10. [CrossRef] [PubMed]
14. Gueguen, C.; Luce, S.; Lombardi, V.; Baron-Bodo, V.; Moingeon, P.; Mascarell, L. IL-10 mRNA levels in whole blood cells correlate with house dust mite allergen immunotherapy efficacy. *Allergy* **2019**, *74*, 2223–2226. [CrossRef] [PubMed]
15. Jutel, M.; Akdis, M.; Budak, F.; Aebischer-Casaulta, C.; Wrzyszcz, M.; Blaser, K.; Akdis, C.A. IL-10 and TGF-beta cooperate in the regulatory T cell response to mucosal allergens in normal immunity and specific immunotherapy. *Eur. J. Immunol.* **2003**, *33*, 1205–1214. [CrossRef]
16. Stringari, G.; Tripodi, S.; Caffarelli, C.; Dondi, A.; Asero, R.; Di Rienzo Businco, A.; Bianchi, A.; Candelotti, P.; Ricci, G.; Bellini, F.; et al. The effect of component-resolved diagnosis on specific immunotherapy prescription in children with hay fever. *J. Allergy Clin. Immunol.* **2014**, *134*, 75–81. [CrossRef]
17. Di Spigna, G.; Ladogana, P.; Covelli, B.; Ricciardone, M.; Salzano, S.; Spalletti Cernia, D.; Mormile, I.; Varriale, G.; Catapano, O.; Spadaro, G.; et al. Component resolved diagnosis by recombinant allergens in patients with allergies to inhalants. *J. Biol. Regul. Homeost. Agents* **2020**, *34*, 1729–1737. [CrossRef]
18. Cohen, J. *Statistical Power Analysis for the Behavioral Sciences*, 2nd ed.; Routledge Academic: New York, NY, USA, 1988; p. 567.
19. Mauer, Y.; Taliercio, R.M. Managing adult asthma: The 2019 GINA guidelines. *Cleve Clin. J. Med.* **2020**, *87*, 569–575. [CrossRef]
20. Fortescue, R.; Kew, K.M.; Leung, M.S.T. Sublingual immunotherapy for asthma. *Cochrane Database Syst. Rev.* **2020**, *9*, CD011293. [CrossRef]
21. Passalacqua, G.; Canonica, G.W. Specific immunotherapy in asthma: Efficacy and safety. *Clin. Exp. Allergy* **2011**, *41*, 1247–1255. [CrossRef]
22. Bernstein, D.I.; Wanner, M.; Borish, L.; Liss, G.M.; Immunotherapy Committee of the American Academy of Allergy, Asthma and Immunology. Twelve-year survey of fatal reactions to allergen injections and skin testing: 1990–2001. *J. Allergy Clin. Immunol.* **2004**, *113*, 1129–1136. [CrossRef] [PubMed]
23. Przybyszowski, M.; Stachura, T.; Szafraniec, K.; Sladek, K.; Bochenek, G. The influence of self-assessment of asthma control on the Asthma Control Test outcome. *J. Asthma* **2021**, *58*, 537–546. [CrossRef] [PubMed]
24. Schatz, M.; Mosen, D.M.; Kosinski, M.; Vollmer, W.M.; Magid, D.J.; O'Connor, E.; Zeiger, R.S. Validity of the Asthma Control Test completed at home. *Am. J. Manag. Care* **2007**, *13*, 661–667. [PubMed]
25. Schatz, M.; Zeiger, R.S.; Drane, A.; Harden, K.; Cibildak, A.; Oosterman, J.E.; Kosinski, M. Reliability and predictive validity of the Asthma Control Test administered by telephone calls using speech recognition technology. *J. Allergy Clin. Immunol.* **2007**, *119*, 336–343. [CrossRef]
26. Ciprandi, G.; La Mantia, I. VAS for assessing the perception of antihistamines use in allergic rhinitis. *Acta Biomed.* **2019**, *90*, 41–44. [CrossRef]
27. Sousa-Pinto, B.; Azevedo, L.F.; Jutel, M.; Agache, I.; Canonica, G.W.; Czarlewski, W.; Papadopoulos, N.G.; Bergmann, K.C.; Devillier, P.; Laune, D.; et al. Development and validation of combined symptom-medication scores for allergic rhinitis. *Allergy* **2021**, *54*. [CrossRef]
28. Bourdin, A.; Bjermer, L.; Brightling, C.; Brusselle, G.G.; Chanez, P.; Chung, K.F.; Custovic, A.; Diamant, Z.; Diver, S.; Djukanovic, R.; et al. ERS/EAACI statement on severe exacerbations in asthma in adults: Facts, priorities and key research questions. *Eur. Respir J.* **2019**, *54*, 1900900. [CrossRef]
29. Chung, K.F.; Wenzel, S.E.; Brozek, J.L.; Bush, A.; Castro, M.; Sterk, P.J.; Adcock, I.M.; Bateman, E.D.; Bel, E.H.; Bleecker, E.R.; et al. International ERS/ATS guidelines on definition, evaluation and treatment of severe asthma. *Eur. Respir J.* **2014**, *43*, 343–373. [CrossRef]
30. Miller, M.K.; Lee, J.H.; Blanc, P.D.; Pasta, D.J.; Gujrathi, S.; Barron, H.; Wenzel, S.E.; Weiss, S.T.; Group, T.S. TENOR risk score predicts healthcare in adults with severe or difficult-to-treat asthma. *Eur. Respir J.* **2006**, *28*, 1145–1155. [CrossRef]
31. Barber, D.; de la Torre, F.; Feo, F.; Florido, F.; Guardia, P.; Moreno, C.; Quiralte, J.; Lombardero, M.; Villalba, M.; Salcedo, G.; et al. Understanding patient sensitization profiles in complex pollen areas: A molecular epidemiological study. *Allergy* **2008**, *63*, 1550–1558. [CrossRef]
32. Ruiz-Garcia, M.; Garcia Del Potro, M.; Fernandez-Nieto, M.; Barber, D.; Jimeno-Nogales, L.; Sastre, J. Profilin: A relevant aeroallergen? *J. Allergy Clin. Immunol.* **2011**, *128*, 416–418. [CrossRef] [PubMed]
33. Rodriguez Del Rio, P.; Diaz-Perales, A.; Sanchez-Garcia, S.; Escudero, C.; Ibanez, M.D.; Mendez-Brea, P.; Barber, D. Profilin, a Change in the Paradigm. *J. Investig. Allergol. Clin. Immunol.* **2018**, *28*, 1–12. [CrossRef] [PubMed]
34. Pfaar, O.; Lou, H.; Zhang, Y.; Klimek, L.; Zhang, L. Recent developments and highlights in allergen immunotherapy. *Allergy* **2018**, *73*, 2274–2289. [CrossRef] [PubMed]

35. Dhami, S.; Nurmatov, U.; Arasi, S.; Khan, T.; Asaria, M.; Zaman, H.; Agarwal, A.; Netuveli, G.; Roberts, G.; Pfaar, O.; et al. Allergen immunotherapy for allergic rhinoconjunctivitis: A systematic review and meta-analysis. *Allergy* **2017**, *72*, 1597–1631. [CrossRef] [PubMed]

36. Kristiansen, M.; Dhami, S.; Netuveli, G.; Halken, S.; Muraro, A.; Roberts, G.; Larenas-Linnemann, D.; Calderon, M.A.; Penagos, M.; Du Toit, G.; et al. Allergen immunotherapy for the prevention of allergy: A systematic review and meta-analysis. *Pediatr. Allergy Immunol.* **2017**, *28*, 18–29. [CrossRef] [PubMed]

37. Roberts, G.; Pfaar, O.; Akdis, C.A.; Ansotegui, I.J.; Durham, S.R.; Gerth van Wijk, R.; Halken, S.; Larenas-Linnemann, D.; Pawankar, R.; Pitsios, C.; et al. EAACI Guidelines on Allergen Immunotherapy: Allergic rhinoconjunctivitis. *Allergy* **2018**, *73*, 765–798. [CrossRef] [PubMed]

38. Agache, I.; Lau, S.; Akdis, C.A.; Smolinska, S.; Bonini, M.; Cavkaytar, O.; Flood, B.; Gajdanowicz, P.; Izuhara, K.; Kalayci, O.; et al. EAACI Guidelines on Allergen Immunotherapy: House dust mite-driven allergic asthma. *Allergy* **2019**, *74*, 855–873. [CrossRef]

39. Ryan, D.; Gerth van Wijk, R.; Angier, E.; Kristiansen, M.; Zaman, H.; Sheikh, A.; Cardona, V.; Vidal, C.; Warner, A.; Agache, I.; et al. Challenges in the implementation of the EAACI AIT guidelines: A situational analysis of current provision of allergen immunotherapy. *Allergy* **2018**, *73*, 827–836. [CrossRef]

40. Bousquet, J.; Pfaar, O.; Togias, A.; Schunemann, H.J.; Ansotegui, I.; Papadopoulos, N.G.; Tsiligianni, I.; Agache, I.; Anto, J.M.; Bachert, C.; et al. 2019 ARIA Care pathways for allergen immunotherapy. *Allergy* **2019**, *74*, 2087–2102. [CrossRef]

41. Borg, M.; Lokke, A.; Hilberg, O. Compliance in subcutaneous and sublingual allergen immunotherapy: A nationwide study. *Respir Med.* **2020**, *170*, 106039. [CrossRef]

42. Musa, F.; Al-Ahmad, M.; Arifhodzic, N.; Al-Herz, W. Compliance with allergen immunotherapy and factors affecting compliance among patients with respiratory allergies. *Hum. Vaccin. Immunother.* **2017**, *13*, 514–517. [CrossRef] [PubMed]

43. Leader, B.A.; Rotella, M.; Stillman, L.; DelGaudio, J.M.; Patel, Z.M.; Wise, S.K. Immunotherapy compliance: Comparison of subcutaneous versus sublingual immunotherapy. *Int. Forum Allergy Rhinol.* **2016**, *6*, 460–464. [CrossRef] [PubMed]

44. Fujimura, T.; Yonekura, S.; Horiguchi, S.; Taniguchi, Y.; Saito, A.; Yasueda, H.; Inamine, A.; Nakayama, T.; Takemori, T.; Taniguchi, M.; et al. Increase of regulatory T cells and the ratio of specific IgE to total IgE are candidates for response monitoring or prognostic biomarkers in 2-year sublingual immunotherapy (SLIT) for Japanese cedar pollinosis. *Clin. Immunol.* **2011**, *139*, 65–74. [CrossRef] [PubMed]

45. Ciprandi, G.; Alesina, R.; De Amici, M. Serum specific IgE: Biomarker for specific immunotherapy responsiveness? *Allergol. Immunopathol.* **2014**, *42*, 369–371. [CrossRef] [PubMed]

46. Tosca, M.; Silvestri, M.; Accogli, A.; Rossi, G.A.; Ciprandi, G. Serum-specific IgE and allergen immunotherapy in allergic children. *Immunotherapy* **2014**, *6*, 29–33. [CrossRef]

47. Matricardi, P.M.; Dramburg, S.; Potapova, E.; Skevaki, C.; Renz, H. Molecular diagnosis for allergen immunotherapy. *J. Allergy Clin. Immunol.* **2019**, *143*, 831–843. [CrossRef]

48. Caruso, M.; Cibella, F.; Emma, R.; Campagna, D.; Tringali, G.; Amaradio, M.D.; Polosa, R. Basophil biomarkers as useful predictors for sublingual immunotherapy in allergic rhinitis. *Int. Immunopharmacol.* **2018**, *60*, 50–58. [CrossRef]

49. Van Overtvelt, L.; Baron-Bodo, V.; Horiot, S.; Moussu, H.; Ricarte, C.; Horak, F.; Zieglmayer, P.; Zieglmayer, R.; Montagut, A.; Galvain, S.; et al. Changes in basophil activation during grass-pollen sublingual immunotherapy do not correlate with clinical efficacy. *Allergy* **2011**, *66*, 1530–1537. [CrossRef]

50. Breiteneder, H.; Peng, Y.Q.; Agache, I.; Diamant, Z.; Eiwegger, T.; Fokkens, W.J.; Traidl-Hoffmann, C.; Nadeau, K.; O'Hehir, R.E.; O'Mahony, L.; et al. Biomarkers for diagnosis and prediction of therapy responses in allergic diseases and asthma. *Allergy* **2020**, *75*, 3039–3068. [CrossRef]

51. Tortajada-Girbes, M.; Mesa Del Castillo, M.; Larramona, H.; Lucas, J.M.; Alvaro Lozano, M.; Tabar, A.I.; Soler Lopez, B.; Martinez-Canavate, A.; Immunotherapy Working Group of the Spanish Society of Pediatric Clinical Immunology and Allergology. Decision-making for pediatric allergy immunotherapy for aeroallergens: A narrative review. *Eur. J. Pediatr.* **2019**, *178*, 1801–1812. [CrossRef]

52. Pitsios, C. Allergen Immunotherapy: Biomarkers and Clinical Outcome Measures. *J. Asthma Allergy* **2021**, *14*, 141–148. [CrossRef] [PubMed]

53. Kouser, L.; Kappen, J.; Walton, R.P.; Shamji, M.H. Update on Biomarkers to Monitor Clinical Efficacy Response During and Post Treatment in Allergen Immunotherapy. *Curr. Treat. Options Allergy* **2017**, *4*, 43–53. [CrossRef] [PubMed]

54. Pfaar, O.; Agache, I.; Bergmann, K.C.; Bindslev-Jensen, C.; Bousquet, J.; Creticos, P.S.; Devillier, P.; Durham, S.R.; Hellings, P.; Kaul, S.; et al. Placebo effects in allergen immunotherapy-An EAACI Task Force Position Paper. *Allergy* **2021**, *76*, 629–647. [CrossRef] [PubMed]

55. Bonertz, A.; Roberts, G.; Slater, J.E.; Bridgewater, J.; Rabin, R.L.; Hoefnagel, M.; Timon, M.; Pini, C.; Pfaar, O.; Sheikh, A.; et al. Allergen manufacturing and quality aspects for allergen immunotherapy in Europe and the United States: An analysis from the EAACI AIT Guidelines Project. *Allergy* **2018**, *73*, 816–826. [CrossRef] [PubMed]

56. Bonertz, A.; Roberts, G.C.; Hoefnagel, M.; Timon, M.; Slater, J.E.; Rabin, R.L.; Bridgewater, J.; Pini, C.; Pfaar, O.; Akdis, C.; et al. Challenges in the implementation of EAACI guidelines on allergen immunotherapy: A global perspective on the regulation of allergen products. *Allergy* **2018**, *73*, 64–76. [CrossRef]

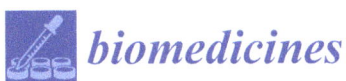

biomedicines

Article

The Mediating Effect of Cytokines on the Association between Fungal Sensitization and Poor Clinical Outcome in Asthma

Ching-Hsiung Lin [1,2,3,4,*], Yi-Rong Li [5], Chew-Teng Kor [6,7], Sheng-Hao Lin [1,4,5], Bin-Chuan Ji [1], Ming-Tai Lin [1] and Woei-Horng Chai [1]

1   Division of Chest Medicine, Department of Internal Medicine, Changhua Christian Hospital, Changhua 500, Taiwan; 112364@cch.org.tw (S.-H.L.); 99257@cch.org.tw (B.-C.J.); 13081@cch.org.tw (M.-T.L.); 80690@cch.org.tw (W.-H.C.)
2   Institute of Genomics and Bioinformatics, National Chung Hsing University, Taichung 402, Taiwan
3   Ph.D. Program in Translational Medicine, National Chung Hsing University, Taichung 402, Taiwan
4   Department of Recreation and Holistic Wellness, MingDao University, Changhua 523, Taiwan
5   Thoracic Medicine Research Center, Changhua Christian Hospital, Changhua 500, Taiwan; 181065@cch.org.tw
6   Big Data Center, Changhua Christian Hospital, Changhua 500, Taiwan; 179297@cch.org.tw
7   Graduate Institute of Statistics and Information Science, National Changhua University of Education, Changhua 500, Taiwan
*   Correspondence: teddy@cch.org.tw; Tel.: +886-4-7238595; Fax: +886-4-7232942

Citation: Lin, C.-H.; Li, Y.-R.; Kor, C.-T.; Lin, S.-H.; Ji, B.-C.; Lin, M.-T.; Chai, W.-H. The Mediating Effect of Cytokines on the Association between Fungal Sensitization and Poor Clinical Outcome in Asthma. *Biomedicines* 2022, 10, 1452. https://doi.org/10.3390/biomedicines10061452

Academic Editor: Stanislawa Bazan-Socha

Received: 2 June 2022
Accepted: 17 June 2022
Published: 19 June 2022

Publisher's Note: MDPI stays neutral with regard to jurisdictional claims in published maps and institutional affiliations.

Abstract: Sensitization to fungal allergens is one of the proposed phenotypes in asthma. An association between fungal sensitization and worse clinical outcomes is apparent. Moreover, fungal sensitization in asthma that is associated with different type of immunological mechanism has been reported. How the role of cytokines mediates the association between fungal sensitization and poorer asthmatic outcomes remains unclear. We aimed to determine role of cytokines in the relationship between fungal sensitization and worse clinical outcomes in asthma. Method: We conducted a prospective study to recruit adult patients with asthma. Data including age, sex, height, weight, smoking history, medication, emergency visit and admission, pulmonary function testing result, and Asthma Control Test (ACT) scores were collected. We used the automated BioIC method to measure fungal allergen sIgE in sera. Serum levels of Interleukin (IL) -4, IL-13, IL-6, IL-9, IL-10, IL-17 A, IL-22, Interferon (IFN) -γ, Immunoglobulin E (IgE), Tumor necrosis factor-α (TNF-α), and Transforming growth factor-β (TGF-β) were measured using ELISA. Result: IL-6 and IL-17A had a significant positive correlation between sensitization and most fungi species compared to IgE. Sensitization to *Candida albicans* had strongly positive association both with IL-6 and IL-17A. However, only IL-17A had significant relationship with ED visit times. The mediation analysis result indicates that IL-17A had a significant positively mediating effect (ME) on the association between *Candida albicans* and ED visit times. Conclusion: IL-17A is a potential mediator to link *Candida albicans* sensitization and ED visits for asthma. We suggest that patients with fungal sensitization, such as *Candida albicans*, have poorer outcomes associated with Th17-mediated immune response rather than Th2.

Keywords: asthma; fungal sensitization; IL-17A; *Candida albicans*; mediation effect

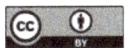

Copyright: © 2022 by the authors. Licensee MDPI, Basel, Switzerland. This article is an open access article distributed under the terms and conditions of the Creative Commons Attribution (CC BY) license (https://creativecommons.org/licenses/by/4.0/).

1. Introduction

Asthma is a chronic inflammatory disease of the airways that significantly impairs quality of life [1]. It is also characterized by a variety of clinical presentations and outcomes, which can be classified into different phenotypes [2]. A previous study has suggested that sensitization to fungal allergens is one of the proposed phenotypes [3]. Cumulative studies demonstrate that fungal sensitization in patients with asthma has been associated with increased asthma severity as well as worse clinical outcomes, including worse asthma control, decreased lung function, increased hospital and intensive care unit (ICU) admissions, respiratory arrest, and asthma-related deaths [4–8]. Although an association between fungal sensitization and worse clinical outcomes is apparent, whether such an association is causal remains unconfirmed.

Fungal sensitization is an immune-mediated response to a fungus without evidence of inflammation or tissue damage [9]. In previous studies, both innate and adaptive immunity related to fungal sensitization in asthma. A review study indicated that allergic sensitization to fungi is mediated by the innate immune response driven by the innate lymphoid cells group 2 and the adaptive immune response driven by TH2 cells [4]. However, immune responses to fungi are mediated by a network of innate and adaptive immune cells, including but not limited to ILC2s and Th2 cells. Fairs A et al. show elevated levels of neutrophils in *A. fumigatus*-IgE–sensitized patients in comparison to non-sensitized patients with asthma, suggesting a Th1- or Th17-mediated immune response [6]. Moreover, an animal model of fungal-sensitized asthma found that IL-1Ra deficiency enhanced Th1 and Th17 immunity, increased neutrophil recruitment, and exacerbated disease [10,11]. Furthermore, a murine acute allergic asthma model demonstrated that sensitization with *A. fumigatus cpe* also elicited a higher percentage of IL-17AF+ eosinophil cells compared with OVA sensitization [12]. These studies reflected that fungal sensitization in asthma are associated with different type of immunological mechanism, including neutrophil, eosinophil, Th1, Th2, and Th17.

Cytokines, or intracellular signaling proteins, target specific cells causing consequences such as cell-mediated immunity and allergic responses [13–15]. Therefore, cytokines were chosen in order to investigate known cytokines of interest in asthma and to also examine the complex groups of Th1, Th2, Tregs, and Th17 representative cytokines. A previous study suggested that Th1, Th2, and Th17 immune responses relate to fungal sensitization in asthma; however, the cytokine profile of asthmatic patients who are sensitized to fungi is rare. Recent study reported that interleukin-33 levels were higher in severe asthmatic patients with fungal sensitization than in those without fungal sensitization. However, the study only analyzed the association between multiple fungal sensitization and cytokine, the relationship between species-specific sensitization to fungi and cytokines was not revealed [16].

To understand the immunological mechanism between fungal sensitization and asthma is vital for devising therapeutic interventions to prevent worse outcomes. In this study, we aimed to determine role of cytokines in the relationship between fungal sensitization and worse clinical outcomes in asthma. Firstly, we analyzed the cytokine profile regarding Th1, Th2, and Th17 immune response associated with sensitization to specific fungi species. Secondly, we evaluate the role of cytokine in the association between fungal sensitization and measures of disease control and worsen outcomes in asthma.

2. Material and Methods

2.1. Study Population

We enrolled patients who were at least 20 years old and presented with asthma; they were recruited from the Changhua Christian Hospital (Changhua, Taiwan) from 2012 through 2019. Patients with pulmonary tuberculosis, bronchiectasis, chronic obstructive pulmonary disease, chronic bronchitis, lung cancer, and cystic fibrosis were excluded from the study. The living environment of the patients registered this study was similar to that of patients who lived in nearly the same area (urban area around Changhua in Taiwan). Therefore, there was no major difference in climate, environment, etc., among patients. The study protocol was approved by the Institutional Review Board of Changhua Christian Hospital (IRB number 120607; approval date: 20/11/2012). The protocol was implemented in compliance with the Declaration of Helsinki. All participants provided written informed consent.

2.2. Collection of Clinical Information

Data including age, sex, height, weight, and smoking history were obtained from a chart review. Medication use and health care utilization, including emergency visits and admissions in the year, were obtained from medical records. The control status of asthma and disease-specific quality of life were determined using Chinese version of the Asthma Control Test (ACT).

2.3. Pulmonary Function Assessment

Pulmonary function, during stable asthma, was measured using a spirometer, which accommodates criteria of the American Thoracic Society. Each participant was required to perform three cycles of inhalation and exhalation, and the best forced expiratory volume in one second (FEV1), PEF, and forced vital capacity (FVC) were selected. GLI-2012-predicted values were used as the reference values for the executed spirometry.

2.4. Detection of Allergen Sensitization

We used the automated microfluidic-based multiplexed immunoassay system (BioIC Allergen-Specific IgE Detection Kit; GENERAL MEDICAL CO., LTD, Taichung, Taiwan) to measure fungal allergen sIgE in sera. The levels equal to or greater than Class 1 ($\geq$1 AU) were considered positive. The sIgE to fungi allergens, including *Aspergillus flavus, Aspergillus niger, Penicillium chrysogenum, Botrytis cinerea, Fusarium solani, Rhodotoeula, Trichophyton rubrum, Saccharomyces, Penicillium, Penicillium notatum, Cladosporium herbarum, Aspergillus fumigatus, Candida albicans,* and *Alternaria alternata* were detected.

2.5. Serum Levels of Cytokines

Serum levels of IL-4, IL-13, IL-6, IL-9, IL-10, IL-17 A, IL-22, IFN-γ, TNF-α, and TGF-β measured using The BioLegend LEGEND MAX™ Enzyme-Linked Immunosorbent Assay kits (Biolegend, San Diego, CA, USA). IL-19 was detected using Quantikine Enzyme-Linked Immunosorbent Assay kits (R&D Systems, Minneapolis, MN, USA).

2.6. Statistical Analysis

Statistical analysis was performed using SPSS 22.0 for Windows (IBM Corporation, Armonk, New York, NY, USA). Data are expressed as mean $\pm$ SD, median, or percentage. Two-way comparisons were performed using the unpaired t-test for parametric variables and the Mann–Whitney test for nonparametric variables. Categorical variables were compared using the χ^2 test or Fisher's exact test. Spearman correlation analysis were used to determine the relationships between fungi, clinical outcomes, and cytokines. Correlation matrix plot were produced in R using the ggplot2 package. We performed mediation analysis using the SPSS PROCESS macro, version 2.16 (model 4), developed by Hayes [17]. All statistical tests were two-sided, with $p < 0.05$ considered to indicate statistical significance.

3. Results
3.1. Clinical Features of Patients with Asthma

As presented in Table 1, 97 patients (42.86% men) with asthma were enrolled in the study. The mean age was 56.71 $\pm$ 12.62 years old. In total, 84.5% of patients were never smokers, and 57.7% of patients had steroid use. The mean of ACT score, FEV1% predicted, and FEV1/FVC were 20.3 $\pm$ 3.9, 71.3 $\pm$ 19.3, and 72.2 $\pm$ 12.9, respectively. Additionally, 7.2% of patients experienced an ED visit and 12.4% of patients had admission.

Table 1. Clinical features of patients with asthma.

	Patients With Asthma (N = 97)
Age (mean ± SD)	49.1 ± 18.2
BMI (kg/m2) (mean ± SD)	24.8 ± 4.2
Gender (N, %)	
Male	39 (40.2%)
Female	58 (59.8%)
Smoking status	
Never smoker	82 (84.5%)
Ever smoker	5 (5.2%)
Current smoker	10 (10.3%)
Steroid use	
No	41 (42.3%)
Yes	56 (57.7%)
ACT (mean ± SD)	20.3 ± 3.9
FEV1% (mean ± SD)	71.3 ± 19.3
FEV1/FVC (mean ± SD)	72.2 ± 12.9
ED visit times (N, %)	
0 times	90 (92.8%)
1 times	6 (6.2%)
2 times	1 (1.0%)
Admission times (N, %)	
0 times	85 (87.6%)
1 times	9 (9.3%)
2 times	3 (3.1%)
Fungal sensitization (N,%)	
Without sensitization	7 (7.2%)
With sensitization	90 (92.8%)
Aspergillus flavus (mean ± SD)	0.4 ± 0.82
Aspergillus niger (mean ± SD)	1.26 ± 1.72
Penicillium chrysogenum (mean ± SD)	0.66 ± 3.32
Botrytis cinerea (mean ± SD)	3.66 ± 31.35
Fusarium solani (mean ± SD)	1.34 ± 1.32
Rhodotoeula (mean ± SD)	2.03 ± 3.46
Trichophyton rubrum (mean ± SD)	1.12 ± 1.95
Saccharomyces (mean ± SD)	0.38 ± 0.86
Penicillium (mean ± SD)	0.22 ± 1
Penicillium notatum (mean ± SD)	0.2 ± 0.6
Cladosporium herbarum (mean ± SD)	1.09 ± 3.41
Aspergillus fumigatus (mean ± SD)	1.6 ± 3.45
Candida albicans (mean ± SD)	2.23 ± 2.15
Alternaria alternata (mean ± SD)	0.19 ± 0.6
IgE (mean ± SD)	394.08 ± 947.1
IL-4 (0.0125–1 ng/mL) (mean ± SD)	0.025 ± 0.096
IL-6 (ng/mL) (mean ± SD)	0.446 ± 0.503
IL-9 (0.04–3 ng/mL) (mean ± SD)	0.258 ± 0.386
IL-10 (0.04–2.5 ng/mL) (mean ± SD)	0.05 ± 0.089
IL-17 A (0.03125–2 ng/mL) (mean ± SD)	0.381 ± 0.501
IL-13 (0.0625–4 ng/mL) (mean ± SD)	0.137 ± 0.394
IL-19 (0.0625–2 ng/mL) (mean ± SD)	0.195 ± 0.147
IL-22 (0.0125–1 ng/mL) (mean ± SD)	0.023 ± 0.092
IFN-γ (0.047–1.5 ng/mL) (mean ± SD)	0.209 ± 0.462
TGF-β (0.03–2 ng/mL) (mean ± SD)	0.091 ± 0.079
TNF-α (0.03125–2 ng/mL) (mean ± SD)	0.408 ± 0.602

3.2. Correlation among Fungi, Clinical Outcome of Asthmatic Patients, and Cytokines

The association between fungal sensitization and worse asthmatic outcomes has previously been reported. We first examined the relationship between fungi species and clinical outcomes. The correlation analysis results found that no significant relationship between fungi species and asthmatic outcomes, including pulmonary function testing result, ACT score, steroid use, ED visit times, and admission times (Figure 1A). Next, we evaluated the association between fungi species and immune markers. The results demonstrated that IL-6 and IL-17A have a positive relation with most fungi species. IL-6 was especially positively associated with *Aspergillus flavus, Aspergillus niger, Botrytis cinerea, Trichophyton rubrum, Cladosporium herbarum, Aspergillus fumigatus*, and *Candida albicans*. IL-17 had a particularly positive association with *Botrytis cinerea, Saccharomyces*, and *Candida albicans* (Figure 1B). However, only IL-17 was positively associated with ED visit times and FEV1 (Figure 1C).

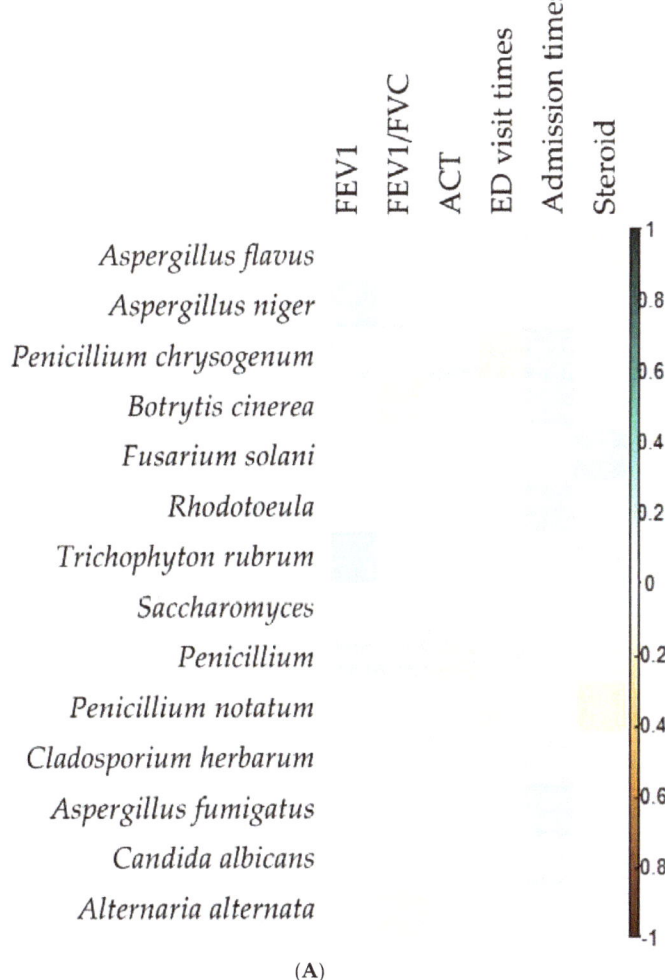

(A)

Figure 1. *Cont.*

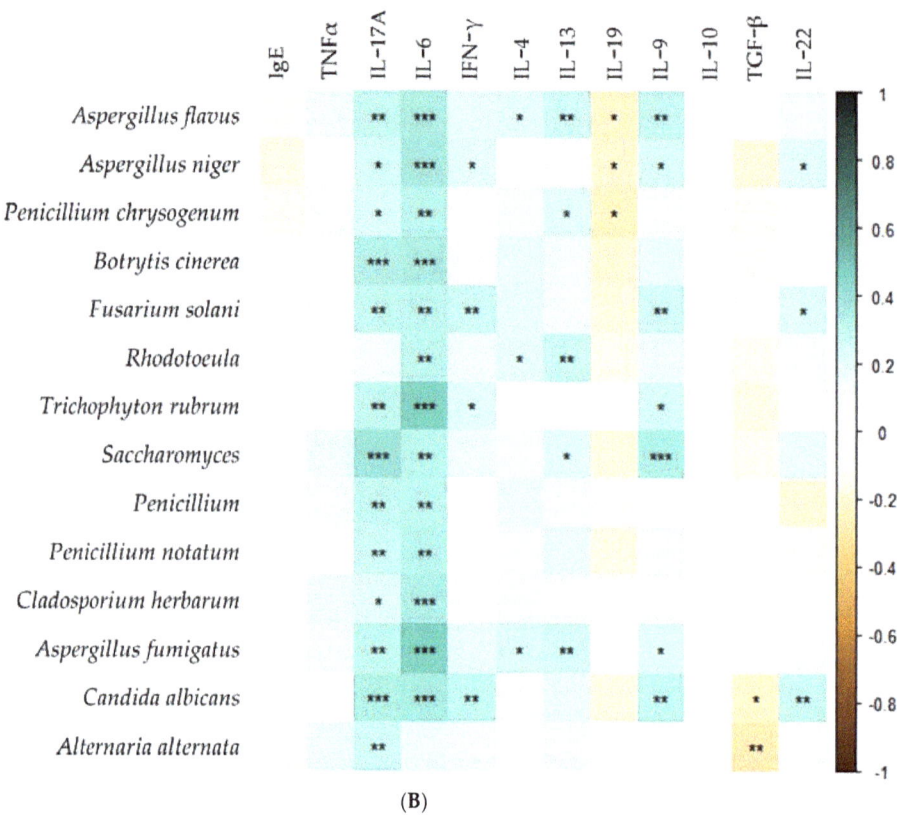

(B)

Figure 1. *Cont.*

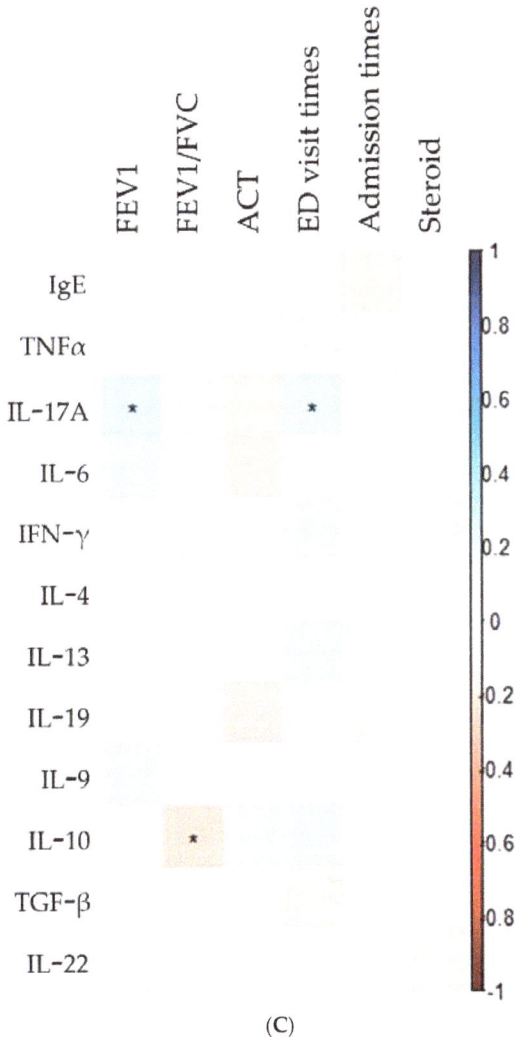

(C)

Figure 1. Correlation matrix plot between (**A**) fungus and asthma-related outcomes, (**B**) inflammatory cytokine and asthma-related outcomes, and (**C**) fungus and inflammatory cytokine. * $p < 0.05$, ** $p < 0.01$, *** $p < 0.001$.

3.3. Correlation among Botrytis cinerea, Saccharomyces, and Candida albicans and ED Times and IL-17A

A strong positive correlation was observed between IL-17A and *Botrytis cinerea*, *Candida albicans*, and *Saccharomyces* (*Botrytis cinerea*: r = 0.34, $p < 0.0001$; *Candida albicans*: r = 0.36, $p < 0.0001$; *Saccharomyces*: r = 0.39, $p < 0.0001$). The correlation between IL-17A and ED visit times was positively significant. ED visit times had no significant correlation with *Botrytis cinerea*, *Candida albicans*, and *Saccharomyces* (Figure 2).

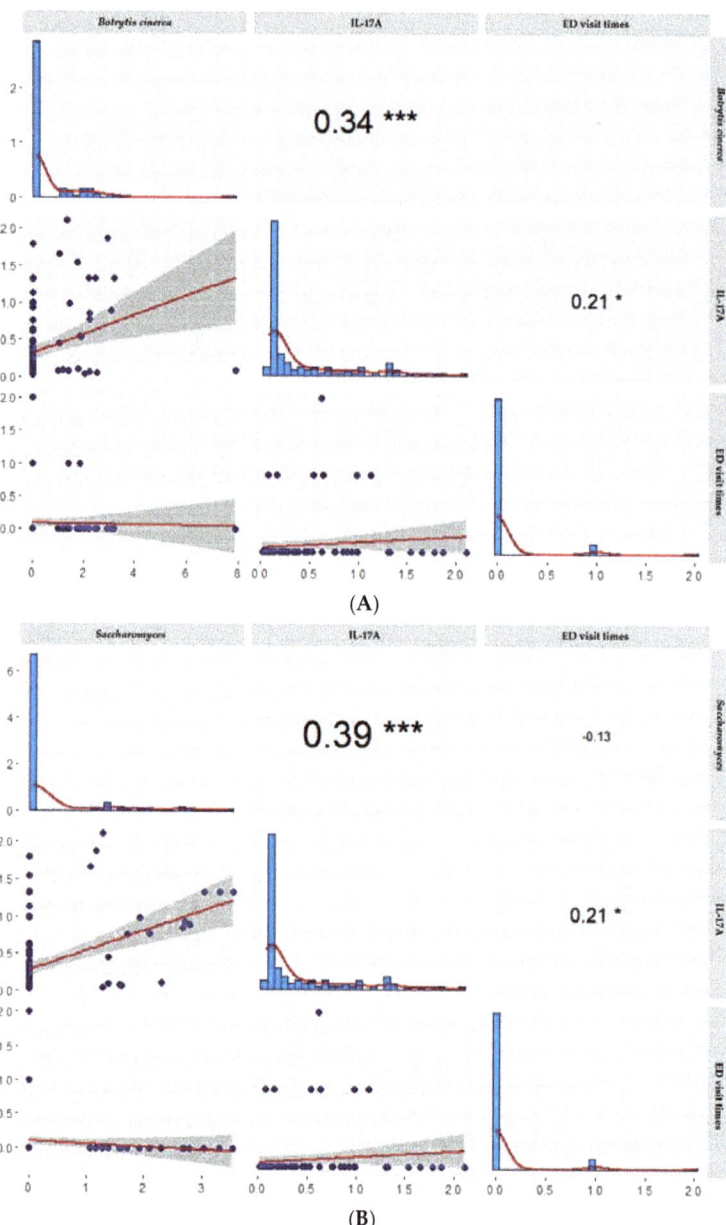

Figure 2. *Cont.*

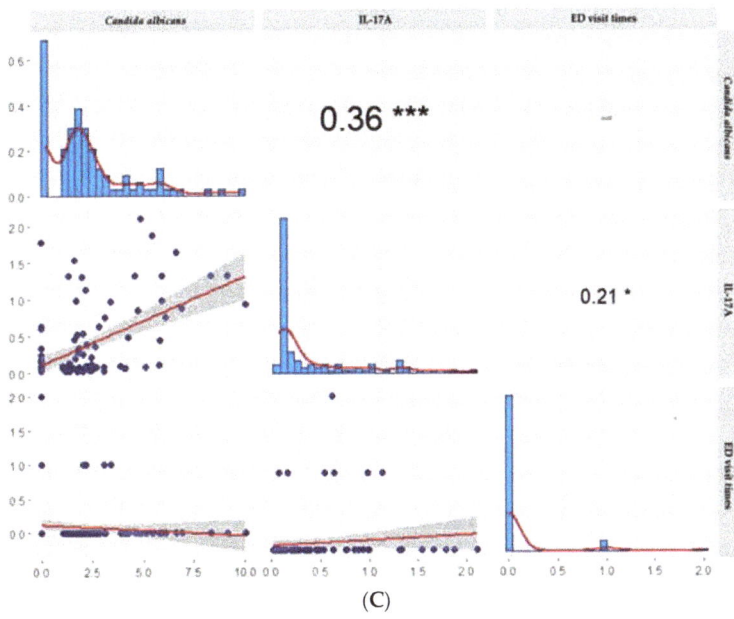

(C)

Figure 2. The scatter matrix, histogram, and Spearman rank correlation matrix among (**A**) *Botrytis cinerea*, (**B**) *Saccharomyces*, and (**C**) *Candida albicans* and ED times and IL-17A. * $p < 0.05$, *** $p < 0.001$.

3.4. IL-17A Levels in Asthmatic Patients with and without Fungal Sensitization Grouped by ED Visit Times

Previous studies indicated that fungal sensitization is associated with increased asthma severity and poorer clinical outcomes. However, we only observed a correlation between IL-17A and sensitized to various fungi (*Botrytis cinerea*, *Saccharomyces*, and *Candida albicans*), as well as between ED visit times and IL-17A, but not between fungal sensitization and ED visit times. Thus, we further investigated the IL-17A Levels in asthmatic patients with or without fungal sensitization stratified by ED visit times. The results show that patients who were sensitized to *Botrytis cinerea* had higher levels of IL-17 than patients without sensitization to *Botrytis cinerea* (Figure 3A). Patients with *Saccharomyces* had no ED visit event (Figure 3B). Conversely, patients with an ED visit (1 time) sensitized to *Candida albicans* had higher IL-17A compared to patients who were not sensitized, but without significant difference (Figure 3C).

3.5. Role of IL-17A in the Associations between Candida albicans and ED Visit Times

To clarify the role of IL-17A in the relationship between *Candida albicans* sensitization and ED visit times. We investigated the role played by IL-17A in transmitting *Candida albicans* sensitization changes to ED visit times in asthmatic patients using mediation analysis. The total effect of *Candida albicans* on ED visit times was −0.106 (95% CI: −0.454, 0.133). IL-17A had a significant positively mediating effect (ME) on the association between *Candida albicans* and ED visit times (ME = 0.0175, 95% CI: 0.012, 0.528) (Figure 4).

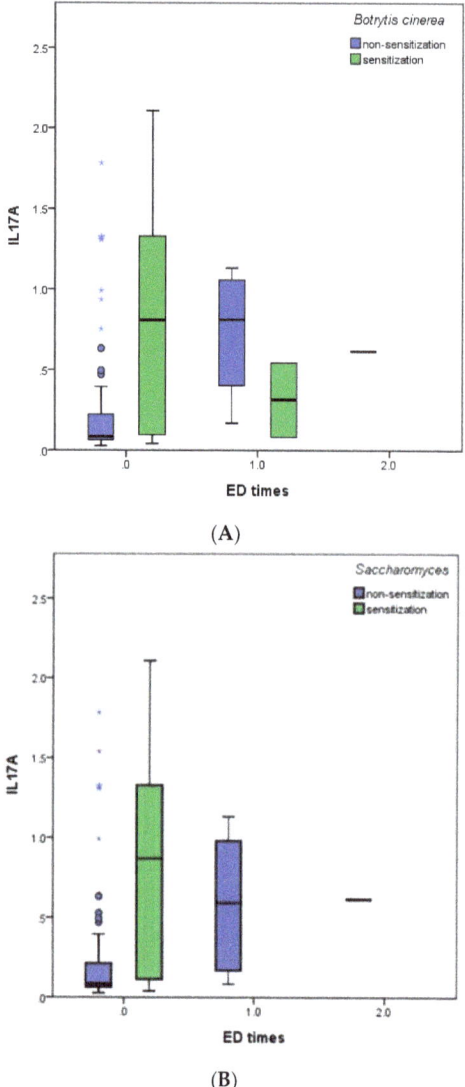

(A)

(B)

Figure 3. *Cont.*

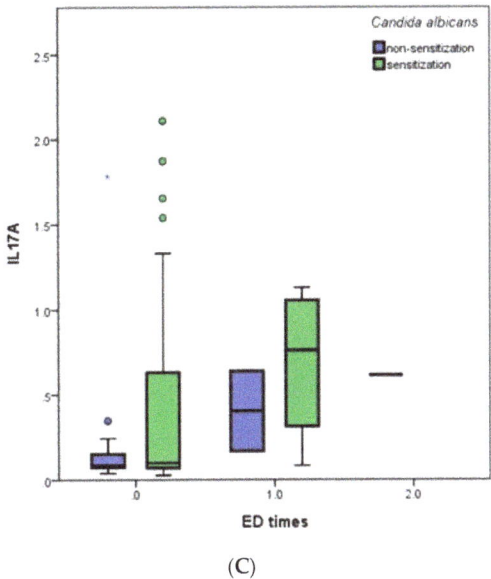

(**C**)

Figure 3. Comparing IL-17A levels in asthmatic patients with fungal sensitization and non-sensitization grouped by ED visit times. *Botrytis cinerea* (**A**); *Saccharomyces* (**B**); *Candida albicans* (**C**). * $p < 0.05$.

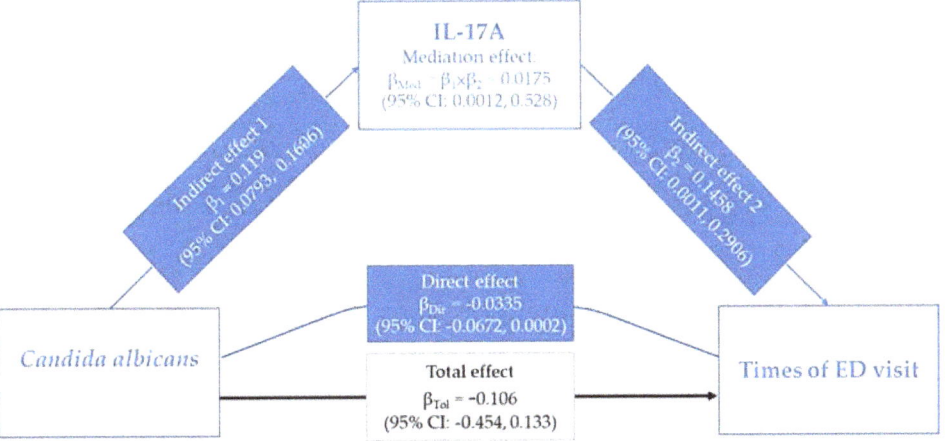

Figure 4. The contribution of IL-17A for the association between *Candida albicans* and ED visits. Single mediation models and regression coefficients (β), with 95% confidence intervals (95% CI) examining potential mediators of IL-17A.

4. Discussion

Being sensitized to fungi is a potential risk factor for worsening asthma outcomes, but the mechanisms underlying the fungal sensitization associated with poorer asthmatic outcomes remain unclear. The present study shows a link between cytokines and fungal sensitization associated with poorer asthmatic outcomes. Firstly, we observed that IL-6 and IL-17A, but no IgE, had a significant association with sensitization to most species of fungi in out testing panel. Only ED visit times were positively associated with IL-17A, and we noticed that the level of IL-17A was higher in patients with *Candida albicans* sensitization who had ED visits compared with those who did not, though the difference is not significant. The mediation analysis revealed that IL-17A had positive mediation effect between *Candida albicans* sensitization and ED visit times. Overall, our finding indicated that sensitization to *Candida albicans* had a positive correlation with IL-17A levels, which were then associated with ED visits in asthmatics. Based on present results, IL-17A could be a biomarker for asthmatics with frequent emergency department visits for *Candida albicans* sensitization.

Sensitization to fungi is associated with increased asthma severity, poorer clinical outcomes, and mortality. In previous studies, the prevalence of fungal sensitization in asthma has varied. According to a UK study, 66% of patients with severe asthma were sensitized to one or more fungi, as determined by SPT or specific serum IgE testing or both [18]. Moreover, asthma patients referred to subspecialty clinics showed that 17.3% were allergic to fungi [19], but another study showed 76.3% to be allergic to at least one fungus [20]. Further, 32% of the 576 patients enrolled in the study with severe eosinophilic asthma demonstrated sensitivity to fungal allergens [21]. In our study, we found that 92.8% of asthmatic patients had fungal sensitization. These results indicate that the exact prevalence of fungal sensitization in patients with asthma remain unclear. It is likely that the large differences seen in the prevalence of fungal sensitization among asthmatic patients are related to differences in patient populations, testing methods, and geographic locations.

Fungal sensitization is associated with worse asthmatic outcomes being reported. For example, the number asthmatic patients with fungus sensitization requiring intensive care unit admission and mechanical ventilation was higher than those without fungus sensitization or nonfungal sensitization [19]. Furthermore, the lung function of patients sensitized to thermotolerant filamentous fungi was lower than that of patients not sensitized to any fungi [20]. Despite this, we were unable to find any association between fungal sensitization with measures of control, severity, or steroid use in our population. However, we found that patients with fungal sensitization had a higher prevalence of ED visits than patients without fungal sensitization (7.78% versus 0%, data not shown). These finding suggest that exposure to inhaled allergens to which patients are sensitized can increase asthma symptoms or precipitate exacerbation. According to GINA guidelines, patients with persistent symptoms and/or exacerbations should undergo allergen testing. It is possible that patients with fungal sensitization were not identified because of lack of testing [19]. Thus, greater awareness of asthmatics at risk for more difficult disease outcomes should support earlier identification of fungal sensitization.

Allergic asthma is defined by the presence of allergic sensitization and a correlation between allergen exposure and asthma symptoms. One biomarker of allergic asthma is total serum IgE level, which is more commonly elevated in allergic compared with nonallergic asthma [22], is inversely associated with lung function in asthmatics [23], and is associated with the prevalence of asthma [24]. A previous study reported that patients with fungal sensitization (*Penicillium chrysogenum*, *Cladosporium herbarum*, *Aspergillus fumigatus*, *Mucor racemosus*, *Stemphylium herbarum*, and *Alternaria alternata*) had a higher total serum IgE concentration than patients with no sensitization or nonfungal sensitization [19]. In present study, our data demonstrate that sensitization to most species of fungi had a positive relationship with IL-6 and IL-17 rather than IgE. In previous study, eosinophils and eosinophilic production of IL-23 and IL-17 were shown to be beneficial in invasive aspergillosis but detrimental in allergic disease in a mice model [12]. In addition, IL-6 is essential for mucus hypersecretion by airway epithelial cells triggered in response to inhaled *Aspergillus fumigatus* extract, which was found in a mouse model of allergic airway inflammation induced by direct airway exposure to extracts of *Aspergillus fumigatus* [25]. These findings suggest that the immune response regarding fungal sensitization is not only associated with IgE, but also other mechanisms involved that are related to IL-6/IL-17A axis. In allergic asthma, B cells may regulate the T cell response by modulating the phenotypic response. For example, in a JH$^{-/-}$ (B cell-deficient) murine model of fungal allergic asthma, levels of the inflammatory cytokines IL-6 and IL-17A were significantly elevated, and there was significantly more robust airway eosinophilia and neutrophilia [26]. The evidence suggests that the IL-6/IL-17A axis is associated with fungal allergic asthma in conditions with B cell deficiency. Thus, the IL-6/IL-17A axis would be a possible mechanism associated with fungal sensitization other than IgE.

Accumulating evidence now suggests that Th17 cells and their related cytokines are also involved in the pathophysiology of allergic asthma. IL-17 expression is increased in the lung, sputum, bronchoalveolar lavage fluid (BALF), and sera in patients with asthma, and the severity of AHR is positively correlated with IL-17 expression levels [27,28]. In our study, IL-17, but not IL-6, had a positive correlation with ED visits and had a significant mediation effect on the association between *Candida albicans* sensitization and ED visit. A previous study found that IL-17 increased in *Aspergillus fumigatus*-sensitized mice [29]. In addition, IL-17A response is associated strongly with acute ABPA, and its specific decline in response to ABPA treatment suggests that this atypical Th17 response plays an active role in manifesting and/or exacerbating disease [30]. The evidence supports the hypothesis that IL-17A has a mediated effect on the relationship between *Candida albicans* sensitization and poorer clinical outcomes, particularly ED visits. A previous study identified the role of IL-17-mediated immunity in Candidiasis, and the implications for clinical therapies for both autoimmune conditions and fungal infections [31]. In asthma, to our best knowledge, our findings firstly provide evidence that IL-17A is a potential mediator to link *Candida albicans* sensitization and poorer clinical outcomes. Despite the underlying cell-mediated mechanism is unclear, a study report that protective lung Th2 and Th17 cell responses against the common mucosa-associated fungus *Candida albicans* are coordinated through lung megakaryocytes and platelets [32]. The findings pointed suggested that Th17, an IL-17-producing cell, may have a protective effect against allergy to *Candida albicans* in the lungs.

Th17 immune responses differ between the sexes due to suppressive and enhancing effects of sex hormones [33]. A previous study indicated testosterone is associated with expansion of Th17 populations in a murine model of experimental autoimmune encephalomyelitis (EAE) [34]. However, a recent study indicated that the increased production of IL-17A by 17β-estradiol and progesterone from TH17 cells may provide a potential mechanism for the increased prevalence of severe asthma in women compared with men [35]. In contrast, estrus levels of estradiol downregulated the Th17 response to *Candida albicans* in in vivo vaginal infection models [36]. In our finding, we found that the IL-17 levels in asthmatic patients were 3.28 and 4.17 in males and females, respectively, but there is no significance between sex differences ($p = 0.369$) (Supplemental Table S1). The correlation between IL-17 and *Candida albicans* was 0.233 and 0.458 in males and females, respectively, but there are no significant differences between males and females in the correlation between IL-17 and *Candida albicans* ($p_{interaction} = 0.166$) (Supplemental Table S1). The finding demonstrates that sex difference has no influence on the correlation between IL-17 and *Candida albicans* in our population. Taken together, we suggest that the influence of sex difference on IL-17 is inconsistent that may depend on disease-specific characteristics or severity; thus, the mediation effect of IL-17 between poor outcomes and *Candida albicans* across sex difference is needs further study.

There are some limitations of our study. Firstly, further evaluation in a multiple center setting is needed to expand the generalizability. Secondly, we lacked information regarding immune cell type; therefore, the cell-mediated immune response related to IL-17A in fungal sensitization, especially in *Candida albicans*, needs to be further investigation. Thirdly, since some of our asthma patients were without ED visits, the causal effect is difficult to clarify due to limitation of statistical method.

5. Conclusions

In present study, we found that both IL-6 and IL-17A have a strong positive correlation with *Candida albicans*. Only IL-17A had significant positive association with ED visit times. There is a significant mediation effect of IL-17A on the association between *Candida albicans* sensitization and ED visit times. Altogether, IL-17A is a potential mediator to link *Candida albicans* sensitization and ED visits for asthma. Patients with fungal sensitization, such as *Candida albicans*, who have worse outcomes may associate with Th17-mediated immune responses rather than Th2.

Supplementary Materials: The following supporting information can be downloaded at: https:// www.mdpi.com/article/10.3390/biomedicines10061452/s1, Table S1: IL-17A level and the correlation between IL-17 and *Candida albicans* in asthmatic patients in males and females.

Author Contributions: Conceptualization, C.-H.L.; Data curation, S.-H.L., B.-C.J., M.-T.L. and W.-H.C.; Formal analysis, Y.-R.L. and C.-T.K.; Funding acquisition, C.-H.L.; Investigation, C.-H.L. and Y.-R.L.; Methodology, Y.-R.L. and C.-T.K.; Project administration, C.-H.L.; Supervision, C.-H.L.; Visualization, Y.-R.L. and C.-T.K.; Writing—original draft, C.-H.L. and Y.-R.L.; Writing—review and editing, C.-H.L. All authors have read and agreed to the published version of the manuscript.

Funding: This research was funded by Changhua Christian Hospital, grant number 110-CCH-MST-122.

Institutional Review Board Statement: The study was conducted in accordance with the Declaration of Helsinki and approved by the Institutional Review Board of Taiwan Changhua Christian Hospital (IRB number 120607; approval date: 20/11/2012)).

Informed Consent Statement: The protocol was implemented in compliance with the Declaration of Helsinki. All participants provided written informed consent.

Data Availability Statement: Due to ethical reasons, these data cannot be made public.

Conflicts of Interest: All authors declare no conflict of interest related to the data collected and procedures in this study.

References

1. Holgate, S.T.; Wenzel, S.; Postma, D.S.; Weiss, S.T.; Renz, H.; Sly, P.D. Asthma. *Nat. Rev. Dis. Primers* **2015**, *1*, 15025. [CrossRef]
2. Levy, B.D.; Noel, P.J.; Freemer, M.M.; Cloutier, M.M.; Georas, S.N.; Jarjour, N.N.; Ober, C.; Woodruff, P.G.; Barnes, K.C.; Bender, B.G.; et al. Future Research Directions in Asthma. An NHLBI Working Group Report. *Am. J. Respir. Crit. Care Med.* **2015**, *192*, 1366–1372. [CrossRef] [PubMed]
3. Denning, D.W.; O'Driscoll, B.R.; Hogaboam, C.M.; Bowyer, P.; Niven, R.M. The link between fungi and severe asthma: A summary of the evidence. *Eur. Respir. J.* **2006**, *27*, 615–626. [CrossRef] [PubMed]
4. Kao, C.C.; Hanania, N.A.; Parulekar, A.D. The impact of fungal allergic sensitization on asthma. *Curr. Opin. Pulm. Med.* **2021**, *27*, 3–8. [CrossRef] [PubMed]
5. Tanaka, A.; Fujiwara, A.; Uchida, Y.; Yamaguchi, M.; Ohta, S.; Homma, T.; Watanabe, Y.; Yamamoto, M.; Suzuki, S.; Yokoe, T. Evaluation of the association between sensitization to common inhalant fungi and poor asthma control. *Ann. Allergy Asthma Immunol.* **2016**, *117*, 163–168.e161. [CrossRef] [PubMed]
6. Fairs, A.; Agbetile, J.; Hargadon, B.; Bourne, M.; Monteiro, W.R.; Brightling, C.E.; Bradding, P.; Green, R.H.; Mutalithas, K.; Desai, D.; et al. IgE sensitization to *Aspergillus fumigatus* is associated with reduced lung function in asthma. *Am. J. Respir. Crit. Care Med.* **2010**, *182*, 1362–1368. [CrossRef]
7. O'Driscoll, B.R.; Hopkinson, L.C.; Denning, D.W. Mold sensitization is common amongst patients with severe asthma requiring multiple hospital admissions. *BMC Pulm. Med.* **2005**, *5*, 4. [CrossRef]
8. O'Hollaren, M.T.; Yunginger, J.W.; Offord, K.P.; Somers, M.J.; O'Connell, E.J.; Ballard, D.J.; Sachs, M.I. Exposure to an aeroallergen as a possible precipitating factor in respiratory arrest in young patients with asthma. *N. Engl. J. Med.* **1991**, *324*, 359–363. [CrossRef] [PubMed]
9. Agarwal, R.; Sehgal, I.S.; Dhooria, S.; Aggarwal, A.N. Challenging cases in fungal asthma. *Med. Mycol.* **2019**, *57* (Suppl. 2), S110–S117. [CrossRef]
10. Godwin, M.S.; Reeder, K.M.; Garth, J.M.; Blackburn, J.P.; Jones, M.; Yu, Z.; Matalon, S.; Hastie, A.T.; Meyers, D.A.; Steele, C. IL-1RA regulates immunopathogenesis during fungal-associated allergic airway inflammation. *JCI Insight* **2019**, *4*, e129055. [CrossRef]
11. Griffiths, J.S.; Camilli, G.; Kotowicz, N.K.; Ho, J.; Richardson, J.P.; Naglik, J.R. Role for IL-1 Family Cytokines in Fungal Infections. *Front. Microbiol.* **2021**, *12*, 633047. [CrossRef] [PubMed]
12. Guerra, E.S.; Lee, C.K.; Specht, C.A.; Yadav, B.; Huang, H.; Akalin, A.; Huh, J.R.; Mueller, C.; Levitz, S.M. Central Role of IL-23 and IL-17 Producing Eosinophils as Immunomodulatory Effector Cells in Acute Pulmonary Aspergillosis and Allergic Asthma. *PLoS Pathog.* **2017**, *13*, e1006175. [CrossRef] [PubMed]
13. Chung, K.F.; Barnes, P.J. Cytokines in asthma. *Thorax* **1999**, *54*, 825–857. [CrossRef] [PubMed]
14. Berger, A. Th1 and Th2 responses: What are they? *BMJ* **2000**, *321*, 424. [CrossRef] [PubMed]

15. Zhang, J.-M.; An, J. Cytokines, inflammation and pain. *Int. Anesthesiol. Clin.* **2007**, *45*, 27–37. [CrossRef]
16. Masaki, K.; Fukunaga, K.; Matsusaka, M.; Kabata, H.; Tanosaki, T.; Mochimaru, T.; Kamatani, T.; Ohtsuka, K.; Baba, R.; Ueda, S.; et al. Characteristics of severe asthma with fungal sensitization. *Ann. Allergy Asthma Immunol.* **2017**, *119*, 253–257. [CrossRef]
17. Hayes, A. PROCESS: A Versatile Computational Tool for Observed Variable Mediation, Moderation, and Conditional Process Modeling. 2012. Available online: http://www.afhayes.com/public/process2012.pdf (accessed on 16 May 2016).
18. O'Driscoll, B.R.; Powell, G.; Chew, F.; Niven, R.; Miles, J.F.; Vyas, A.; Denning, D. Comparison of skin prick tests with specific serum immunoglobulin e in the diagnosis of fungal sensitization in patients with severe asthma. *Clin. Exp. Allergy.* **2009**, *39*, 1677–1683. [CrossRef]
19. Medrek, S.K.; Kao, C.C.; Yang, D.H.; Hanania, N.A.; Parulekar, A.D. Fungal sensitization is associated with increased risk of life-threatening asthma. *J. Allergy Clin. Immunol. Pract.* **2017**, *5*, 1025–1031.e2. [CrossRef]
20. Woolnough, K.F.; Richardson, M.; Newby, C.; Craner, M.; Bourne, M.; Monteiro, W.; Siddiqui, S.; Bradding, P.; Pashley, C.; Wardlaw, A.J. The relationship between biomarkers of fungal allergy and lung damage in asthma. *Clin. Exp. Allergy* **2017**, *47*, 48–56. [CrossRef]
21. Wardlaw, A.; Howarth, P.H.; Israel, E.; Taillé, C.; Quirce, S.; Mallett, S.; Bates, S.; Albers, F.C.; Kwon, N. Fungal sensitization and its relationship to mepolizumab response in patients with severe eosinophilic asthma. *Clin. Exp. Allergy* **2020**, *50*, 869–872. [CrossRef]
22. Virchow, J.C., Jr.; Kroegel, C.; Walker, C.; Matthys, H. Cellular and immunological markers of allergic and intrinsic bronchial asthma. *Lung* **1994**, *172*, 313–334. [CrossRef] [PubMed]
23. Sherrill, D.L.; Lebowitz, M.D.; Halonen, M.; Barbee, R.A.; Burrows, B. Longitudinal evaluation of the association between pulmonary function and total serum IgE. *Am. J. Respir. Crit. Care Med.* **1995**, *152*, 98–102. [CrossRef]
24. Burrows, B.; Martinez, F.D.; Halonen, M.; Barbee, R.A.; Cline, M.G. Association of asthma with serum IgE levels and skin-test reactivity to allergens. *N. Engl. J. Med.* **1989**, *320*, 271–277. [CrossRef]
25. Neveu, W.A.; Allard, J.B.; Dienz, O.; Wargo, M.J.; Ciliberto, G.; Whittaker, L.A.; Rincon, M. IL-6 is required for airway mucus production induced by inhaled fungal allergens. *J. Immunol.* **2009**, *183*, 1732–1738. [CrossRef]
26. Ghosh, S.; Hoselton, S.A.; Asbach, S.V.; Steffan, B.N.; Wanjara, S.B.; Dorsam, G.P.; Schuh, J.M. B lymphocytes regulate airway granulocytic inflammation and cytokine production in a murine model of fungal allergic asthma. *Cell Mol. Immunol.* **2015**, *12*, 202–212. [CrossRef] [PubMed]
27. Chakir, J.; Shannon, J.; Molet, S.; Fukakusa, M.; Elias, J.; Laviolette, M.; Boulet, L.; Hamid, Q. Airway remodeling-associated mediators in moderate to severe asthma: Effect of steroids on TGF-beta, IL-11, IL-17, and type I and type III collagen expression. *J. Allergy Clin. Immunol.* **2003**, *111*, 1293–1298. [CrossRef] [PubMed]
28. Molet, S.; Hamid, Q.; Davoine, F.; Nutku, E.; Tahaa, R.; Pagé, N.; Olivenstein, R.; Elias, J.; Chakir, J. IL-17 is increased in asthmatic airways and induces human bronchial fibroblasts to produce cytokines. *J. Allergy Clin. Immunol.* **2001**, *108*, 430–438. [CrossRef] [PubMed]
29. Matsuse, H.; Yamagishi, T.; Kodaka, N.; Nakano, C.; Fukushima, C.; Obase, Y.; Mukae, H. Therapeutic modality of plasmacytoid dendritic cells in a murine model of *Aspergillus fumigatus* sensitized and infected asthma. *AIMS Allergy Immunol.* **2017**, *1*, 232–241. [CrossRef]
30. Bacher, P.; Hohnstein, T.; Beerbaum, E.; Röcker, M.; Blango, M.G.; Kaufmann, S.; Röhmel, J.; Eschenhagen, P.; Grehn, C.; Seidel, K.; et al. Human Anti-fungal Th17 Immunity and Pathology Rely on Cross-Reactivity against Candida albicans. *Cell* **2019**, *176*, 1340–1355.e15. [CrossRef]
31. Conti, H.R.; Gaffen, S.L. IL-17-Mediated Immunity to the Opportunistic Fungal Pathogen Candida albicans. *J. Immunol.* **2015**, *195*, 780–788. [CrossRef]
32. Lagree, K.; Underhill, D.M. Candida-induced asthma steps up to the plate-lets. *Immunity* **2021**, *54*, 2442–2444. [CrossRef] [PubMed]
33. Sandquist, I.; Kolls, J. Update on regulation and effector functions of Th17 cells. *F1000Res* **2018**, *7*, 205. [CrossRef]
34. Zhang, M.A.; Rego, D.; Moshkova, M.; Kebir, H.; Chruscinski, A.; Nguyen, H.; Akkermann, R.; Stanczyk, F.Z.; Prat, A.; Steinman, L.; et al. Peroxisome proliferator-activated receptor (PPAR)α and -γ regulate IFNγ and IL-17A production by human T cells in a sex-specific way. *Proc. Natl. Acad. Sci. USA* **2012**, *109*, 9505–9510. [CrossRef] [PubMed]
35. Newcomb, D.C.; Cephus, J.Y.; Boswell, M.G.; Fahrenholz, J.M.; Langley, E.W.; Feldman, A.S.; Zhou, W.; Dulek, D.E.; Goleniewska, K.; Woodward, K.B.; et al. Estrogen and progesterone decrease let-7f microRNA expression and increase IL-23/IL-23 receptor signaling and IL-17A production in patients with severe asthma. *J. Allergy Clin. Immunol.* **2015**, *136*, 1025–1034.e11. [CrossRef] [PubMed]
36. Lasarte, S.; Elsner, D.; Guía-González, M.; Ramos-Medina, R.; Sánchez-Ramón, S.; Esponda, P.; Muñoz-Fernández, M.A.; Relloso, M. Female sex hormones regulate the Th17 immune response to sperm and Candida albicans. *Hum. Reprod.* **2013**, *28*, 3283–3291. [CrossRef]

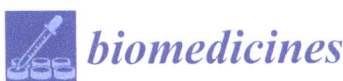

Article

Increased Oxidative Stress in Asthma—Relation to Inflammatory Blood and Lung Biomarkers and Airway Remodeling Indices

Stanisława Bazan-Socha [1,*,†,‡], Krzysztof Wójcik [1,†,‡], Magdalena Olchawa [2], Tadeusz Sarna [2], Jakub Pięta [3], Bogdan Jakieła [1,‡], Jerzy Soja [1,§], Krzysztof Okoń [4], Jacek Zarychta [1,5,‡], Lech Zaręba [6], Michał Stojak [7], Daniel P. Potaczek [8], Jan G. Bazan [6] and Magdalena Celińska-Lowenhoff [1,‡]

1   Department of Internal Medicine, Faculty of Medicine, Jagiellonian University Medical College, Skawinska 8, 31-066 Krakow, Poland; krzysztof.wojcik@uj.edu.pl (K.W.); b.jakiela@uj.edu.pl (B.J.); jerzy.soja@uj.edu.pl (J.S.); jzar@mp.pl (J.Z.); magdalena.celinska-lowenhoff@uj.edu.pl (M.C.-L.)
2   Department of Biophysics, Faculty of Biochemistry, Biophysics and Biotechnology, Jagiellonian University, Gronostajowa 7, 30-387 Krakow, Poland; magdalena.olchawa@uj.edu.pl (M.O.); tadeusz.sarna@uj.edu.pl (T.S.)
3   Institute of Applied Radiation Chemistry, Faculty of Chemistry, Lodz University of Technology, Zeromskiego 116, 90-924 Lodz, Poland; jakub.pieta@p.lodz.pl
4   Department of Pathology, Faculty of Medicine, Jagiellonian University Medical College, Grzegorzecka 16, 31-531 Krakow, Poland; k.okon@uj.edu.pl
5   Pulmonary Hospital, Gladkie 1, 34-500 Zakopane, Poland
6   Institute of Computer Science, College of Natural Sciences, University of Rzeszow, Pigonia 1, 35-310 Rzeszow, Poland; lzareba@ur.edu.pl (L.Z.); bazan@ur.edu.pl (J.G.B.)
7   Department of Plant Product Technology and Nutrition Hygiene, Faculty of Food Technology, University of Agriculture in Krakow, Balicka 122, 30-149 Krakow, Poland; michal.stojak@urk.edu.pl
8   Translational Inflammation Research Division & Core Facility for Single Cell Multiomics, Philipps-University Marburg, 35043 Marburg, Germany; danppot@gmail.com
*   Correspondence: stanislawa.bazan-socha@uj.edu.pl; Tel.: +48-12-424-8023
†   These authors contributed equally to this work.
‡   Skawinska 8, 31-066 Krakow, Poland.
§   Jakubowskiego 2, 30-688 Krakow, Poland.

Citation: Bazan-Socha, S.; Wójcik, K.; Olchawa, M.; Sarna, T.; Pięta, J.; Jakieła, B.; Soja, J.; Okoń, K.; Zarychta, J.; Zaręba, L.; et al. Increased Oxidative Stress in Asthma—Relation to Inflammatory Blood and Lung Biomarkers and Airway Remodeling Indices. *Biomedicines* **2022**, *10*, 1499. https://doi.org/10.3390/biomedicines10071499

Academic Editor: Shaker A. Mousa

Received: 12 April 2022
Accepted: 22 June 2022
Published: 24 June 2022

Publisher's Note: MDPI stays neutral with regard to jurisdictional claims in published maps and institutional affiliations.

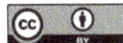

Copyright: © 2022 by the authors. Licensee MDPI, Basel, Switzerland. This article is an open access article distributed under the terms and conditions of the Creative Commons Attribution (CC BY) license (https:// creativecommons.org/licenses/by/ 4.0/).

Abstract: Airway inflammation in asthma is related to increased reactive oxygen species generation, potentially leading to tissue injury and subsequent airway remodeling. We evaluated oxidative stress in peripheral blood from asthmatic subjects ($n = 74$) and matched controls ($n = 65$), using recently developed real-time monitoring of the protein hydroperoxide (HP) formation by the coumarin boronic acid (CBA) assay. We also investigated the relation of the systemic oxidative stress response in asthma to disease severity, lung function, airway remodeling indices (lung computed tomography and histology), and blood and bronchoalveolar lavage fluid (BAL) inflammatory biomarkers. We documented enhanced systemic oxidative stress in asthma, reflected by 35% faster and 58% higher cumulative fluorescent product generation in the CBA assay ($p < 0.001$ for both). The dynamics of HP generation correlated inversely with lung function but not with asthma severity or histological measures of airway remodeling. HP generation was associated positively with inflammatory indices in the blood (e.g., C-reactive protein) and BAL (e.g., interleukin [IL]-6, IL-12p70, and neutrophil count). Bronchial obstruction, thicker airway walls, increased BAL IL-6, and citrullinated histone 3 in systemic circulation independently determined increased HP formation. In conclusion, a real-time CBA assay showed increased systemic HP generation in asthma. In addition, it was associated with inflammatory biomarkers, suggesting that proper disease control can also lead to a decrease in oxidative stress.

Keywords: asthma; oxidative stress; CBA assay; airway remodeling

1. Introduction

Asthma is a chronic disease of the airways that is characterized by variable bronchial obstruction and hyperresponsiveness, often accompanied by structural remodeling [1]. Disease pathogenesis involves various cell types and mediators that participate in airway inflammation, trigger asthma symptoms, and contribute to disease progression. Airway inflammation can be exacerbated by viral infections and exposure to inhaled allergens or airway pollutants. Epidemiological studies demonstrate a clear relationship between air quality and control of asthma symptoms. Exposure to tobacco smoke, ozone, and environmental pollution, such as diesel exhaust, generates reactive oxygen species (ROS) and other oxidative stressors, initiating and augmenting inflammation and sensitizing the airways to other triggers of symptoms [1,2]. Additionally, the inflammatory cells present in the asthmatic airways are considered the primary local source of ROS [3]. Furthermore, ROS itself may play a role in asthma pathogenesis, as they promote type-2 (T2) responses in the lungs and activate nuclear factor (NF)-$\kappa\beta$, a potent pro-inflammatory gene inducer [4].

ROS are produced continuously in a small amount by all cells. Still, if delivered in higher amounts, for example, during inflammation, they alter the pro/antioxidant balance, causing oxidative stress and tissue damage [5]. One signature of increased oxidative stress is the hydroperoxides of amino acid residues (HP), unstable derivatives formed during exposure of proteins to ROS [6]. Previous experimental studies confirmed that oxidative damage to proteins, lipids, or nucleic acids might lead to pathological changes in airway epithelial cells, resulting in increased permeability, mucus secretion, and enhanced airway hyperresponsiveness [5,7–9].

In asthmatic airways, many cell types enhance ROS production, including epithelial and endothelial cells and infiltrating leukocytes; therefore, ROS are necessary components of the innate immune system [5]. However, the lungs and blood provide an efficient defense system against oxidative stress, mediated by two essential elements. The first contains nonenzymatic dietary antioxidants, including tocopherols, carotenes, and lycopene. The second refers to the endogenous system of antioxidant enzymes, such as superoxide dismutase, catalase, and lipoprotein-associated phospholipase A_2 (Lp-PLA$_2$), which combat biochemically oxidative stress [10]. Despite these mechanisms, asthma patients show increased lung oxidative stress, as evidenced by elevated nitric oxide and carbon monoxide concentrations in the exhaled air [3]. Therefore, it has been suggested that asthma is characterized by a decreased ability to respond to oxidative stress [5,10]. For example, patients with severe asthma show decreased plasma activity of Lp-PLA$_2$ [11]. On the contrary, others point to the upregulation of antioxidative mechanisms, albeit with still an overwhelming prooxidative capacity [3,12,13]. Nevertheless, the role of oxidative stress in asthma pathology and airway remodeling has not been comprehensively studied, including how it impacts endothelial injury and early atherosclerosis [14] and increases the risk of prothrombotic and cardiovascular events, as previously reported in that disease [15–17].

Numerous studies on asthma indicate an increased prooxidative potential of peripheral blood leukocytes, mainly neutrophils, and upregulation of oxidative biomarkers in airways, e.g., nitric oxide, or in circulation, e.g., malondialdehyde and uric acid [3,5,13,18]. However, scarcer data analyzed oxidative stress globally in circulating blood, probably due to the lack of reliable research methods that could be successfully applied to serum or plasma samples. Current assays are based mainly on the oxidation of ferrous ions, monitored with orange xylenol or the iodometric test [19,20], and are demanding from a technical point of view. Additionally, they cannot be used in real-time measurements. However, recently Michalski et al. [21] developed and validated a novel real-time fluorescent assay that fits this purpose. In this assay, the profluorescent coumarin boronic acid (CBA) probe reacts with amino acid and protein hydroperoxides to form the corresponding fluorescent product, 7-hydroxycoumarin, which is easily detectable by a fluorescent reader.

Considering the available data on the possible link between airway inflammation, local oxidative stress, premature atherosclerosis, and increased risk of cardiovascular events in asthma, we sought to evaluate the CBA assay in the circulating blood of those subjects. We also examined its relation to asthma severity; lung function and morphometry; blood and bronchoalveolar lavage fluid (BAL) inflammatory biomarkers; and histological measures of airway remodeling, including reticular basement membrane (RBM) thickness and collagen I deposits.

To date, such studies have not yet been performed.

2. Materials and Methods

2.1. Study Participants

We investigated 74 asthma patients enrolled at the Outpatient Clinic of the Allergy and Clinical Immunology Department, University Hospital, Krakow, Poland. Diagnosis of asthma and disease severity (mild, moderate, and severe disease) was established based on the current Global Initiative for Asthma (GINA) guideline [1]. In addition, asthma symptom control was assessed based on the Asthma Control Test (ACT) result (well-controlled, not well-controlled, and very poorly controlled asthma). More details on that issue, including definitions of asthma severity and symptom control grading, are provided in the Supplementary Table S1.

The study was carried out while following the Declaration of Helsinki and the Ethics Committee of Jagiellonian University approved the protocol (approval number: KBET/151/B/2013). Furthermore, all subjects gave written informed consent to participate in the study.

2.2. Spirometry and Lung Computed Tomography (CT)

Spirometry and bronchial reversibility test (after 400 μg of albuterol) were assessed according to the standards of the American Thoracic Society [22], using a Jaeger MasterLab spirometer (Jaeger-Toennies GmbH, Hochberg, Germany). Persistent airflow limitation was defined as an FEV_1/VC index below 0.7 or FEV_1 less than 0.8 of the predicted value after the bronchodilator.

Lung computed tomography (CT) was performed after 400 μg albuterol administration, using 64-raw multidetector computed tomography (Aquilion TSX-101A, Toshiba Medical Systems Corporation, Otawara, Japan) in helical scanning mode (CT parameters: 64×0.5 mm collimation, the helical pitch of 53 and 0.5 s per rotation with standard radiation dose (150 ± 50 mAs and 120 kVp)). The automated AW Server program (Thoracic VCAR, General Electric Healthcare, Wauwatosa, WI, USA) was applied to quantify the cross-sectional geometry of the airways at the site of the right upper lobe apical segmental bronchus (RB1) and the right lower lobe basal posterior bronchus (RB10), including the lumen and wall area, average wall thickness, wall area ratio (WAR, i.e., average difference between the outer and inner areas divided by the outer area), and wall thickness ratio (WTR, i.e., wall thickness divided by the outer diameter) [23]. Spirometry and lung CT measurements were performed only in subjects with asthma.

2.3. Bronchofiberoscopy and Airway Sample Collection

Bronchofiberoscopy was also carried out in asthma patients only, according to the guidelines of the American Thoracic Society [24], using the bronchofiberoscope BF 1T180 (Olympus, Shinjuku, Japan) with local anesthesia (2% lidocaine) and with mild sedation (2.5–5 mg of midazolam, 0.05–0.1 mg of fentanyl i.v.). Bronchoalveolar lavage (BAL) was performed with 200 mL of 0.9% saline administered to the right middle lobe bronchus, and 2 or 3 endobronchial biopsies were taken from the right lower lobe (the carina between B9 and B10) during the procedure. The differential of BAL fluid cells was analyzed by using May–Grunwald–Giemsa-stained cytospin preparations (Thermo Scientific, Walthman, MA, USA; 1000 cells counted). The results were shown as a percentage of all inflammatory cells (except for epithelial cells). The BAL fluid supernatant was aliquoted and stored at $-70\,^\circ C$ until analyzed.

Endobronchial biopsy specimens were formalin-fixed (Sigma-Aldrich, Saint Luis, MO, USA) and prepared for histological examination (e.g., hematoxylin-and-eosin staining) as previously described [23]. The microscope slides were photographed with a Nikon D5300 camera attached to the Zeiss Axioscope microscope with a $100\times$ oil immersion lens. Images were analyzed by AnalySIS 3.2 software (Soft Imaging System GmbH, Muenster, Germany). The RBM thickness was measured along the airway epithelium layer, according to the orthogonal intercept method suggested by Ferrando et al. [25], using arbitrary distance units. For each patient, at least 30 individual RBM measurements were evaluated at intervals of 9.5 μm. The results were expressed as a harmonic mean, as defined in our previous publication [23].

2.4. Laboratory Investigations

2.4.1. Basic Laboratory Tests

The complete blood cell count, the plasma concentration of fibrinogen, serum C-reactive protein (CRP), and immunoglobulin E (IgE) were measured in fasting blood samples by routine laboratory techniques. Serum and plasma samples were aliquoted and stored at $-70\,^{\circ}$C until analysis. Interleukin (IL)-4, IL-5, IL-6, IL-10, IL-12p70, IL-17A, and interferon (INF)-γ in serum and BAL samples were assessed by using commercially available high-sensitivity ELISA assays (eBiosciencea, Vienna, Austria). Periostin (a renowned marker of T2-immune response) was evaluated only in BAL by ELISA (Phoenix Pharmaceuticals, Burlingame, CA, USA). Similarly, citrullinated histone 3 (H3cit), a marker of neutrophil trap formation, was measured in serum, using an ELISA kit (Cayman Chemicals, Ann Arbor, MI, USA). Most BAL cytokine measurements were below the assay threshold (results are not shown in the tables).

2.4.2. Coumarin Boronic Acid (CBA) Assay

To assess the oxidative potential of proteins in serum, we applied the real-time monitoring of HP formation, using the CBA-based assay, as previously described [21,26]. Briefly, 50 μL of serum sample was transferred to 96-microwell black plates and mixed with 150 μL phosphate buffer (50 mM, pH 7.4) containing catalase (100 units/mL), DTPA (diethylenetriaminepentaacetic acid; 0.1 mM), and non-fluorescent CBA as a substrate (0.8 mM). The fluorescence intensity of the reaction product, that is, the 4-hyroxycoumarin (COH), was measured (Ex/Em: 360 nm/465 nm) at 10 min intervals, using a plate reader (ClarioStar, BMG Labtech, Ortenberg, Germany), for 20 h. Each serum sample was analyzed in duplicates, and the arithmetic means presented the experiment's outcome. In each case, the proper background fluorescence was subtracted, and the sample fluorescence was adjusted to the total protein concentration in the serum.

The intensity of fluorescent product generation demonstrated exponential growth that was fitted to the logistic growth model. The resulting sigmoidal logistic growth curve and growth dynamics were described by the three parameters: (1) saturation level, 'K concentration', representing a numerical upper limit of growth; (2) rate factor, 'R', which describes the velocity of the fluorescent product growth; and (3) the area under the curve until saturation level, representing a cumulative generation of the CBA fluorescent product over time.

2.5. Statistical Analysis

Statistical analysis was performed with Statistica TIBCO 13.3 software (TIBCO Software Inc., Palo Alto, CA, USA) and R (version 3.6.1). We used the Shapiro–Wilk test to verify the distribution of the data. As appropriate, continuous variables were reported as a median with 0.25–0.75 quartiles or as a mean with standard deviation. They were compared by using the Mann–Whitney U test or unpaired t-test, respectively. Categorical variables were given as percentages and compared by χ^2 test. The variables of the CBA assay were Box-Cox transformed, and one-way covariance analysis (ANCOVA) was performed to adjust for potential confounders, including age, sex, and BMI. To evaluate the relationship between continuous variables, a Spearman rank correlation test or Pearson correlation tests were performed as applied. The cutoff points for the oxidative stress parameters were calculated based on the receiver operating characteristic (ROC) curve to estimate the odds ratio (OR) with a 95% confidence interval (CI). Independent determinants of cumulative in time concentration, K concentration, and rate factor R were established in multivariate linear regression models, built using a stepwise forward selection procedure, verified by Snedecor's F-distribution; R^2 was evaluated as a measure of variance. Unconditional multivariate logistic regression model and one-way variance analysis (ANOVA) were used to analyze the independent impact of comorbidities, including hypertension, diabetes mellitus, hypercholesterolemia, and oral steroid and statin therapy on evaluating oxidative stress, respectively. Results that had a *p*-value less than 0.05 were considered statistically significant.

3. Results

3.1. Study Participants

Asthma patients and control subjects were well matched according to the demographic variables, including age, sex, body mass index (BMI), and the area of residence, i.e., rural vs. urban area (Table 1). Likewise, the prevalence of other chronic comorbidities (such as arterial hypertension or diabetes mellitus) was similar. Finally, all study participants were current nonsmokers (>5 years).

Table 1. Demographic characteristics and comorbidities in asthmatic patients and control individuals.

Variables	Patients $n = 74$	Controls $n = 65$	*p*-Value
Age, years	53.5 ± 13.1	51.4 ± 12.3	0.63
Male gender, $n(\%)$	19 (26)	23 (35)	0.22
Body mass index, kg/m^2	26.9 ± 4.6	25.9 ± 3.4	0.1
Past smoking, $n(\%)$	13 (18)	15 (23)	0.3
Pack-years of smoking, n	0 (0–0)	0 (0–0)	0.59
Living primarily in inner-city environments, $n(\%)$	39 (53)	38 (58)	0.57
Internal medicine comorbidities			
Hypertension, $n(\%)$	34 (46)	25 (38)	0.67
Diabetes mellitus, $n(\%)$	11 (15)	8 (12)	0.68
Hypercholesterolemia, $n(\%)$	21 (28)	15 (23)	0.52

Categorical variables are presented as *n*-numbers (percentages); continuous variables are presented as median and interquartile range, or mean and standard deviation, as appropriate.

3.2. Clinical Characteristics and Airway Remodeling in Asthma Patients

Among the 74 asthma patients included, 29 (39%) had severe disease (Table 2), and 37 (50%) had persistent airflow limitation. The median duration of asthma was 10 years, and about half of the patients were atopic. Only one-third of the subjects enrolled evaluated their asthma as well-controlled based on the asthma control test, while one-fourth had a very poorly controlled disease.

Based on the BAL cell differential count data (Table 2), 26% of asthma patients showed eosinophilic inflammation (that is, ≥2% of eosinophils), including 15% with neutrophil admixture (mixed inflammation); 28% had a pure neutrophilic (≥4% neutrophils), and 46% had a pauci-granulocytic variant.

In the Supplementary Materials, we provided the clinical characteristics of asthma patients with the division into mild, moderate, and severe disease staging.

Table 2. Clinical characteristics of asthmatic patients, including airway imaging and histo(cyto)logy.

Asthma duration, years	10 (5–20)
Atopy, n(%)	39 (53%)
Severe asthma, n(%)	29 (39%)
Asthma severity (GINA)	
Mild, n(%)	18 (24%)
Moderate, n(%)	27 (36%)
Severe, n(%)	29 (39%)
Asthma symptom control [§]	
Well-controlled asthma, n(%)	22 (30%)
Not-well controlled asthma, n(%)	33 (44%)
Very-poorly controlled asthma, n(%)	19 (26%)
Spirometry values	
FEV_1 before bronchodilator, % of the predicted value	81.8 (66.6–99.4)
FEV_1 after bronchodilator, % of the predicted value	91.9 (73.2–104.1)
VC before bronchodilator, L	3.2 (2.6–3.97)
VC after bronchodilator, L	3.36 (2.7–4)
FEV_1/VC (before bronchodilator)	65.8 (57.4–72.6)
FEV_1/VC (after bronchodilator)	69.9 (63.2–77.5)
Computed tomography airway remodeling indices	
The right upper lobe apical segmental bronchus (RB1)	
Lumen area, mm^2	12.5 (10–16)
Wall area, mm^2	34.8 (27.9–45.4)
Wall thickness, mm	1.9 (1.7–2.1)
Wall thickness ratio (WTR)	24.1 ± 2.7
Wall area ratio (WAR)	73.2 ± 5.6
The right lower lobe basal posterior bronchus (RB10)	
Lumen area, mm^2	12.5 (9–18)
Wall area, mm^2	35.1 ± 12.3
Wall thickness, mm	1.8 (1.6–2.1)
Wall thickness ratio (WTR)	23.6 (22–25.9)
Wall area ratio (WAR)	72.3 (68.5–76.9)
Bronchial biopsy histology	
Reticular basement membrane (RBM) thickness, μm [¥]	6.49 (5.3–7.86)
Collagen I staining, % of the stroma showing reactivity	30 (20–60)
Bronchoalveolar lavage fluid (BAL) cellularity [#]	
Macrophages, %	85 (72–93)
Lymphocytes, %	8 (4–15)
Neutrophils, %	3 (2–5)
Eosinophils, %	1 (0.1–2)
Eosinophils ≥2% in BAL, n(%)	17 (37.5%)
Neutrophils ≥4% in BAL, n(%)	29 (43.3%)
Bronchoalveolar lavage fluid biomarkers [†]	
Periostin, ng/mL	0.85 (0.75–0.97)
Interleukin-6, pg/mL	0.75 (0.1–1.19)
Interleukin-12(p70), pg/mL	0.078 (0.05–0.12)
Asthma therapy	
Oral corticosteroids	14 (19%)
Inhaled corticosteroids (persistent use)	68 (92%)
Long-acting β_2-agonists (persistent use)	54 (73%)
Antileukotrienes	10 (14%)
Theophylline	8 (11%)
Long-acting anticholinergics (persistent use)	5 (7%)

Categorical variables are presented as numbers (percentages); continuous variables are presented as median and 0.25–0.75 quartiles, or mean and standard deviation, as appropriate. Abbreviations and references: BAL—bronchoalveolar lavage fluid, FEV_1—forced expiratory volume in one second, GINA—Global Initiative for Asthma, L—liter, VC—vital capacity; [§] asthma symptom control (assessed based on Asthma Control Test results); [#] BAL cell differential data available in 67 asthma subjects; [†] BAL fluid levels of interleukin (IL)-4, IL-5, IL-10, and IL-17A and interferon γ were below the detection threshold (data not shown); [¥] RBM available in 45 asthma subjects.

Table 2 also summarizes essential measures of structural airway remodeling, as evidenced by CT imaging and airway biopsy specimens. Unfortunately, in this study, we did not collect those data in the control group. However, compared to control datasets in our previous report [27], which was conducted by using a similar methodology, CT imaging parameters suggest mild-to-moderate changes in airway geometry (10% difference on average, $p < 0.05$), whereas RBM thickness is ~30% thicker in asthmatics compared to controls ($p < 0.001$). In Figure 1, we depict representative pictures of RBM measures in control and asthma individuals.

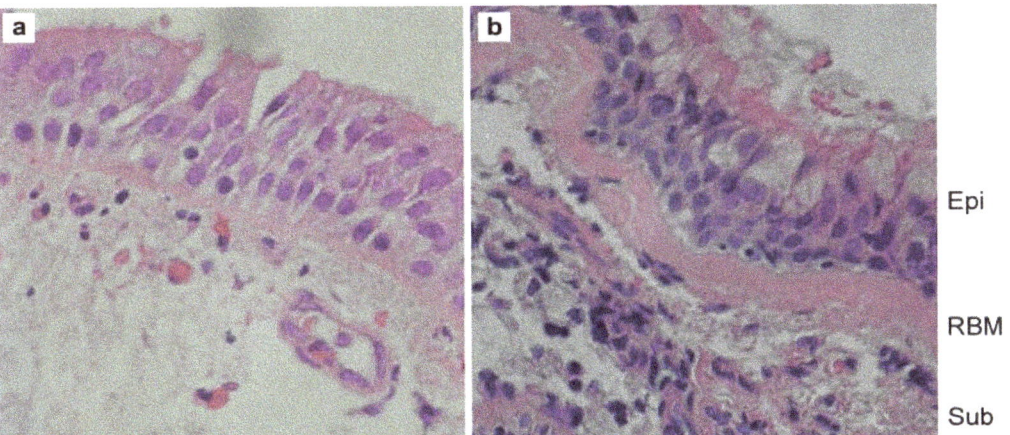

Figure 1. Representative pictures of endobronchial biopsy specimens in a control subject (**a**) and asthma patient (**b**); the reticular basement membrane (RBM) is thicker in asthma. Other abbreviations: Epi—epithelium, Sub—subepithelium.

As expected, the referenced airway CT measures in RB1 and RB10 correlated well with each other (e.g., WTR: r = 0.4, $p < 0.001$) and with spirometry values (e.g., FEV_1: r = −0.34, $p = 0.007$ and r = −0.3, $p = 0.01$, for WTR of RB1 and RB10, respectively).

At the same time, neither CT nor spirometry values were linked with RBM thickness.

3.3. Increased Systemic Generation of Protein Hydroperoxides in Asthma

The fluorescent intensity of the CBA-assay product, reflecting HP generation, increased quickly both in the asthmatics and controls (Figure 2a). However, the velocity of fluorescence growth, reflected by the factor R, was 35% higher, and the saturating concentration (K) increased by 23% more in asthmatics than in controls ($p < 0.001$, using the Mann–Whitney U test; $p = 0.01$ and $p = 0.009$, respectively, using ANCOVA after adjustment for age, sex, and BMI) (Figure 2b).

Compared to the control subjects, asthma patients showed an odds ratio (OR) of 3.14 (95%CI: 1.98–4.97; $p < 0.001$) for having a higher R factor, defined as values above the cut-off point of 42.4 fluorescence (FL) unit (U)/mL/min. Similarly, asthma patients had an OR of 2.57 (95%CI: 1.7–3.88; $p < 0.001$) for having increased K concentration, using a cutoff point of 322 FLU/mL.

Furthermore, we demonstrated a 58% higher cumulative in time HP generation (area under the curve) (Figure 2b, $p < 0.001$, using Mann–Whitney U test; $p = 0.01$, using ANCOVA after adjustment for age, sex, and BMI).

In the asthma group, the dynamics of HP generation were ~20% higher, and K concentration was increased by ~15% in females (Figure 3).

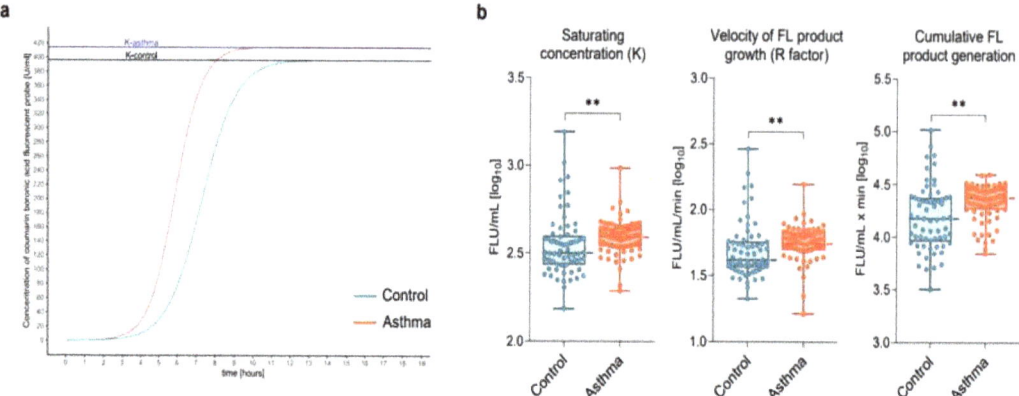

Figure 2. (**a**) Representative curve of fluorescent product generation in the real-time coumarin boronic acid (CBA) assay of asthma patient and control individual (K—saturating concentration). (**b**) Saturating concentration (K), growth velocity (R factor), and cumulative fluorescent (FL) product generation in the real-time coumarin boronic acid (CBA) assay in asthma and control subjects. Abbreviations: FL—fluorescent, FLU—fluorescent unit, K—saturating concentration, R—velocity of fluorescent product growth, ** $p < 0.001$.

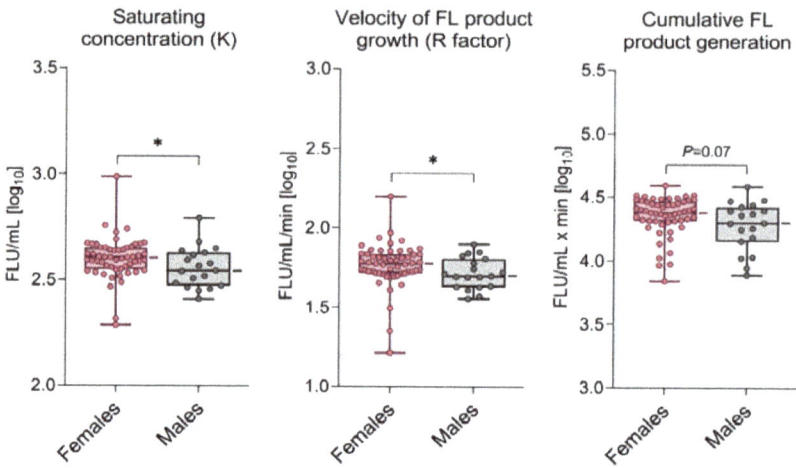

Figure 3. Hydroperoxides' generation in the coumarin boronic acid (CBA) assay was higher in females than males in the asthma group; * $p < 0.05$; for other abbreviations, see legend in Figure 1.

Other demographic variables and comorbidities had no impact on the CBA assay results.

3.4. Systemic Protein Hydroperoxides Generation Was Related to Bronchial Obstruction, Airway Geometry, and Bronchoalveolar Lavage Fluid Biomarkers

Next, we analyzed associations of systemic oxidative stress measures with clinical characteristics of asthma, lung function, airway remodeling indices, and BAL biomarkers.

Surprisingly, the dynamics of HP generation were not related to the severity of asthma, symptom control, or asthma medications used. However, we detected a weak inverse correlation with airway obstruction spirometry indices (Figure 4).

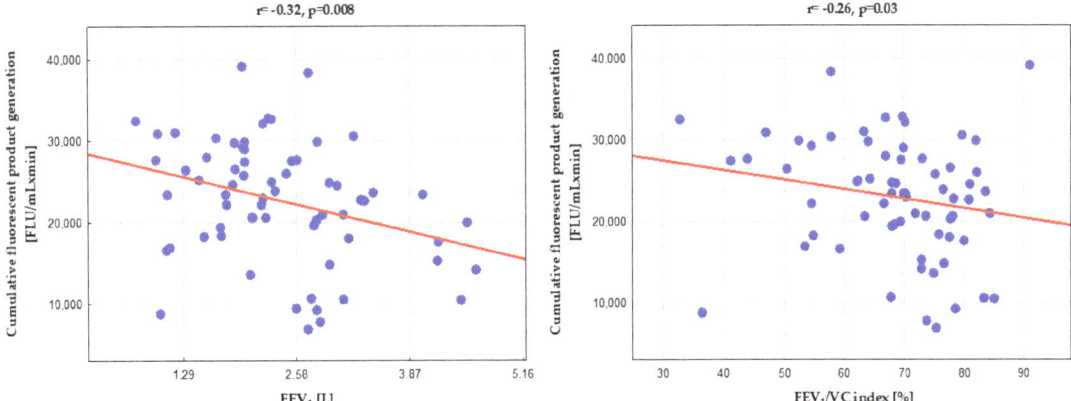

Figure 4. Inverse correlation between hydroperoxide generation in coumarin boronic acid (CBA) assay and lung function; for abbreviations, see the legend in Figure 2 and Table 2.

Furthermore, asthma patients with persistent airflow limitation showed a 19% increase in cumulative HP formation ($p = 0.02$).

Oxidative stress measures were not associated with RBM thickness or collagen I deposit in bronchial biopsy specimens. They were also not directly associated with lung CT parameters. However, multiple regression models showed that WAR or WTR in RB1 could be an independent determinant of higher HP formation dynamics, as presented in Table 3 (a model for the R factor).

Table 3. Multiple linear regression model for a relative increase of fluorescent product growth velocity (R factor) in the real-time CBA assay in asthma patients. Presented variables are documented as independent determinants; however, they explain only 16% of the R factor variability.

Fluorescent Product Growth Velocity (R Factor)		
	β (95% CI)	R^2
FEV$_1$, %	−0.18 (−0.31 to −0.04)	
Wall thickness ratio (WTR), RB1	0.22 (0.08 to 0.36)	0.16
Interleukin 6, BAL, pg/mL	0.28 (0.14 to 0.41)	
Adjustment statistics	F = 2.9, $p < 0.001$	

The resulting standardized regression coefficient (β) with 95% confidence interval (95% CI) for a factor (independent variable) indicates the increase/decrease in standard deviations (SDs) of a dependent variable (R factor) when that particular factor increases by 1 SD and all other variables in the model remain unchanged. Abbreviations: RB1—the right upper lobe apical segmental bronchus; for other abbreviations, see footnote to Table 2.

Among BAL biomarkers, the HP generation was weakly positively associated with the IL-6 and IL-12(p70) concentrations and neutrophil count (Figure 5). Additionally, BAL IL-6 appears to be an independent determinant of higher HP formation, as shown in Table 3.

3.5. Complex Regulation of Circulating Protein Hydroperoxides Generation by Peripheral Blood Biomarkers

Then we investigated the relation of HP generation in asthma to laboratory variables measured in the systemic circulation, including blood cell counts, inflammatory biomarkers, and atherosclerosis risk factors, such as glucose level and lipid profile.

As expected, asthma patients were characterized by increased blood eosinophilia and serum IgE compared to the controls (Table 4). Interestingly, the serum CRP concentration was also marginally elevated in the patients ($p = 0.04$). On the other hand, glucose and total cholesterol levels and blood cytokines were comparable in both study groups, except for

IL-10, which was higher in asthmatics. Similarly, the concentration of H3cit was increased in patients, suggesting neutrophil activation and the formation of extracellular traps [28].

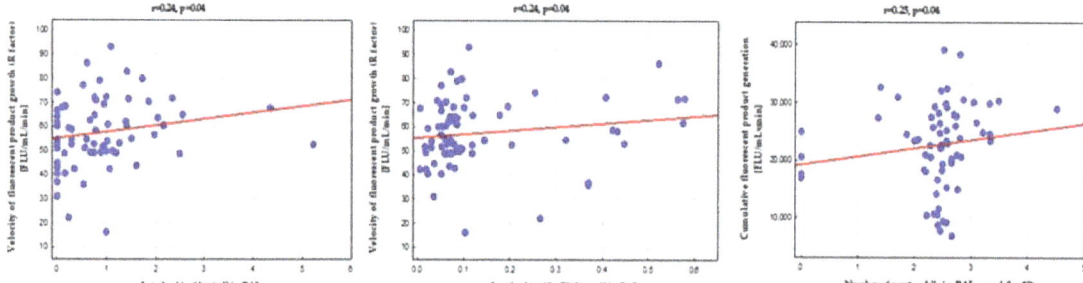

Figure 5. Positive correlations between dynamics in hydroperoxide generation in the real-time coumarin boronic acid (CBA) assay and bronchoalveolar lavage fluid biomarkers (interleukin [IL]-6, IL-12, and BAL neutrophilia); for abbreviations, see the legend in Figure 2 and Table 2.

Table 4. Laboratory parameters in asthmatic patients and control subjects.

	Patients n = 74	Controls n = 65	p-Value
Basic laboratory tests			
Hemoglobin, g/dL	13.5 (13–14.4)	13.9 ± 1.28	0.09
Red blood cell count, $10^6/\mu L$	4.61 ± 0.43	4.6 ± 0.38	0.83
White blood cell count, $10^3/\mu L$	6.68 (5.6–7.96)	5.48 (4.82–6.64)	<0.001 **
Eosinophils, $10^3/\mu L$	275 (135–470)	15 (9–80)	<0.001 **
Monocytes, $10^3/\mu L$	600 (485–815)	480 (430–670)	<0.001 **
Blood platelets, $10^3/\mu L$	218 (191–247)	232 (203–293)	0.01 *
C-reactive protein, mg/L	2.55 (0.58–8.67)	1 (0.9–1.7)	0.04 *
Immunoglobulin E, IU/mL	71.5 (29.4–380)	22.6 (18.5–53.5)	0.001 *
Glucose, mmol/L	5 (4.65–5.55)	5.17 ± 0.54	0.63
Total cholesterol, mmol/L	4.83 ± 0.98	4.8 (4.25–5.35)	0.74
Low-density lipoprotein cholesterol, mmol/L	2.61 ± 0.76	3.38 ± 0.96	<0.001 **
High-density lipoprotein cholesterol, mmol/L	1.34 (1.09–1.61)	1.58 ± 0.41	0.01 *
Triglycerides, mmol/L	1.4 (1–2)	1.09 (0.82–1.42)	<0.001 **
Biomarkers in serum §			
Interleukin-6, pg/mL	0.78 (0.45–2.09)	0.73 ± 0.52	0.31
Interleukin-10, pg/mL	0.57 (0.25–0.97)	0.005 (0.005–0.01)	<0.001 **
Interleukin-12(p70), pg/mL	0.005 (0.005–1.3)	0.005 (0.005–1.69)	0.75
Interleukin-17A, pg/mL	0.005 (0.005–0.12)	0.005 (0.005–0.06)	0.87
Interferon-γ, pg/mL	0.005 (0.005–0.28)	0.11 (0.005–0.27)	0.66
Citrullinated histone H3, ng/mL	16.3 (10.7–19.8)	12.8 (8.2–17.6)	0.04 *

Variables are presented as median and interquartile range, or mean and standard deviation, as appropriate. References: § all serum measurements of interleukin (IL)-4 and IL-5 were below the assay threshold (data not shown); ** $p < 0.001$; * $p < 0.05$ and $p \geq 0.001$.

Interestingly, systemic HP generation in asthma showed a clear negative association with the red blood cell (RBC) count (Figure 6a) and hemoglobin level. This relationship applied to all CBA assay parameters and was not seen in the control grroup.

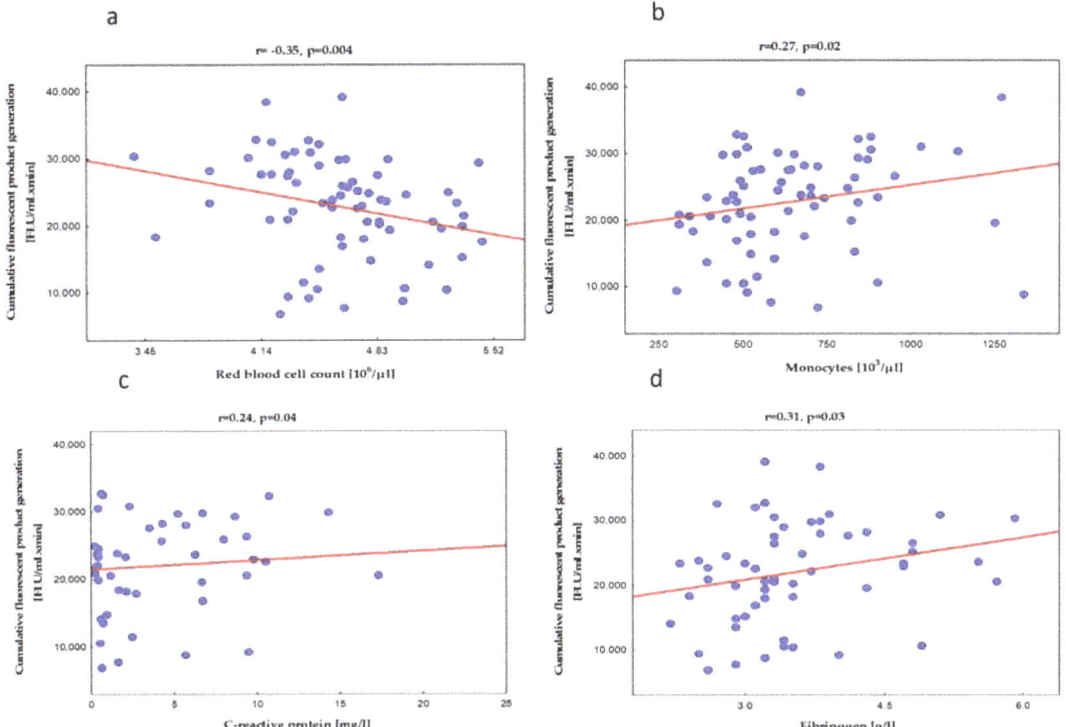

Figure 6. Relationships between cumulative hydroperoxide generation in the real-time coumarin boronic acid (CBA) assay and red blood cell count (**a**) peripheral blood monocyte count (**b**), circulating C-reactive protein (**c**), and fibrinogen (**d**); for abbreviations, see the legend in Figure 2 and Table 2.

Furthermore, we demonstrated a weak positive association between HP formation dynamics and blood monocyte count (Figure 6b) and some nonspecific markers of inflammation, such as serum CRP (Figure 6c) or plasma fibrinogen (Figure 6d). In contrast, it was not directly related to renowned T2 immune response measures in blood, such as eosinophilia.

In Table 5, we demonstrate the independent determinants among the measured blood biomarkers of increased susceptibility to HP formation (R factor) in a multiple regression model. Interestingly, various variables predicted an increase in the dynamics of systemic HP generation, including blood monocyte count, H3cit, and IL-17A, as well as total cholesterol levels. At the same time, the RBC count and, to a much lesser extent, the blood eosinophil count inversely impacted the R factor.

Eventually, we performed a combined analysis by using a multivariable stepwise regression model, considering both the airway and systemic measures investigated in the study that could impact HP generation. As presented in Table 6, susceptibility to increased HP formation was determined best by lower spirometry values (e.g., FEV_1), elevated IL-6 in BAL, and higher circulating H3cit. As expected, the RBC count had a substantial negative contribution to that analysis.

Table 5. Multiple linear regression model for a relative increase of fluorescent product growth velocity (R factor) in the real-time CBA assay in asthma patients. Presented variables were documented as independent determinants; they explain 33% of R factor variability.

Fluorescent Product Growth Velocity (R Factor)		
	β (95% CI)	R^2
Monocyte count, $10^3/\mu L$	0.14 (0.02 to 0.28)	
Red blood cell count, $10^6/\mu L$	−0.58 (−0.73 to −0.43)	
Blood eosinophilia, $10^3/\mu L$	−0.23 (−0.41 to −0.06)	
Citrulinated histone 3, ng/mL	0.22 (0.07 to 0.37)	0.33
Interleukin 17A, pg/mL	0.26 (0.13 to 0.4)	
Total cholesterol, mmol/L	0.22 (0.08 to 0.37)	
Adjustment statistics	F = 3.3, *p* = 0.01	

For data interpretation, see footnote to Table 3.

Table 6. Multiple linear regression model for a relative increase of fluorescent product growth velocity (R factor) in the real-time CBA assay in asthma patients, considering all study variables.

Fluorescent Product Growth Velocity (R Factor)		
	β (95% CI)	R^2
FEV_1, %	−0.21 (−0.34 to −0.07)	
Red blood cell count, $10^6/\mu L$	−0.26 (−0.39 to −0.12)	
Citrulinated histone 3, ng/mL	0.35 (0.23 to 0.47)	0.26
Interleukin 6, BAL, pg/mL	0.19 (0.08 to 0.31)	
Adjustment statistics	F = 5.04, *p* = 0.002	

For data interpretation, see footnote to Table 3. For the abbreviations, see footnote to Table 2.

4. Discussion

The present study demonstrates an increase in the generation of amino acid HP in the peripheral blood of asthmatic patients, reflecting an enhanced systemic oxidative stress response in that disease. In asthma, increased ROS formation by inflammatory cells has already been described in both the airways and systemic circulation [5,13,18]. Here, we show that it can be assessed reliably in the peripheral blood by using a recently developed technically undemanding real-time CBA assay [21,29,30]. Furthermore, we have investigated whether elevated oxidative stress in asthma, related to increased HP generation, is determined by clinical manifestations of the disease, inflammatory patterns, and various measures of airway remodeling.

In our study, increased systemic oxidative stress was associated with different variables related to asthma, including bronchial obstruction, airway geometry, and unspecific inflammatory biomarkers analyzed in the lungs and blood. Nevertheless, it was not associated with asthma severity score and symptom control, suggesting that higher blood oxidative stress in asthma is a feature of that disease per se. That is an unexpected finding since asthma is an inflammatory disease of the airways. However, many reports, including our previous research, have indicated that asthma is associated with higher inflammatory biomarkers in circulation [31]. In addition, this low-grade systemic response was related to the prothrombotic state [32] that was documented previously in that disease, as well as in the epidemiological studies [15–17]. Thus, local airway inflammation is likely associated with a variable degree of systemic response in asthma, activating blood leukocytes further and leading to higher HP production.

On the other hand, lower FEV_1/VC values, reflecting more advanced airway obstruction and thicker bronchial walls in RB1, were independent determinants of higher susceptibility to HP generation. This observation suggests that objective indicators of more severe disease forms may be related, indeed, to the higher circulating oxidative stress capacity. At the same time, various laboratory variables in peripheral blood and

BAL predicted higher HP formation. Among them, the most important were those related to innate immunity and unspecific inflammation, such as BAL neutrophilia and blood monocyte count, as well as circulating CRP, fibrinogen, IL-17A, and H3cit. The latter is a novel biomarker of neutrophil activation and extracellular trap formation [28]. The relation of circulating oxidative stress to CRP in asthmatics is not surprising. A similar association was previously shown in other conditions, e.g., in healthy heavy workers [33]. Conversely, in controls, we did not record such a relationship. However, the six control subjects who had HP generation very high, above the fourth-quartile cutoff point in the asthmatics (Figure 2b), were characterized by the highest CRP values (all within the normal range), as compared to the remaining control subjects (2.65 [1.4–4.6] vs. 1 [1–1.7] mL/L, $p = 0.006$). Interestingly, those six controls have not reported any chronic inflammatory or acute disease or significant clinical symptoms and did not differ in the prevalence of internal comorbidities or other laboratory variables, except for CRP. Therefore, they were not excluded from the control group.

Interestingly, in our study, a higher oxidative stress response in asthma was determined by an increased total cholesterol level in serum. Since hypercholesterolemia and oxidative stress are well-known factors leading to endothelial dysfunction and atherosclerosis [9,14], we speculate that elevated HP generation in asthma might unfavorably affect the cardiovascular system. However, advanced observational and experimental studies are needed to verify this hypothesis.

On the other hand, the negative association of HP generation with blood eosinophilia in a multiple regression model suggests that oxidative stress in asthma is not related to the T2 response [1,12]. Thus, our report is consistent with several epidemiological studies that indicate that an increased risk of cardiovascular diseases in asthma occurs primarily in the late-onset asthma phenotype [34,35] or even in women with adult asthma [17], more frequently representing the non-T2 phenotype [36,37].

The lack of a relationship between HP formation and the histological characteristics of airway remodeling is another surprising finding that deserves a comment. Protein and lipid oxidation were previously linked to pro-inflammatory airway epithelial and endothelial cell modification [5]. Therefore, increased oxidative stress could lead to airway structural changes in the airways, such as the thickening of the RBM. However, the characteristics and role of structural alterations of the bronchial wall in asthma remain unknown. Previously, we have shown that RBM thickening did not depend on the asthma duration or lung function [12]. The current study likewise documents that it is also not linked to asthma severity. Notably, our reports align with former data, such as those published by Payne et al. [38]. They demonstrated that RBM thickening was present even in young children with asthma to a similar extent as seen in milder adult asthmatics and independently of asthma duration, severity, and lung function [38]. Therefore, it seems that changes in RBM occur early during the disease, e.g., as a response to ongoing airway inflammation, and do not progress further, due to the implemented anti-inflammatory treatment. Therefore, airway inflammation may promote ROS overproduction during a stable course of asthma but not further RBM thickening.

One of the strongest associations in our study is a clear inverse relationship between the potential for oxidative stress and RBC count. It indicates a substantial contribution of the antioxidant system of RBCs in balancing enhanced ROS generation. In the systemic circulation, the RBCs are continuously exposed to exogenous and endogenous sources of ROS, e.g., released from activated locally inflammatory cells. However, they possess an extensive antioxidant system, involving nonenzymatic antioxidants, for example, glutathione and enzymes, such as superoxide dismutase, catalase, glutathione peroxidase, and peroxiredoxin-2 [39]. Our data suggest that the antioxidative potential of RBC could diminish the lung-originated oxidative stress in asthma by counteracting ROS, at least to some extent. Therefore, it might be particularly insufficient in asthma patients with anemia.

Whether enhanced oxidative stress in asthma requires any therapeutic modifications is still unknown. However, some interventions have been suggested, including dietary changes, antioxidant vitamins, other antioxidant drugs and supplements, and even radon exposure, with varying results [40]. For example, nutritional studies suggest that asthmatic children with low dietary intake of vitamins C and E and other antioxidants have worse asthma symptoms; however, therapy with these vitamins was ineffective [40]. Another large epidemiological study prospectively documented the lower prevalence of asthma in those with higher α-tocopherol and Lp-PLA$_2$ activity in peripheral blood at baseline [10]. At the same time, two longitudinal studies of dietary intake demonstrated inconsistent results with asthma risk. The Nurses' Health Study showed a higher asthma rate in those with a lower dietary intake of vitamin E [41], while in the E3N study, no such association was documented [42].

Finally, GINA [1] does not recommend any antioxidant supplements to decrease asthma-induced oxidative stress. Therefore, proper disease control, dietary intake of natural antioxidants in fruits and vegetables, and minimizing exposure to environmental pollution and tobacco smoke remain paramount.

Study Limitation

The main limitation of this study is the analysis focused only on HP products in proteins but not lipids or nucleic acids. Furthermore, we did not analyze endogenous or exogenous antioxidants, including genetic polymorphisms [5,10]. However, our study, a pilot in nature, relied on complex analysis, estimating the total harmful effects of ROS on proteins and considering the impacts of all available pro- and antioxidant factors in circulating blood. Furthermore, the CBA assay was measured once; therefore, we cannot assess its variability over time, depending on the course of asthma. Finally, we did not analyze the airway parameters in controls, obviously due to ethical reasons. However, since asthma is a chronic inflammatory lung disease, we believe that our research is valuable and worth publishing. Those factors limit the depth of the investigation but not the study's main findings.

5. Conclusions

We have shown increased levels of amino acid and protein hydroperoxides measured in the serum of asthmatic patients, using a recently developed technically undemanding real-time CBA assay. Furthermore, estimated oxidative stress was related to BAL and blood inflammatory biomarkers, spirometry values, and CT airway geometry measures, but not asthma severity or histological indices of airway remodeling. More prospective and experimental studies are needed to verify the biological role of increased circulating oxidative stress in the clinical course of asthma and extrapulmonary complications.

Supplementary Materials: The following supporting information can be downloaded at https://www.mdpi.com/article/10.3390/biomedicines10071499/s1. Table S1: Clinical characteristics of asthmatic patients divided into mild, moderate, and severe disease stages, including airway imaging and histo(cyto)logy.

Author Contributions: Conceptualization, S.B.-S. and K.W.; funding acquisition, S.B.-S.; patient recruitment, S.B.-S., M.C.-L. and K.W.; CBA assay, J.P., M.O., T.S. and K.W.; bronchoscopy, J.S.; lung CT, J.Z.; histopathological examination, K.O.; validation, S.B.-S., M.S., J.G.B. and B.J.; CBA assay parameters analysis, L.Z. and J.G.B.; statistical Analysis, L.Z.; writing—original draft preparation, S.B.-S., B.J., M.C.-L. and D.P.P.; writing—review, critical revision, and final approval, all authors. All authors have read and agreed to the published version of the manuscript.

Funding: This project was funded by the National Science Centre, Poland, based on decision No. DEC-2013/09/B/NZ5/00758 (to S.B.-S.).

Institutional Review Board Statement: The study was conducted in accordance with the Declaration of Helsinki, and the protocol was approved by the Ethics Committee of the Jagiellonian University approved the study (approval number: KBET/151/B/2013).

Informed Consent Statement: Informed consent was obtained from all subjects involved in the study.

Data Availability Statement: The data presented in this study are available upon request from the corresponding author. The data are not publicly available due to patients' origin.

Conflicts of Interest: The authors declare no conflict of interest.

References

1. Global Initiative for Asthma—Global Initiative for Asthma—GINA. Available online: https://ginasthma.org/ (accessed on 26 September 2018).
2. Hellings, P.W.; Steelant, B. Epithelial barriers in allergy and asthma. *J. Allergy Clin. Immunol.* **2020**, *145*, 1499–1509. [CrossRef] [PubMed]
3. Nadeem, A.; Siddiqui, N.; Alharbi, N.O.; Alharbi, M.M. Airway and systemic oxidant-antioxidant dysregulation in asthma: A possible scenario of oxidants spill over from lung into blood. *Pulm. Pharmacol. Ther.* **2014**, *29*, 31–40. [CrossRef] [PubMed]
4. Liu, X.; Yi, M.; Jin, R.; Feng, X.; Ma, L.; Wang, Y.; Shan, Y.; Yang, Z.; Zhao, B. Correlation between oxidative stress and NF-κB signaling pathway in the obesity-asthma mice. *Mol. Biol. Rep.* **2020**, *47*, 3735–3744. [CrossRef] [PubMed]
5. Kleniewska, P.; Pawliczak, R. The participation of oxidative stress in the pathogenesis of bronchial asthma. *Biomed. Pharmacother.* **2017**, *94*, 100–108. [CrossRef]
6. Morgan, P.E.; Pattison, D.I.; Davies, M.J. Quantification of hydroxyl radical-derived oxidation products in peptides containing glycine, alanine, valine, and proline. *Free Radic. Biol. Med.* **2012**, *52*, 328–339. [CrossRef]
7. Aihua, B.; Yuqing, C.; Zhang, M.; Feng, L.; Xin, Z. Effects of ozone oxidative stress on the airway hyperresponsiveness and mucus production in mice with acute allergic airway inflammation. *Zhonghua Jie He He Hu Xi Za Zhi* **2015**, *38*, 179–184.
8. Casalino-Matsuda, S.M.; Monzón, M.E.; Forteza, R.M. Epidermal Growth Factor Receptor Activation by Epidermal Growth Factor Mediates Oxidant-Induced Goblet Cell Metaplasia in Human Airway Epithelium. *Am. J. Respir. Cell Mol. Biol.* **2012**, *34*, 581–591. [CrossRef] [PubMed]
9. Salisbury, D.; Bronas, U. Reactive oxygen and nitrogen species: Impact on endothelial dysfunction. *Nurs. Res.* **2015**, *64*, 53–66. [CrossRef]
10. Larkin, E.K.; Gao, Y.-T.; Gebretsadik, T.; Hartman, T.J.; Wu, P.; Wen, W.; Yang, G.; Bai, C.; Jin, M.; Roberts, L.J., II; et al. New Risk Factors for Adult-Onset Incident Asthma. A Nested Case–Control Study of Host Antioxidant Defense. *Am. J. Respir. Crit. Care Med.* **2014**, *191*, 45–53. [CrossRef]
11. Kuczia, P.; Mastalerz, L.; Potaczek, D.P.; Cybulska, A.; Zareba, L.; Bazan-Socha, S.; Undas, A. Increased activity of lipoprotein-associated phospholipase A2 in non-severe asthma. *Allergol. Int.* **2019**, *68*, 450–455. [CrossRef]
12. Bazan-Socha, S.; Buregwa-Czuma, S.; Jakiela, B.; Zareba, L.; Zawlik, I.; Myszka, A.; Soja, J.; Okon, K.; Zarychta, J.; Kozlik, P.; et al. Reticular Basement Membrane Thickness Is Associated with Growth- and Fibrosis-Promoting Airway Transcriptome Profile-Study in Asthma Patients. *Int. J. Mol. Sci.* **2021**, *22*, 998. [CrossRef] [PubMed]
13. Abboud, M.M.; Al-Rawashde, F.A.; Al-Zayadneh, E.M. Alterations of serum and saliva oxidative markers in patients with bronchial asthma. *J. Asthma* **2021**. Epub ahead of print. [CrossRef] [PubMed]
14. Pacholczak-Madej, R.; Kuszmiersz, P.; Iwaniec, T.; Zaręba, L.; Zarychta, J.; Walocha, J.; Dropiński, J.; Bazan-Socha, S. Endothelial dysfunction and pentraxin-3 in clinically stable adult asthma patients. *J. Investig. Allergol. Clin. Immunol.* **2021**, *31*, 417–425. [CrossRef]
15. Tattersall, M.; Guo, M.; Korcarz, C. Asthma predicts cardiovascular disease events: The multi-ethnic study of atherosclerosis. *Arter. Thromb Vasc Biol.* **2015**, *35*, 1520–1525. [CrossRef] [PubMed]
16. Strand, L.B.; Tsai, M.K.; Wen, C.P.; Chang, S.; Brumpton, B.M. Is having asthma associated with an increased risk of dying from cardiovascular disease? A prospective cohort study of 446 346 Taiwanese adults. *BMJ Open* **2018**, *8*, e019992. [CrossRef]
17. Onufrak, S.J.; Abramson, J.L.; Austin, H.D.; Holguin, F.; McClellan, W.M.; Vaccarino, L.V. Relation of Adult-Onset Asthma to Coronary Heart Disease and Stroke. *Am. J. Cardiol.* **2008**, *101*, 1247–1252. [CrossRef]
18. Nadeem, A.; Chhabra, S.K.; Masood, A.; Raj, H.G. Increased oxidative stress and altered levels of antioxidants in asthma. *J. Allergy Clin. Immunol.* **2003**, *111*, 72–78. [CrossRef]
19. Bou, R.; Codony, R.; Tres, A.; Decker, E.A.; Guardiola, F. Determination of hydroperoxides in foods and biological samples by the ferrous oxidation–xylenol orange method: A review of the factors that influence the method's performance. *Anal. Biochem.* **2008**, *377*, 1–15. [CrossRef]
20. Gay, C.; Collins, J.; Gebicki, J.M. Hydroperoxide Assay with the Ferric–Xylenol Orange Complex. *Anal. Biochem.* **1999**, *273*, 149–155. [CrossRef]
21. Michalski, R.; Zielonka, J.; Gapys, E.; Marcinek, A.; Joseph, J.; Kalyanaraman, B. Real-time measurements of amino acid and protein hydroperoxides using coumarin boronic acid. *J. Biol. Chem.* **2014**, *289*, 22536–22553. [CrossRef]
22. Culver, B.H.; Graham, B.L.; Coates, A.L.; Wanger, J.; Berry, C.E.; Clarke, P.K.; Hallstrand, T.S.; Hankinson, J.L.; Kaminsky, D.A.; MacIntyre, N.R.; et al. Recommendations for a Standardized Pulmonary Function Report. An Official American Thoracic Society Technical Statement. *Am. J. Respir. Crit. Care Med.* **2017**, *196*, 1463–1472. [CrossRef] [PubMed]
23. Kozlik, P.; Zuk, J.; Bartyzel, S.; Zarychta, J.; Okon, K.; Zareba, L.; Bazan, J.G.; Kosalka, J.; Soja, J.; Musial, J.; et al. The relationship of airway structural changes to blood and bronchoalveolar lavage biomarkers, and lung function abnormalities in asthma. *Clin. Exp. Allergy* **2020**, *50*, 15–28. [CrossRef] [PubMed]

24. Sokolowski, J.W.; Burgher, L.W.; Jones, F.L.; Patterson, J.R.; Selecky, P.A. Position Paper on Guidelines for Fiberoptic Bronchoscopy in Adults. *Am. Rev. Respir. Dis.* **1987**, *136*, 1066. [CrossRef] [PubMed]
25. Ferrando, R.E.; Nyengaard, J.R.; Hays, S.R.; Fahy, J.V.; Woodruff, P.G. Applying stereology to measure thickness of the basement membrane zone in bronchial biopsy specimens. *J. Allergy Clin. Immunol.* **2003**, *112*, 1243–1245. [CrossRef]
26. Olchawa, M.M.; Szewczyk, G.M.; Zadlo, A.C.; Krzysztynska-Kuleta, O.I.; Sarna, T.J. The effect of aging and antioxidants on photoreactivity and phototoxicity of human melanosomes: An in vitro study. *Pigment. Cell Melanoma Res.* **2021**, *34*, 670–682. [CrossRef]
27. Bazan-Socha, S.; Jakiela, B.; Zuk, J.; Zarychta, J.; Soja, J.; Okon, K.; Dziedzina, S.; Zareba, L.; Dropinski, J.; Wojcik, K.; et al. Interactions via α 2 β 1 Cell Integrin May Protect against the Progression of Airway Structural Changes in Asthma. *Int. J. Mol. Sci.* **2021**, *22*, 6315. [CrossRef]
28. Kuczia, P.; Zuk, J.; Iwaniec, T.; Soja, J.; Dropinski, J.; Malesa-Wlodzik, M.; Zareba, L.; Bazan, J.G.; Undas, A.; Bazan-Socha, S. Citrullinated histone H3, a marker of extracellular trap formation, is increased in blood of stable asthma patients. *Clin. Transl. Allergy* **2020**, *10*, 31. [CrossRef]
29. Olchawa, M.M.; Krzysztynska-Kuleta, O.I.; Mokrzynski, K.T.; Sarna, P.M.; Sarna, T.J. Quercetin protects ARPE-19 cells against photic stress mediated by the products of rhodopsin photobleaching. *Photochem. Photobiol. Sci.* **2020**, *19*, 1022–1034. [CrossRef]
30. Olchawa, M.; Krzysztynska-Kuleta, O.; Duda, M.; Pawlak, A.; Pabisz, P.; Czuba-Pelech, B.; Sarna, T. In vitro phototoxicity of rhodopsin photobleaching products in the retinal pigment epithelium (RPE). *Free Radic. Res.* **2019**, *53*, 456–471. [CrossRef]
31. Bazan-Socha, S.; Mastalerz, L.; Cybulska, A.; Zareba, L.; Kremers, R.; Zabczyk, M.; Pulka, G.; Iwaniec, T.; Hemker, C.; Undas, A. Prothrombotic State in Asthma Is Related to Increased Levels of Inflammatory Cytokines, IL-6 and TNFα, in Peripheral Blood. *Inflammation* **2017**, *40*, 1225–1235. [CrossRef]
32. Bazan-Socha, S.; Mastalerz, L.; Cybulska, A.; Zareba, L.; Kremers, R.; Zabczyk, M.; Pulka, G.; Iwaniec, T.; Hemker, C.; Undas, A. Asthma is associated with enhanced thrombin formation and impaired fibrinolysis. *Clin. Exp. Allergy* **2016**, *46*, 932–944. [CrossRef] [PubMed]
33. Zelzer, S.; Tatzber, F.; Herrmann, M.; Wonisch, W.; Rinnerhofer, S.; Kundi, M.; Obermayer-Pietsch, B.; Niedrist, T.; Cvirn, G.; Wultsch, G.; et al. Work Intensity, Low-Grade Inflammation, and Oxidative Status: A Comparison between Office and Slaughterhouse Workers. *Oxid. Med. Cell. Longev.* **2018**, *2018*, 2737563. [CrossRef] [PubMed]
34. Lee, H.M.; Truong, S.T.; Wong, N.D. Association of adult-onset asthma with specific cardiovascular conditions. *Respir. Med.* **2012**, *106*, 948–953. [CrossRef] [PubMed]
35. Tattersall, M.C.; Barnet, J.H.; Korcarz, C.E.; Hagen, E.W.; Peppard, P.E.; Stein, J.H. Late-Onset Asthma Predicts Cardiovascular Disease Events: The Wisconsin Sleep Cohort. *J. Am. Heart Assoc.* **2016**, *5*, e003448. [CrossRef] [PubMed]
36. Ricciardolo, F.L.M.; Sprio, A.E.; Baroso, A.; Gallo, F.; Riccardi, E.; Bertolini, F.; Carriero, V.; Arrigo, E.; Ciprandi, G. Characterization of t2-low and t2-high asthma phenotypes in real-life. *Biomedicines* **2021**, *9*, 1648. [CrossRef]
37. Miethe, S.; Guarino, M.; Alhamdan, F.; Simon, H.U.; Renz, H.; Dufour, J.F.; Potaczek, D.P.; Garn, H. Effects of obesity on asthma: Immunometabolic links. *Polish Arch. Intern. Med.* **2018**, *128*, 469–477. [CrossRef]
38. Payne, D.N.R.; Rogers, A.V.; Ädelroth, E.; Bandi, V.; Guntupalli, K.K.; Bush, A.; Jeffery, P.K. Early thickening of the reticular basement membrane in children with difficult asthma. *Am. J. Respir. Crit. Care Med.* **2003**, *167*, 78–82. [CrossRef]
39. Mohanty, J.G.; Nagababu, E.; Rifkind, J.M. Red blood cell oxidative stress impairs oxygen delivery and induces red blood cell aging. *Front. Physiol.* **2014**, *5*, 84. [CrossRef]
40. Dozor, A.J. The role of oxidative stress in the pathogenesis and treatment of asthma. *Ann. N. Y. Acad. Sci.* **2010**, *1203*, 133–137. [CrossRef]
41. Troisi, R.J.; Willett, W.C.; Weiss, S.T.; Trichopoulos, D.; Rosner, B.; Speizer, F.E. A prospective study of diet and adult-onset asthma. *Am. J. Respir. Crit. Care Med.* **2012**, *151*, 1401–1408. [CrossRef]
42. Varraso, R.; Kauffmann, F.; Leynaert, B.; Le Moual, N.; Boutron-Ruault, M.C.; Clavel-Chapelon, F.; Romieu, I. Dietary patterns and asthma in the E3N study. *Eur. Respir. J.* **2009**, *33*, 33–41. [CrossRef] [PubMed]

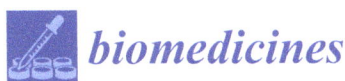

Article

Bcl10 Regulates Lipopolysaccharide-Induced Pro-Fibrotic Signaling in Bronchial Fibroblasts from Severe Asthma Patients

Rakhee K. Ramakrishnan [1], Khuloud Bajbouj [1], Maha Guimei [2], Surendra Singh Rawat [3], Zaina Kalaji [1], Mahmood Y. Hachim [3], Bassam Mahboub [1,4], Saleh M. Ibrahim [1,5], Rifat Hamoudi [1,6,*], Rabih Halwani [1,7,*] and Qutayba Hamid [1,8,*]

[1] Sharjah Institute for Medical Research, College of Medicine, University of Sharjah, Sharjah P.O. Box 27272, United Arab Emirates; rramakrishnan@sharjah.ac.ae (R.K.R.); kbajbouj@sharjah.ac.ae (K.B.); u21105961@sharjah.ac.ae (Z.K.); bhmahboub@dha.gov.ae (B.M.); saleh.ibrahim@sharjah.ac.ae (S.M.I.)
[2] Department of Pathology, Faculty of Medicine, Alexandria University, Alexandria 21526, Egypt; maha.guimei@alexmed.edu.eg
[3] College of Medicine, Mohammed Bin Rashid University, Dubai P.O. Box 505055, United Arab Emirates; surendrasingh.rawat@mbru.ac.ae (S.S.R.); mahmood.almashhadani@mbru.ac.ae (M.Y.H.)
[4] Rashid Hospital, Dubai Health Authority, Dubai P.O. Box 4545, United Arab Emirates
[5] Lübeck Institute of Experimental Dermatology (LIED), University of Lübeck, 23562 Lübeck, Germany
[6] Division of Surgery and Interventional Science, University College London, London WC1E 6BT, UK
[7] Immunology Research Lab, College of Medicine, King Saud University, Riyadh P.O. Box 145111, Saudi Arabia
[8] Meakins-Christie Laboratories, McGill University, Montreal, QC H3A 0G4, Canada
* Correspondence: rhamoudi@sharjah.ac.ae (R.H.); rhalwani@sharjah.ac.ae (R.H.); qalheialy@sharjah.ac.ae (Q.H.)

Citation: Ramakrishnan, R.K.; Bajbouj, K.; Guimei, M.; Rawat, S.S.; Kalaji, Z.; Hachim, M.Y.; Mahboub, B.; Ibrahim, S.M.; Hamoudi, R.; Halwani, R.; et al. Bcl10 Regulates Lipopolysaccharide-Induced Pro-Fibrotic Signaling in Bronchial Fibroblasts from Severe Asthma Patients. *Biomedicines* **2022**, *10*, 1716. https://doi.org/10.3390/biomedicines10071716

Academic Editor: Stanislawa Bazan-Socha

Received: 31 May 2022
Accepted: 30 June 2022
Published: 15 July 2022

Publisher's Note: MDPI stays neutral with regard to jurisdictional claims in published maps and institutional affiliations.

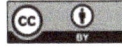

Copyright: © 2022 by the authors. Licensee MDPI, Basel, Switzerland. This article is an open access article distributed under the terms and conditions of the Creative Commons Attribution (CC BY) license (https://creativecommons.org/licenses/by/4.0/).

Abstract: Subepithelial fibrosis is a characteristic hallmark of airway remodeling in asthma. Current asthma medications have limited efficacy in treating fibrosis, particularly in patients with severe asthma, necessitating a deeper understanding of the fibrotic mechanisms. The NF-κB pathway is key to airway inflammation in asthma, as it regulates the activity of multiple pro-inflammatory mediators that contribute to airway pathology. Bcl10 is a well-known upstream mediator of the NF-κB pathway that has been linked to fibrosis in other disease models. Therefore, we investigated Bcl10-mediated NF-κB activation as a potential pathway regulating fibrotic signaling in severe asthmatic fibroblasts. We demonstrate here the elevated protein expression of Bcl10 in bronchial fibroblasts and bronchial biopsies from severe asthmatic patients when compared to non-asthmatic individuals. Lipopolysaccharide (LPS) induced the increased expression of the pro-fibrotic cytokines IL-6, IL-8 and TGF-β1 in bronchial fibroblasts, and this induction was associated with the activation of Bcl10. Inhibition of the Bcl10-mediated NF-κB pathway using an IRAK1/4 selective inhibitor abrogated the pro-fibrotic signaling induced by LPS. Thus, our study indicates that Bcl10-mediated NF-κB activation signals increased pro-fibrotic cytokine expression in severe asthmatic airways. This reveals the therapeutic potential of targeting Bcl10 signaling in ameliorating inflammation and fibrosis, particularly in severe asthmatic individuals.

Keywords: severe asthma; bronchial fibroblasts; fibrosis; Bcl10; NF-κB pathway; cytokines

1. Introduction

Asthma is a chronic respiratory disease that is usually associated with inflammation and remodeling of the airways. Subepithelial fibrosis is a characteristic hallmark of airway remodeling in asthma, particularly in patients with severe asthma [1]. Unfortunately, current asthma medications cannot sufficiently target and ameliorate subepithelial fibrosis. Therefore, a deeper understanding of the fibrotic mechanisms in action is essential to identify novel therapeutic targets. This could aid in ameliorating fibrosis and improving the airway dynamics in asthma patients.

The Nuclear factor (NF)-kappaB (NF-κB) signaling pathway is a highly versatile pathway that plays a vital role in multiple biological processes, including cell growth, survival, development, immune response and inflammation [2]. NF-κB is a key signaling pathway in asthma pathogenesis, particularly in airway inflammation. Persistent activation of the NF-κB pathway was noted in peripheral blood mononuclear cells isolated from patients with severe uncontrolled asthma [3]. As a result, increased levels of pro-inflammatory mediators were secreted by these cells despite continuous systemic glucocorticoid treatment. At the same time, activation of NF-κB signaling has also been noted in lung fibroblasts during fibrogenesis [4]. Furthermore, NF-κB activation induces the expression of pro-fibrotic cytokines such as IL-6, IL-8 and TGF-β [5–7].

B-cell lymphoma/leukemia 10 (Bcl10) is an adaptor protein associated with the constitutive activation of canonical NF-κB in mucosa-associated lymphoid tissue (MALT) B cell lymphoma [8]. Bcl10 has been largely studied in antigen receptor-mediated lymphocyte activation, where it was found to interact with CARMA/CARD-containing scaffold proteins and MALT1 paracaspase to form the three-component CBM signalosome that sets in motion a cascade of events that eventually lead to NF-κB induction [9,10]. Depending on the cell-specific chromatin landscape accessible to NF-κB or other transcription factors, the activation of this pathway through CBM complex signaling results in the inducible expression of numerous inflammatory cytokines, chemokines and factors that control cellular functions, including survival, proliferation and differentiation [11]. Thus, CBM signaling is essential for host defense and tissue homeostasis. However, alterations in the signaling components, including Bcl10, have been implicated in diseases such as autoinflammatory diseases, lymphoproliferative disorders and immunodeficiencies, as well as cancers [12].

Bcl10 signaling plays an important role in establishing the inflammatory environment associated with asthma. Bcl10 is involved in FcεRI-mediated NF-κB activation, pro-inflammatory cytokine release and degranulation of mast cells [13]. IgE-mediated allergic inflammatory response was found to be impaired in Bcl10-deficient mast cells [13,14], indicating Bcl10 as a key regulator of immune signaling in mast cells. Furthermore, Bcl10 also complexes with CARMA3/CARD10 and MALT1 to form the CBM-3 signalosome as a result of G-protein-coupled receptor (GPCR) activation to induce pro-inflammatory gene expression in non-immune cells such as fibroblasts and endothelial cells [15].

Interestingly, studies also indicate Bcl10 to be an important mediator of fibrotic remodeling. Angiotensin II (Ang II)-induced fibrotic signaling, such as extracellular matrix (ECM) synthesis and myofibroblast proliferation, was mediated by Bcl10 via the CBM-3 signalosome [16,17]. Bcl10 also regulated lipopolysaccharide (LPS)-induced activation of NF-κB and IL-8 in human intestinal epithelial cells [18], suggesting a role for Bcl10 in epithelial inflammation. Moreover, NF-κB-regulated genes in the airway epithelium contributed to allergen-induced peribronchial fibrosis and mucus production [19].

NF-κB activation is increasingly recognized in the pathogenesis of asthma and Bcl10-mediated NF-κB signaling has widely been studied as an inflammatory pathway in immune cells [20]. However, the role of Bcl10-driven NF-κB activation is yet to be explored in the context of airway remodeling in asthma. Since Bcl10 is an important mediator of fibrotic remodeling in other disease models, we hypothesized that the Bcl10-mediated NF-κB pathway promotes fibrotic signaling in severe asthmatic fibroblasts.

2. Materials and Methods

2.1. Cell Culture and Treatment of Primary Human Bronchial Fibroblasts

The primary bronchial fibroblasts were isolated from endobronchial tissue biopsies obtained from patients with severe asthma or healthy volunteers. These fibroblasts were archived at Quebec Respiratory Health Research Network Tissue Bank (McGill University Health Centre (MUHC)/Meakins-Christie Laboratories Tissue Bank, Montreal, QC, Canada), as previously described [21]. The original study was approved by the MUHC Research Ethics Board (REB) with reference number 2003–1879 and the subjects had provided written informed consent in accordance with the Declaration of Helsinki. The fibroblasts were age-matched with a mean age of 43.4 ± 8.3 years for the severe asthmatics and 43.7 ± 12.5 years for the non-asthmatics. Furthermore, cells were chosen from subjects who were non-smokers, as smoking patients with severe asthma demonstrated a distinct gene expression profile compared to non-smoking severe asthmatics and non-smoking individuals without asthma [22].

The cells were revived in Dulbecco's modified Eagle's medium (DMEM)—high glucose supplemented with 10% fetal bovine serum (FBS), 2 mM L-glutamine, 100 units/mL of penicillin, and 100 ng/mL streptomycin in 75-cm^2 flasks. The cells were maintained at 37 °C in 5% CO_2 with medium change performed every 2–3 days. They were harvested when 80–90% confluent using 0.1% trypsin-ethylenediaminetetraacetic acid (EDTA) solution and seeded into multiwell tissue culture plates for experiments.

The cells were seeded into 6- or 12-well plates at approximate cell density/well of 10×10^4, and 5×10^4, respectively. At ~70% confluency, they were serum-starved in FBS-free DMEM complete medium for a period of 24 h before experiments. For baseline measurements, the cells were cultured in DMEM complete medium thereafter. For LPS stimulation experiments, the cells were stimulated with 10 μg/mL of LPS (Sigma-Aldrich, Burlington, MA, USA, Cat. No. L8643) for the specified amount of time. Selective inhibition of Interleukin 1b Receptor-associated Kinase (IRAK) 1/4 was carried out to block the Bcl10 upstream signaling. Accordingly, the cells were pre-treated with 50 μM of IRAK 1/4 Inhibitor I (R&D Systems, Minneapolis, MN, USA, Cat. No. 5665/50) for 1 h prior to LPS stimulation for 2 h.

2.2. Quantitative Real-Time Polymerase Chain Reaction (qRT-PCR)

In order to investigate the mRNA expression of the different components of the NF-κB activation pathway and fibrotic markers in bronchial fibroblasts, qRT-PCR was performed. Total RNA was extracted from cell pellets using Trizol Reagent (Invitrogen, Waltham, MA, USA, Cat. No. 15596018), according to manufacturer instructions. RNA quality and yield were determined by Nanodrop (Thermo Scientific, Waltham, MA, USA) spectrophotometric measurements. cDNA synthesis was performed from 200 ng of total RNA using the High-Capacity cDNA Reverse Transcription Kit (Applied Biosystems, Waltham, MA, USA, Cat. No. 4368814) in the Veriti Thermal Cycler (Applied Biosystems, Waltham, MA, USA). qRT-PCR reactions were set up using the 5× Hot FirePol EvaGreen qRT-PCR SuperMix (Solis Biodyne, Tartu, Estonia, Cat. No. 08-36-00001) in QuantStudio 3 Real-Time PCR System (Applied Biosystems, Waltham, MA, USA). The primers used are listed in Table 1. Gene expression was analyzed using the Comparative CT (ΔΔCT) method after normalization to the housekeeping gene 18s RNA. All results are presented as fold expression change compared to non-asthmatic healthy controls in baseline experiments or untreated controls in LPS stimulation experiments.

Table 1. List of primer sequences.

Gene Name	Forward Primer (5′–3′)	Reverse Primer (5′–3′)
TLR4	GCAGTTTCTGAGCAGTCGTGC	CGTCTCCAGAAGATGTGCCGC
BCL10	GAAGTGAAGAAGGACGCCTTAG	AGATGATCAAAATGTCTCTCAGC
MALT1	CTCCGCCTCAGTTGCCTAGA	CAACCTTTTTCACCCATTAACTTCA
CARMA3/CARD10	GGAGCCTCAGACCCTACAGTT	GCAGGTCTAGCAGGTTACGG
IκBα	CTGGGCATCGTGGAGCTTTTGG	TCTGTTGACATCAGCCCCACAC
A20	AATGGCTTCCACAGACACACC	CAAAGGGGCGAAATTGGAACC
RELA	GCCGAGTGAACCGAAACTCTGG	TTGTCGGTGCACATCAGCTTGC
IL-6	GAAAGCAGCAAAGAGGCAC	GCACAGCTCTGGCTTGTTCC
IL-8	CCACACTGCGCCAACACAG	CTTCTCCACAACCCTCTGC

Table 1. *Cont.*

Gene Name	Forward Primer (5′–3′)	Reverse Primer (5′–3′)
TGF-β1	AAATTGAGGGCTTTCGCCTTA	GAACCCGTTGATGTCCACTTG
COL1A1	GATTGACCCCAACCAAGGCTG	GCCGAACCAGACATGCCTC
COL5A1	GTCGATCCTAACCAAGGATGC	GAACCAGGAGCCCGGGTTTTC
FN1	CTGGGAACACTTACCGAGTGGG	CCACCAGTCTCATGTGGTCTCC
TBK1	AGCGGCAGAGTTAGGTGAAA	CCAGTGATCCACCTGGAGAT
IRF3	TCTGCCCTCAACCGCAAAGAAG	TACTGCCTCCATTGGTGTC
IRF7	GCTGGACGTGACCATCATGTA	GGGCCGTATAGGAACGTGC
IFNβ1	CCTGTGGCAATTGAATGGGAGGC	AGATGGTCAATGCGGCGTCCTC
18S	TGACTCAACACGGGAAACC	TCGCTCCACCAACTAAGAAC

2.3. Western Blotting

In order to investigate the protein expression of Bcl10, western blotting was performed. The cell pellets were lysed in 10X RIPA buffer (abcam, Cambridge, UK, Cat. No. ab156034) diluted to 1X and supplemented with $1\times$ Protease Inhibitor Cocktail (Sigma-Aldrich, Burlington, MA, USA, Cat. No. P2714) and 1 mM PMSF (Sigma-Aldrich, Burlington, MA, USA, Cat. No. P7626). The protein lysates were quantified using the Protein Assay Kit II (Bio-Rad, Hercules, CA, USA, Cat. No. 5000002) with bovine serum albumin (BSA) as standard. The lysates were boiled in $10\times$ Laemmli Sample Buffer diluted to $1\times$, and total protein was separated using 4–20% Mini-PROTEAN TGX Precast Protein Gels (Biorad, Hercules, CA, USA, Cat. No. 4561095-6). Post electrophoresis, the proteins were transferred onto a 0.2 μm nitrocellulose membrane (Bio-Rad, Hercules, CA, USA, Cat. No. 1620112) and blocked in 5% non-fat dry milk for at least an hour at room temperature (RT) before incubating the membrane overnight at 4 °C with anti-Bcl10 antibody (331.3) (Santa Cruz, TX, USA, Cat. No. sc-5273). The membrane was subsequently incubated for 1 h at RT with the respective horseradish peroxidase (HRP)-linked secondary antibody. The blots were developed using the Clarity™ Western ECL Substrate (Bio-Rad, Hercules, CA, USA, Cat. No. 170-5060) in the ChemiDoc™ Touch Gel and Western Blot Imaging System (Bio-Rad, Hercules, CA, USA). Anti-β-actin (Sigma-Aldrich, Burlington, MA, USA, Cat. No. Cat# A5441) was used as the loading control. Image Lab software (Bio-Rad, Hercules, CA, USA) was used to detect and quantify the protein bands. Protein levels were normalized to β-actin and thereafter to healthy controls.

2.4. Immunohistochemistry

Formalin-fixed paraffin-embedded (FFPE) sections of bronchial biopsy tissues on slides were obtained from non-asthmatic control individuals, mild asthma, moderate asthma and severe asthma subjects. These slides were archived at the Biobank of the Quebec Respiratory Health Research Network Canada with MUHC REB number BMB-02-039-t [23]. According to retrieved data, patients had been classified into mild, moderate and severe based on frequency of exacerbations, lung function and medication usage, as previously described [23]. Immunohistochemical staining was performed to determine the expression and distribution of Bcl10 as previously described [24]. Briefly, routine deparaffinization in xylene and rehydration steps in decreasing concentrations of ethanol were performed. Heat-activated antigen retrieval was carried out using Tris EDTA buffer at pH 9.0 for Bcl10, as per manufacturer recommendations. The sections were incubated in hydrogen peroxidase blocking solution for 30 min to block the endogenous peroxidase activity. The slides were then blocked in 1% BSA for 20 min at RT and immunostained using mouse monoclonal anti-Bcl10 (Santa Cruz, TX, USA, Cat. No. sc-5273) antibody overnight at 4 °C. The slides were developed using HRP/DAB (ABC) Detection IHC kit (Abcam, Cambridge, UK, Cat. No. ab64264), according to manufacturer recommendations. The primary antibody was omitted to serve as technical negative control and appropriate positive control tissue was used. Nuclei were counterstained blue with hematoxylin (Thermo Scientific Shandon, Waltham, MA, USA). The stained slides were then examined and analyzed by a histopathologist.

2.5. Paraffin Embedding and Immunocytochemistry of Human Bronchial Cells

Human bronchial fibroblasts (HBFs) and human bronchial epithelial cells (HBE) were clotted, processed and immunostained. Briefly, 5×10^5 cells were centrifuged at 1200 rpm for 5 min and placed on ice immediately after centrifugation. 120 µL of plasma was then added dropwise to the cell pellet, followed by gentle vortexing for 10 s. 80 µL of thrombin (Sigma-Aldrich, Burlington, MA, USA, Cat. No. T4393) was then added and mixed so as to clot the cells together. The clotted cells were then transferred to a sheet of Speci-wrap paper, which was folded and secured inside a formalin cassette. The clotted cells were then processed using Excelsior AS Tissue Processor (Thermo Fisher Scientific, Waltham, MA, USA) to generate FFPE blocks of the clotted cells, which were then immunostained as described above.

2.6. Statistical Analysis

All data are presented as mean ± standard error of the mean (SEM) of 2–4 independent experiments using GraphPad Prism 6.0 software (GraphPad, San Diego, CA, USA). Data analyses were performed using unpaired two-tailed Student's *t*-test while comparing NHBF and DHBF, one-way ANOVA followed by Tukey's multiple comparison tests or two-way ANOVA followed by Sidak's multiple comparison tests for statistical analysis of the data. A p value < 0.05 was considered statistically significant.

3. Results

3.1. Activation of Bcl10-Mediated NF-κB in Severe Asthmatic Fibroblasts

Persistent activation of the NF-κB signaling pathway characterized the peripheral blood mononuclear cells isolated from patients with severe asthma [3]. We therefore first examined the expression of various components of this pathway in bronchial fibroblasts from severe asthmatics (S-As) and healthy subjects. To compare the basal expression levels, normal human bronchial fibroblasts (NHBF) and asthmatic diseased human bronchial fibroblasts (DHBF) in culture were pelleted and lysed for qRT-PCR analysis. The mRNA expression of TLR4 ($p = 0.0056$), MALT1 ($p = 0.0006$) and CARMA3 ($p = 0.0067$) was significantly upregulated in DHBF relative to NHBF (Figure 1A). IKBα gene expression was significantly downregulated in DHBF ($p = 0.0116$). Furthermore, A20 deubiquitinase, another negative regulator of NF-κB that terminates downstream signaling events [25], was also lowered in DHBF compared to NHBF (Figure 1A). Increased mRNA levels of RELA subunit were also found in DHBF compared to NHBF, albeit without any statistical significance ($p = 0.09$). Since increased expression of the intermediates of the NF-κB pathway was noted, we next measured the expression of NF-κB-target genes, including IL-6 and IL-8. While a significant increase in IL-8 expression was observed in DHBF ($p = 0.0231$), IL-6 transcript levels showed an increased trend in DHBF when compared to NHBF. Bcl10 being a critical mediator of NF-κB signaling, we next investigated the protein expression of Bcl10 in these fibroblasts at basal levels. It was interesting to note a trend of 3-fold increase in the relative protein expression of Bcl10 in DHBF in comparison to NHBF ($p = 0.0524$) (Figure 1B).

The elevated expression of Bcl10 in bronchial fibroblasts from severe asthmatic subjects and the increased signature of key NF-κB genes at baseline suggest activation of the Bcl10-mediated NF-κB pathway in S-As fibroblasts.

3.2. Increased Cytoplasmic Bcl10 Expression in Subepithelial Fibroblasts from Severe Asthma Patients

In order to validate the increased protein expression of Bcl10 in severe asthma, we evaluated its immunohistochemical expression and distribution in bronchial biopsies obtained from normal individuals and asthma patients of varying severities. Bcl10 protein was variably expressed in the airways of both normal and asthma patients.

Expression of Bcl10 was strong and more pronounced in the subepithelial fibroblasts in severe asthmatic patients compared to weak to moderate expression noted in mild and moderate asthmatics, respectively (Figure 2C–F). The non-asthmatic healthy individuals showed almost no expression of Bcl10 in subepithelial fibroblasts (Figure 2A,B). On the other hand, the mucosal bronchial epithelial cells showed variable nuclear and cytoplasmic staining for Bcl10 in both healthy and asthmatic patients.

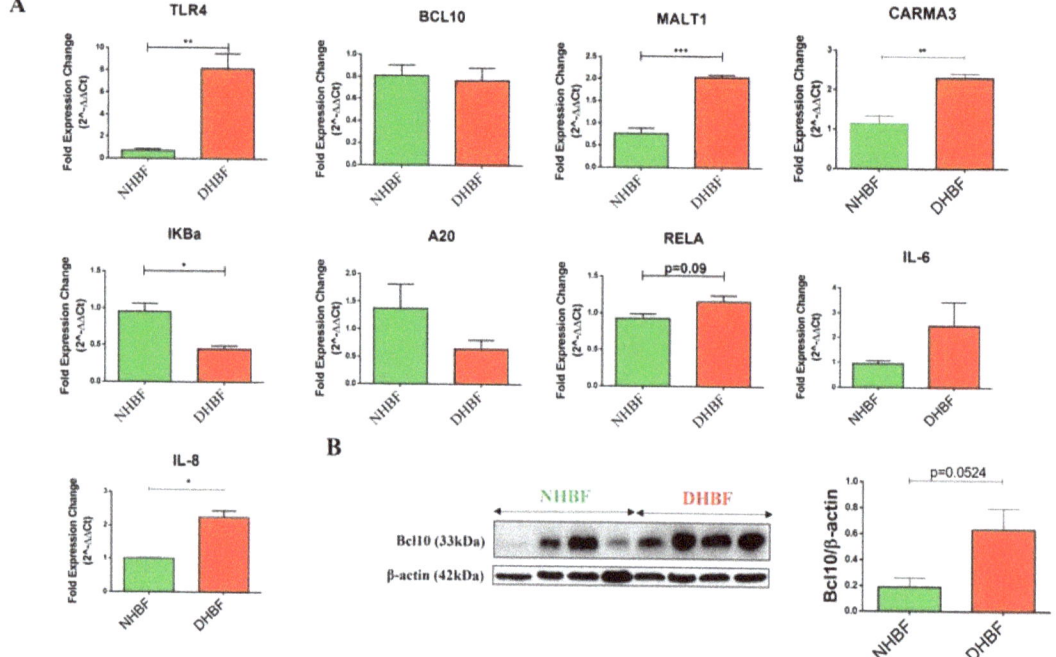

Figure 1. Activation of NF-κB in severe asthmatic fibroblasts. NHBF and DHBF were cultured in DMEM complete medium post serum-starvation. (**A**) Under basal conditions, mRNA expression of NF-κB pathway members, TLR4, BCL10, MALT1, CARMA3, IκBα, A20, RELA, IL-6 and IL-8, in NHBF and DHBF was analyzed by qRT-PCR and expressed as fold expression change relative to NHBF post normalization to housekeeping gene 18s rRNA. (**B**) Whole cell lysates were subjected to immunoblot analysis of Bcl10 protein levels. β-actin was used as loading control. Data are represented as mean ± SEM from at least 3 unique donors in each group. * $p < 0.05$, ** $p < 0.01$, *** $p < 0.001$ determined by unpaired two-tailed Student *t*-test.

In the control biopsies, the surface epithelium showed positive Bcl10 expression in both the cytoplasm and the nuclei whereas the subepithelial fibroblasts were mostly negative for Bcl10 (Figure 2A,B). Biopsies from mild and moderate cases of asthma displayed moderate Bcl10 expression in both the epithelium and subepithelium with very few subepithelial fibroblasts staining positively for Bcl10 (Figure 2C,D). Biopsies from severe asthmatic subjects showed an increased number of fibroblasts in the subepithelium with intense Bcl10 staining (Figure 2E,F). These findings suggest that the intensity of positive Bcl10 staining as well as the distribution of Bcl10-positive cells increased with increasing severity of asthma.

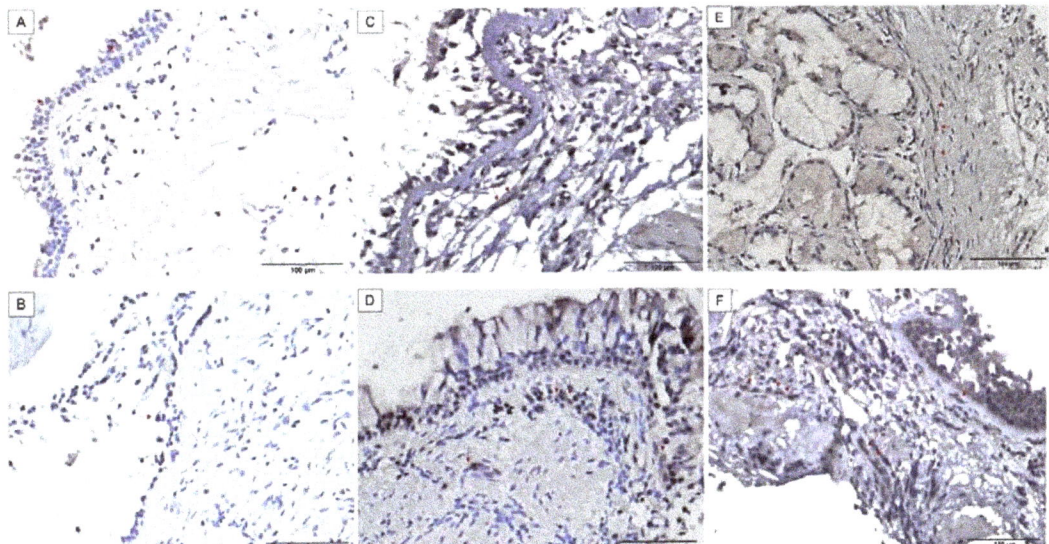

Figure 2. Increased cytoplasmic Bcl10 expression in subepithelial fibroblasts of bronchial biopsies from asthma patients with increasing severity. Representative images taken at 400X magnification showing Bcl10 expression. Representative bronchial biopsy sections from (**A,B**) healthy control showing positive Bcl10 staining in surface epithelium and no Bcl10 staining in subepithelial fibroblasts, (**C,D**) mild and moderate asthma patients showing minimal and weak Bcl10 cytoplasmic expression in subepithelial fibroblasts, (**E,F**) severe asthmatic patients showing numerous subepithelial fibroblasts with strong Bcl10 expression. (Red arrows indicate Bcl10-positive cells).

3.3. Subcellular Localization of Bcl10 in Bronchial Fibroblasts and Bronchial Epithelial Cells

Subcellular localization of Bcl10 correlated with the development of MALT lymphoma, with strong nuclear Bcl10 expression seen in MALT lymphomas with t(1;14)(p22;q32) translocation [26]. To understand the potential role of Bcl10 in fibroblast function, we next assessed their subcellular localization in human bronchial fibroblasts (HBF) and bronchial epithelial cells (HBE) from severe asthmatic and healthy subjects. We clotted the HBFs and HBEs, and stained them for Bcl10 using immunocytochemistry. In bronchial fibroblasts, Bcl10 expression was highly intense in DHBF when compared to NHBF (Figure 3A). Strong and more pronounced cytoplasmic Bcl10 expression was noted in DHBF compared to NHBF. Similarly, in bronchial epithelial cells, a greater number of Bcl10-positive cells were detected in DHBE relative to NHBE (Figure 3B). Taken together, these findings confirm constitutively higher Bcl10 expression in asthma, particularly in severe asthma, and its localization predominantly in the cytoplasmic compartment in bronchial fibroblasts.

3.4. Bcl10 Mediates LPS-Induced Pro-Fibrotic Cytokine Signaling in Bronchial Fibroblasts

In order to assess the role of Bcl10 in pro-fibrotic signaling, the bronchial fibroblasts were stimulated with LPS and the level of pro-fibrotic cytokines, IL-6, IL-8 and TGFβ1, was analyzed. The fibroblasts were serum-starved for 24 h and then exposed to 10 μg/mL of LPS for different time-points. We then studied the effect of LPS stimulation on the gene expression of BCL10 using qRT-PCR. LPS stimulation was observed to significantly upregulate the expression of BCL10 in both NHBF and DHBF in comparison to their respective unexposed controls and this increase was found to be time-dependent (Figure 4A).

A

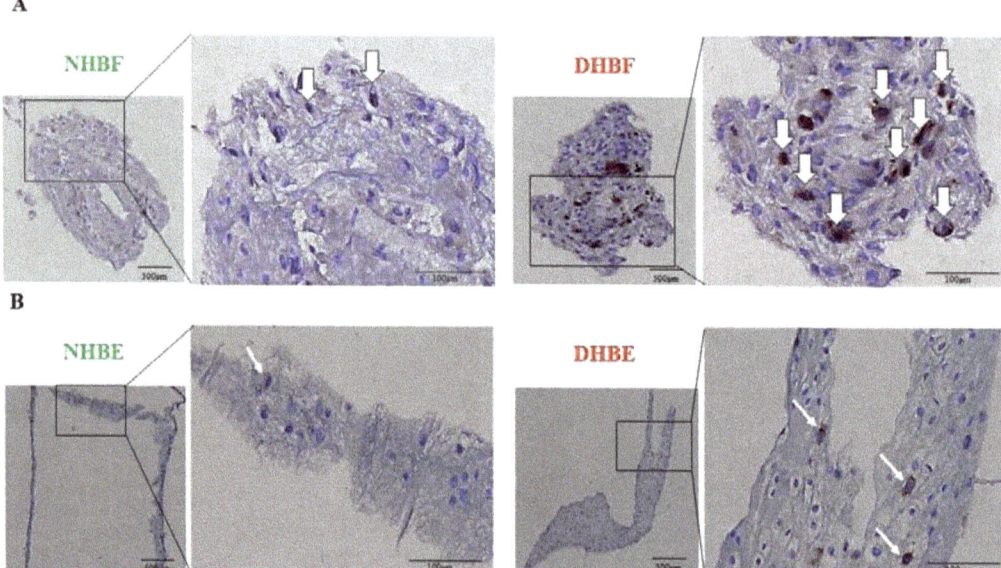

B

Figure 3. Subcellular localization of Bcl10 in bronchial fibroblasts and bronchial epithelial cells. NHBF and DHBF were cultured in DMEM complete medium, and NHBE and DHBE were cultured in Pneumacult complete medium. (**A**) Cellular clots of NHBF and DHBF, and (**B**) NHBE and DHBE were immunostained for Bcl10 and the white arrows indicate Bcl10-positive cells.

Since cross-linking of Toll-like receptor 4 (TLR4) with LPS induces the synthesis and secretion of pro-inflammatory and pro-fibrotic cytokines [27], we next examined the expression of IL-6, IL-8 and TGFβ1 in NHBF and DHBF upon LPS stimulation for 2 h. LPS strongly induced IL-6 gene expression in both NHBF and DHBF, whereas IL-8 and TGFβ1 was induced to a lower extent when compared to their unexposed control (Figure 4C). The induction of collagen expression by LPS in primary cultured mouse lung fibroblast [28] led us to next assess the expression of collagen markers, COL1A1 and COL5A1, and fibronectin in NHBF and DHBF. No significant alteration in the expression of these markers was observed in NHBF and DHBF upon LPS stimulation for 2 h (Figure 4D).

To further confirm the role of Bcl10 in LPS-induced pro-fibrotic cytokine signaling, we blocked the activity of IRAK1 and IRAK4, upstream adaptors that are responsible for recruiting Bcl10 to the TLR4 signaling complex and further signaling to NF-κB [29] using an IRAK1/4 inhibitor. In addition to restoring Bcl10 levels, the LPS-induced upregulation of IL-6, IL-8 and TGFβ1 was reversed upon exposure to the IRAK inhibitor (Figure 4B,C). The IRAK inhibitor suppressed the elevated gene expression of Bcl10 and IL-6 in both NHBF and DHBF. Interestingly, a reduction in COL5A1 expression and a reducing trend in COL1A1 and FN1 expression was noted in LPS-stimulated NHBF in the presence of IRAK1/4 inhibition (Figure 4D).

TLR4 can signal via the MyD88-dependent as well as the TRIF-dependent pathways, both of which, in turn, activate the canonical NF-κB pathway [30]. Bcl10-mediated signaling is a part of the MyD88-dependent pathway, which represents the early phase of activation of NF-κB. The TRIF-dependent pathway involves signaling through TBK1 and IRF complexes culminating in IFN-β expression and represents the late phase activation of NF-κB. Since TBK1 was reported to stimulate NF-κB and mediate the induction of inflammatory cytokine genes [31,32], we examined the expression of intermediates of the TRIF-dependent pathway upon stimulation with LPS and in the presence of IRAK1/4 inhibition. IRAK1/4 inhibition disrupts Bcl10 signaling, and therefore, Bcl10-mediated NF-κB signaling, but not TBK1-

mediated NF-κB signaling. Therefore, as expected, LPS induced the expression of TBK1, IRF3, IRF7 and IFN-β in both NHBF and DHBF, with a statistically significant increase noted in IRF3 (Figure 5). IRAK1/4 inhibition led to a further increase in IRF3 expression but the expression of TBK1, IRF7 and IFNβ was unaffected. The inhibition of LPS-induced expression of IL-6, IL-8 and TGFβ1 upon inhibiting Bcl10 signaling and not TRIF or TBK1 thus confirms that Bcl10-mediated signaling regulates pro-fibrotic cytokine expression in bronchial fibroblasts.

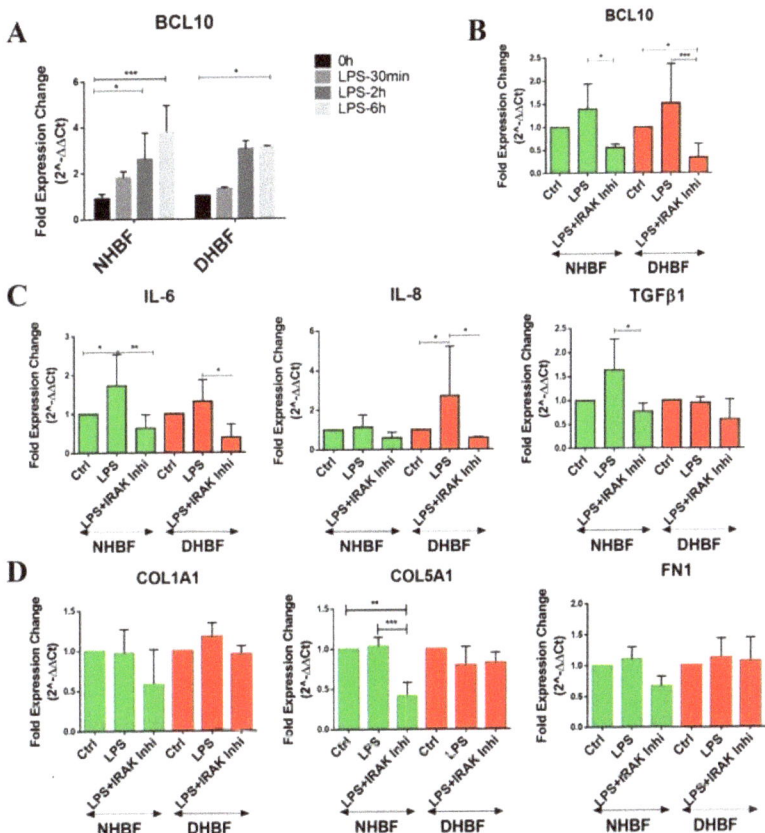

Figure 4. Bcl10 mediates LPS-induced pro-fibrotic cytokine signaling in bronchial fibroblasts. (**A**) NHBF and DHBF were serum-starved for 24 h, and thereafter, exposed to LPS (10 μg/mL) for the indicated time points for mRNA analysis. The effect of LPS treatment on the mRNA expression of BCL10 in NHBF and DHBF was analyzed by qRT-PCR and expressed as fold expression change relative to the respective untreated control at 0 h post normalization to housekeeping gene 18s rRNA. NHBF and DHBF were serum-starved for 24 h, and thereafter, pre-treated with IRAK 1/4 Inhibitor I (50 μM) for 1 h prior to LPS (10 μg/mL) stimulation for 2 h for mRNA analysis. The effect of LPS treatment and IRAK1/4 inhibition on the mRNA expression of (**B**) BCL10, (**C**) pro-fibrotic cytokines, IL-6, IL-8 and TGF-β1, and (**D**) ECM components, COL1A1, COL5A1 and FN1, in NHBF and DHBF was analyzed by qRT-PCR and expressed as fold expression change relative to the respective untreated control post normalization to housekeeping gene 18s rRNA. Data representative of at least 3 independent experiments. Data presented as mean ± SEM after normalization to untreated control. * $p < 0.05$, ** $p < 0.01$, *** $p < 0.001$, statistical significance assessed by one-way ANOVA with Tukey's multiple comparison tests.

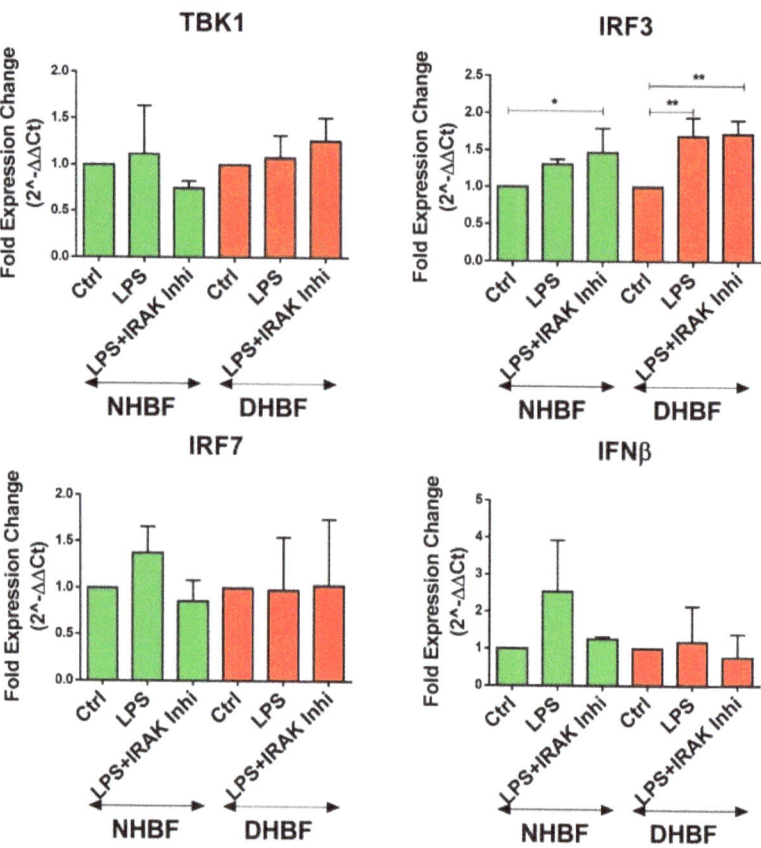

Figure 5. TRIF-dependent pathway not involved in LPS-induced pro-fibrotic cytokine signaling in bronchial fibroblasts. NHBF and DHBF were serum-starved for 24 h, and thereafter, pre-treated with IRAK 1/4 Inhibitor I (50 μM) for 1 h prior to LPS (10 μg/mL) stimulation for 2 h for mRNA analysis. The effect of LPS treatment and IRAK1/4 inhibition on the mRNA expression of TBK1, IRF3, IRF7 and IFN-β in NHBF and DHBF was analyzed by qRT-PCR and expressed as fold expression change relative to the respective untreated control post normalization to housekeeping gene 18s rRNA. Data presented as mean ± SEM after normalization to untreated control. * $p < 0.05$, ** $p < 0.01$, statistical significance assessed by one-way ANOVA with Tukey's multiple comparison tests.

4. Discussion

Human studies as well as in vivo animal models have reported increased activation of the classical and alternative NF-κB pathways in asthmatic airway tissues and in inflammatory cells [3,33]. As such, NF-κB signaling intermediates are attractive therapeutic targets for airway diseases such as asthma, as the underlying inflammation is independent of stimuli [34] and is mediated at least in part by NF-κB mediated signaling in bronchial fibroblasts (Figure 1). Bcl10 being a critical mediator of NF-κB signaling prompted us to explore its role in fibrotic remodeling in bronchial fibroblasts from severe asthma. To the best of our knowledge, this is the first report providing evidence of elevated protein expression of Bcl10 in the pathogenesis of severe asthma as well as the role of Bcl10-mediated signaling in the LPS-induced pro-fibrotic cytokine expression in bronchial fibroblasts.

NF-κB is a key component of the inflammatory network that controls cytokine production in airway pathology [20]. Overexpression of Bcl10 is an indicator of constitutive

NF-κB activation in tumors including MALT lymphoma [8,35], and persistent NF-κB activation is known to characterize severe uncontrolled asthma [3]. At baseline, the S-As fibroblasts demonstrated differential gene expression of various intermediates of the NF-κB pathway when compared to their healthy counterparts, supporting the notion of activation of NF-κB in severe asthma (Figure 1A). This was further confirmed by the increased protein expression of Bcl10 at basal levels in S-As fibroblasts (Figure 1B). We have also previously reported the increased expression of pro-fibrotic and pro-inflammatory mediators associated with the NF-κB activation, such as IL-6, IL-8, IL-11 and GROα (CXCL1) in these S-As fibroblasts [36]. Thus, the increased Bcl10 expression in S-As fibroblasts appears to signify the activation of the Bcl10-mediated NF-κB pathway in severe asthma. The observation that complete Bcl10 deficiency severely impaired fibroblast function in an immunodeficient individual [37] is testament to its importance in fibroblast response. Numerous lymphoid malignancies are characterized by the constitutive aberrant activation of the NF-κB pro-inflammatory pathway. Here, we demonstrated a similar pattern of Bcl10-mediated NF-κB activation in airway structural fibroblasts.

Furthermore, Bcl10 was differentially expressed in the sub-epithelial fibroblasts among the varying severities of asthma, ranging from weak expression in control biopsies to moderate expression in mild-to-moderate asthma and strong expression in severe asthma (Figure 2A–F). Just as in the case of MALT lymphoma, high Bcl10 expression in fibrotic airway tissues is paradoxical, considering that Bcl10 is a pro-apoptotic CARD-containing adaptor molecule [38]. However, certain cellular contexts in vivo may influence Bcl10 to behave as an anti-apoptotic molecule. For instance, overexpression of Bcl10 conferred a survival advantage to activated primary B cells even after withdrawal of the activating stimuli [39]. Alternately, the subcellular localization of Bcl10 may be a pre-determining factor in explaining this paradox. Bcl10 was predominantly expressed in the cytoplasm of subepithelial fibroblasts irrespective of the disease severity (Figure 2). However, Bcl10 nuclear expression was detected in the bronchial epithelium of non-asthmatic and asthmatic individuals (Figure 2). The different subcellular localization pattern of Bcl10 between the bronchial fibroblasts and epithelial cells (Figure 3A,B), indicates cell-dependent functional role of Bcl10. Here, it is interesting to note that the NF-κB-independent functions of Bcl10 include actin remodeling. For instance, Bcl10 regulates TCR-induced actin polymerization and cell spreading in T cells, and FcγR-induced actin polymerization and phagocytosis in monocytes/macrophages [40]. Subsequently, the role of Bcl10 in actin dynamics, cytoskeletal and membrane remodeling in macrophages was found to entail phagosome formation [11] This may perhaps explain the cytoplasmic expression of Bcl10 in S-As fibroblasts indicating Bcl10-dependent actin polymerization in addition to its role in NF-κB activation. Actin dynamics and polymerization are key to the contractile property of fibroblasts [42]. Thus, the presence of Bcl10 in the cytoplasmic compartment of S-As fibroblasts may signify its role in regulating actin dynamics and contraction of bronchial fibroblasts, and by this means, contributing to airway hyperresponsiveness in severe asthma. However, further studies are required to completely understand the physiological relevance of this subcellular localization.

Toll-like receptors (TLRs) such as TLR4 and TLR2 are important for the adaptive Th2-cytokine-driven inflammatory response in asthma [43,44]. Engagement of the TLR initiates the recruitment and activation of several adaptor molecules resulting in the activation of multiple signaling cascades, including NF-κB. TLR activation of the NF-κB pathway regulates the expression of immunomodulatory and inflammatory mediators. For instance, LPS binding to the TLR4 initiates an inflammatory cascade that climaxes in the release of cytokines such as IL-8 and IL-6, and the recruitment of an inflammatory infiltrate of lymphocytes, macrophages and polymorphonuclear leukocytes [45,46]. However, the signal transduction of the TLR4-Bcl10-NF-κB axis in asthmatic fibroblasts is far from understood, and the role of Bcl10 in TLR4-mediated fibroblast function is largely unknown.

Since the basal expression of TLR4, CARMA3, BCL10 and MALT1 was elevated in DHBF when compared to NHBF (Figure 1), we speculated that the TLR4-BCL10-NF-κB axis responds to LPS stimulation in bronchial fibroblasts and stays upregulated in S-As fibroblasts contributing to the activation of NF-κB in these cells. Here, we show that Bcl10 is a mediator of LPS-induced increase in pro-fibrotic cytokine expression (Figure 4). While LPS stimulation for 2 h boosted the expression of Bcl10, IL-6, IL-8 and TGF-β1 in bronchial fibroblasts, IRAK1/4 inhibition reversed the LPS-induced increase in all components, indicating increased Bcl10-mediated signaling contributed to pro-fibrotic cytokine expression upon LPS exposure in bronchial fibroblasts. Although LPS stimulation was previously reported to induce collagen expression in lung fibroblasts [28], there was no increase in COL1A1, COL5A1 and FN1 expression in NHBF and DHBF with LPS stimulation (Figure 4D). This could be attributed to the short exposure to LPS. While 2 h of LPS stimulation was sufficient to induce pro-fibrotic cytokine signaling in these fibroblasts, longer exposure may pave way to increased ECM secretion via activation of phosphoinositide3-kinase-Akt (PI3K-Akt) pathway [28] as well as autocrine signaling from IL-6 and TGF-β1 [47,48].

Since TLR4 signaling activates the canonical NF-κB pathway via the MyD88-dependent as well as the TRIF-dependent pathways [30], we next aimed to verify which of these pathways contributed to pro-fibrotic signaling. While IRAK1/4 inhibition had no effect on the TRIF-dependent pathway, the LPS-induced increase in Bcl10 was abolished and this was accompanied by a corresponding decrease in IL-6, IL-8 and TGF-β1 expression (Figure 5). This indicates Bcl10 signaling directly to its downstream mediators, including IL-6, IL-8 and TGF-β1 in response to LPS in bronchial fibroblasts. Furthermore, since Bcl10 inhibition was not accompanied by alterations in the TRIF-dependent induction of type I interferons, anti-viral signaling and immune defense against viral infections will be sustained in these cells. Considering the activated status of NF-κB pathway in S-As fibroblasts, an exaggerated response to LPS may cause greater extent of inflammatory damage and remodeling changes in severe asthmatic airways.

Increased levels of IL-6 were detected in the sputum of asthmatic subjects when compared to healthy controls, which correlated with impaired lung function in allergic asthma [49]. Further, high circulating levels of IL-6 increased the risk of exacerbations by 10% for each 1-pg/μL increase in baseline IL-6 level [50]. IL-6 is a pleiotropic cytokine with both pro-inflammatory and pro-fibrotic functions [51]. Severe asthma is also characterized by elevated IL-8 levels and associated neutrophilia [52,53]. We have previously reported the upregulation of IL-6 and IL-8 expression at basal levels in S-As fibroblasts when compared to non-asthmatic fibroblasts [36]. The ability of these fibroblasts to produce increased levels of ECM proteins as well as pro-inflammatory and pro-fibrotic cytokines have implicated them in remodeling and inflammation, two key processes involved in the pathogenesis of asthma. IL-8 is known to contribute to the pathogenesis of severe asthma by facilitating various features of airway remodeling, including neutrophil recruitment, epithelial-to-mesenchymal transition [54], angiogenesis [55] and proliferation and migration of ASM cells [56]. TGF-β is the central mediator of fibrotic tissue remodeling in asthma [57]. TGF-β gene polymorphisms were recently reported as a risk factor for asthma control [58]. The persistently high levels of TGF-β in severe asthma may contribute to increased collagen secretion from severe asthmatic fibroblasts despite treatment with oral corticosteroids [59]. Here, we showed that Bcl10 mediated the LPS-induced expression of IL-6, IL-8 and TGF-β1 in bronchial fibroblasts, highlighting the pathogenic role of Bcl10-mediated signaling in promoting airway remodeling in severe asthma.

Although extensively studied in immune cells, Bcl10-mediated NF-κB activation is emerging as an important pathway in non-immune cells as well. For instance, angiotensin II promotes liver fibrosis by activating the CBM-3-dependent NF-κB pathway in hepatocytes [16]. Lysophosphatidic acid-induced NF-κB activation and IL-6 production in murine embryonic fibroblasts involves signaling through adapter proteins Bcl10 and Malt1 [60]. In one study, Bcl10 was found to be an essential component of TLR4 response in human primary fibroblasts [37] and Bcl10 deficiency was found to abolish TLR4 signaling in response to LPS stimuli and subsequent production of IL-6 and IL-8. Our results are consistent with the observations made in this study.

We identified the Bcl10-mediated NF-κB pathway as a mechanism contributing to fibrotic remodeling and inflammation in severe asthma (Figure 6). Further studies are, however, essential to delineate the molecular interactions of Bcl10 to develop a more complete understanding to explain the signal transduction in bronchial fibroblasts. Another interesting option is to explore the kinetics of CBM-3 formation in S-As fibroblasts taking into account the activation of the Bcl10-mediated NF-κB pathway in these fibroblasts.

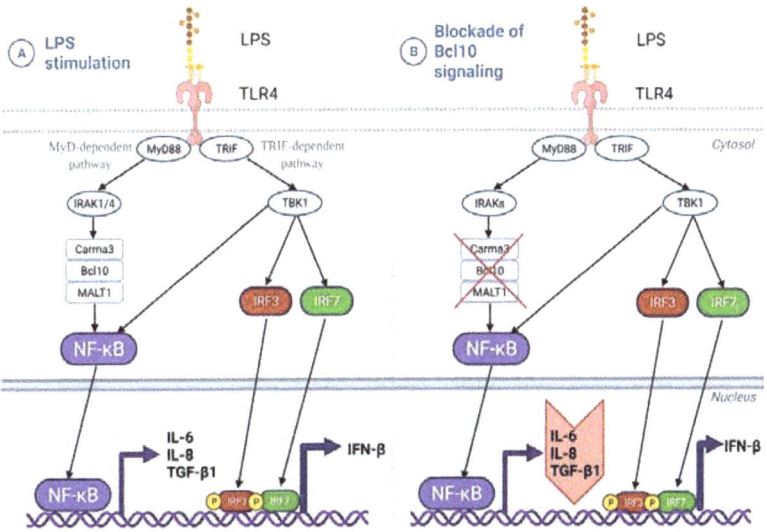

Figure 6. Induction of Bcl10-mediated pro-fibrotic cytokine signaling by LPS in bronchial fibroblasts. (**A**) In bronchial fibroblasts, LPS stimulation of TLR4 receptor activates both the MyD88-dependent and TRIF-dependent pathways. Bcl10-mediated NF-κB activation has downstream effects on airway inflammation and remodeling through the secretion of IL-6, IL-8 and TGF-β1 cytokines. (**B**) Blockade of this Bcl10 signaling cascade may ameliorate both inflammation and fibrosis by impeding the expression of IL-6, IL-8 and TGF-β1 cytokines.

Some of the limitations of our study include the lack of specific Bcl10 inhibition that would demonstrate the direct causal relationship between BCL10 and NF-κB pathway activation and could be addressed by using BCL10 siRNA/CRISPR and NF-κB dual luciferase reporter assay. However, we were able to show that an IRAK1/4 selective inhibitor that inhibits the signaling upstream of Bcl10 abrogated the pro-fibrotic signaling induced by LPS. Since the S-As fibroblasts were derived from patients on medications such as glucocorticosteroids and biologics, the results need to be interpreted with caution, as these medications are known to alter inflammatory cell signaling events in asthmatic airways [61]. Nevertheless, the enhanced signature of key NF-κB genes at baseline in the S-As fibroblasts suggest refractoriness to steroids in these patients. Another shortcoming of our study is the lack of in vivo investigation that we aim to explore in future studies.

5. Conclusions

Although NF-κB signaling is a well-characterized pathway in airway inflammation, we, for the first time, show activation of Bcl10-mediated NF-κB pathway in severe asthmatic fibroblasts. Furthermore, Bcl10 immunoreactivity in the subepithelium of airway tissues varied in intensity and distribution with increasing severity of asthma, relaying its importance in asthma severity. We further identified Bcl10 as a mediator of signal transduction from TLR4 to the activation of NF-κB inducible genes, including of IL-6, IL-8 and TGF-β1, in bronchial fibroblasts. This allows us to selectively target Bcl10 to impede its pathological signaling in severe asthma. Current asthma medications, including corticosteroid therapy, are not completely effective against airway remodeling, necessitating the identification of new therapeutic targets. Targeted therapy aimed at targeting key molecular signaling pathways is emerging as a novel strategy to treat asthma [62]. Bcl10 may serve as a potential biomarker for testing the activation of NF-kB pathway in asthmatic patients and for asthma targeted therapy, taking into account its role in both airway inflammation and remodeling.

Author Contributions: Conceptualization, R.K.R., R.H. (Rifat Hamoudi), R.H. (Rabih Halwani) and Q.H.; Data curation, R.K.R., M.G. and Z.K.; Formal analysis, R.K.R., K.B. and R.H. (Rabih Halwani); Funding acquisition, B.M., R.H. (Rifat Hamoudi) and Q.H.; Investigation, R.K.R., K.B., M.G., M.Y.H., S.M.I. and R.H. (Rabih Halwani); Methodology, R.K.R., K.B., M.G., S.S.R., Z.K., M.Y.H., R.H. (Rifat Hamoudi) and R.H. (Rabih Halwani); Project administration, R.K.R., K.B. and Q.H.; Resources, R.H. (Rifat Hamoudi) and Q.H.; Supervision, K.B., B.M., S.M.I., R.H. (Rifat Hamoudi), R.H. (Rabih Halwani) and Q.H.; Validation, R.K.R., M.G., S.S.R. and Z.K.; Visualization, R.K.R. and S.S.R.; Writing—original draft, R.K.R.; Writing—review & editing, K.B., M.G., S.S.R., Z.K., M.Y.H., B.M., S.M.I., R.H. (Rifat Hamoudi), R.H. (Rabih Halwani) and Q.H. All authors have read and agreed to the published version of the manuscript.

Funding: This study was supported by the targeted research grant (2101090295), collaborative research grant (22010902103), and competitive research grant (1901090263) from the University of Sharjah, as well as the Tissue Injury and Repair group operational grant (150317), COVID-19 research grant (CoV19-0307) and collaborative research grant (2001090278) to R.H. (Rabih Halwani) from the University of Sharjah. The funders had no role in study design, data collection and analysis, decision to publish, or preparation of the manuscript.

Institutional Review Board Statement: The samples used in this study were collected from the original study that was conducted in accordance with the Declaration of Helsinki, and approved by the MUHC Research Ethics Board with reference number 2003–1879 and BMB-02-039-t.

Informed Consent Statement: Informed consent was obtained from all subjects involved in the study.

Data Availability Statement: The data presented in this study are available within the article.

Acknowledgments: We would like to thank Bushra Mdkhana and Swati Goel for their technical help and valuable support.

Conflicts of Interest: The authors declare no conflict of interest.

References

1. Minshall, E.M.; Leung, D.Y.; Martin, R.J.; Song, Y.L.; Cameron, L.; Ernst, P.; Hamid, Q. Eosinophil-associated TGF-beta1 mRNA expression and airways fibrosis in bronchial asthma. *Am. J. Respir. Cell Mol. Biol.* **1997**, *17*, 326–333. [CrossRef]
2. Vallabhapurapu, S.; Karin, M. Regulation and function of NF-kB transcription factors in the immune system. *Annu. Rev. Immunol.* **2009**, *27*, 693–733. [CrossRef] [PubMed]
3. Gagliardo, R.; Chanez, P.; Mathieu, M.; Bruno, A.; Costanzo, G.; Gougat, C.; Vachier, I.; Bousquet, J.; Bonsignore, G.; Vignola, A.M. Persistent activation of nuclear factor-kappaB signaling pathway in severe uncontrolled asthma. *Am. J. Respir. Crit. Care Med.* **2003**, *168*, 1190–1198. [CrossRef] [PubMed]
4. Dong, J.; Ma, Q. In Vivo Activation and Pro-Fibrotic Function of NF-κB in Fibroblastic Cells during Pulmonary Inflammation and Fibrosis Induced by Carbon Nanotubes. *Front. Pharmacol.* **2019**, *10*, 1140. [CrossRef] [PubMed]
5. McFarland, B.C.; Hong, S.W.; Rajbhandari, R.; Twitty, G.B.; Gray, G.K., Jr.; Yu, H.; Benveniste, E.N.; Nozell, S.E. NF-κB-induced IL-6 ensures STAT3 activation and tumor aggressiveness in glioblastoma. *PLoS ONE* **2013**, *8*, e78728. [CrossRef]
6. Kunsch, C.; Rosen, C.A. NF-kB subunit-specific regulation of the interleukin-8 promoter. *Mol. Cell. Biol.* **1993**, *13*, 6137–6146.
7. Rameshwar, P.; Narayanan, R.; Qian, J.; Denny, T.N.; Colon, C.; Gascon, P. NF-kB as a central mediator in the induction of TGF-beta in monocytes from patients with idiopathic myelofibrosis: An inflammatory response beyond the realm of homeostasis. *J. Immunol.* **2000**, *165*, 2271–2277. [CrossRef]
8. Willis, T.G.; Jadayel, D.M.; Du, M.Q.; Peng, H.; Perry, A.R.; Abdul-Rauf, M.; Price, H.; Karran, L.; Majekodunmi, O.; Wlodarska, I.; et al. Bcl10 is involved in t(1;14)(p22;q32) of MALT B cell lymphoma and mutated in multiple tumor types. *Cell* **1999**, *96*, 35–45. [CrossRef]

9. Lucas, P.C.; Yonezumi, M.; Inohara, N.; McAllister-Lucas, L.M.; Abazeed, M.E.; Chen, F.F.; Yamaoka, S.; Seto, M.; Nunez, G. Bcl10 and MALT1, independent targets of chromosomal translocation in malt lymphoma, cooperate in a novel NF-kB signaling pathway. *J. Biol. Chem.* **2001**, *276*, 19012–19019. [CrossRef]
10. Gaide, O.; Martinon, F.; Micheau, O.; Bonnet, D.; Thome, M.; Tschopp, J. Carma1, a CARD-containing binding partner of Bcl10, induces Bcl10 phosphorylation and NF-kB activation. *FEBS Lett.* **2001**, *496*, 121–127. [CrossRef]
11. Bhatt, D.; Ghosh, S. Regulation of the NF-kB-Mediated Transcription of Inflammatory Genes. *Front. Immunol.* **2014**, *5*, 71. [CrossRef] [PubMed]
12. Ruland, J.; Hartjes, L. CARD-BCL-10-MALT1 signalling in protective and pathological immunity. *Nat. Rev. Immunol.* **2019**, *19*, 118–134. [CrossRef]
13. Chen, Y.; Pappu, B.P.; Zeng, H.; Xue, L.; Morris, S.W.; Lin, X.; Wen, R.; Wang, D. B cell lymphoma 10 is essential for FcepsilonR-mediated degranulation and IL-6 production in mast cells. *J. Immunol.* **2007**, *178*, 49–57. [CrossRef] [PubMed]
14. Klemm, S.; Gutermuth, J.; Hultner, L.; Sparwasser, T.; Behrendt, H.; Peschel, C.; Mak, T.W.; Jakob, T.; Ruland, J. The Bcl10-Malt1 complex segregates Fc epsilon RI-mediated nuclear factor kappa B activation and cytokine production from mast cell degranulation. *J. Exp. Med.* **2006**, *203*, 337–347. [CrossRef] [PubMed]
15. Wang, D.; You, Y.; Lin, P.C.; Xue, L.; Morris, S.W.; Zeng, H.; Wen, R.; Lin, X. Bcl10 plays a critical role in NF-kB activation induced by G protein-coupled receptors. *Proc. Natl. Acad. Sci. USA* **2007**, *104*, 145–150. [CrossRef]
16. McAllister-Lucas, L.M.; Ruland, J.; Siu, K.; Jin, X.; Gu, S.; Kim, D.S.; Kuffa, P.; Kohrt, D.; Mak, T.W.; Nunez, G.; et al. CARMA3/Bcl10/MALT1-dependent NF-kB activation mediates angiotensin II-responsive inflammatory signaling in nonimmune cells. *Proc. Natl. Acad. Sci. USA* **2007**, *104*, 139–144. [CrossRef]
17. Marko, L.; Henke, N.; Park, J.K.; Spallek, B.; Qadri, F.; Balogh, A.; Apel, I.J.; Oravecz-Wilson, K.I.; Choi, M.; Przybyl, L.; et al. Bcl10 mediates angiotensin II-induced cardiac damage and electrical remodeling. *Hypertension* **2014**, *64*, 1032–1039. [CrossRef]
18. Bhattacharyya, S.; Borthakur, A.; Pant, N.; Dudeja, P.K.; Tobacman, J.K. Bcl10 mediates LPS-induced activation of NF-kB and IL-8 in human intestinal epithelial cells. *Am. J. Physiol. Gastrointest. Liver Physiol.* **2007**, *293*, G429–G437. [CrossRef]
19. Broide, D.H.; Lawrence, T.; Doherty, T.; Cho, J.Y.; Miller, M.; McElwain, K.; McElwain, S.; Karin, M. Allergen-induced peribronchial fibrosis and mucus production mediated by IkB kinase beta-dependent genes in airway epithelium. *Proc. Natl. Acad. Sci. USA* **2005**, *102*, 17723–17728. [CrossRef]
20. Schuliga, M. NF-kB Signaling in Chronic Inflammatory Airway Disease. *Biomolecules* **2015**, *5*, 1266–1283. [CrossRef]
21. Panariti, A.; Baglole, C.J.; Sanchez, V.; Eidelman, D.H.; Hussain, S.; Olivenstein, R.; Martin, J.G.; Hamid, Q. Interleukin-17A and vascular remodelling in severe asthma; lack of evidence for a direct role. *Clin. Exp. Allergy* **2018**, *48*, 365–378. [CrossRef] [PubMed]
22. Bigler, J.; Boedigheimer, M.; Schofield, J.P.R.; Skipp, P.J.; Corfield, J.; Rowe, A.; Sousa, A.R.; Timour, M.; Twehues, L.; Hu, X.; et al. A Severe Asthma Disease Signature from Gene Expression Profiling of Peripheral Blood from U-BIOPRED Cohorts. *Am. J. Respir. Crit. Care Med.* **2017**, *195*, 1311–1320. [CrossRef] [PubMed]
23. Poon, A.H.; Choy, D.F.; Chouiali, F.; Ramakrishnan, R.K.; Mahboub, B.; Audusseau, S.; Mogas, A.; Harris, J.M.; Arron, J.R.; Laprise, C.; et al. Increased Autophagy-Related 5 Gene Expression Is Associated with Collagen Expression in the Airways of Refractory Asthmatics. *Front. Immunol.* **2017**, *8*, 355. [CrossRef] [PubMed]
24. Ichikawa, T.; Panariti, A.; Audusseau, S.; Mogas, A.K.; Olivenstein, R.; Chakir, J.; Laviolette, M.; Allakhverdi, Z.; Al Heialy, S.; Martin, J.G.; et al. Effect of bronchial thermoplasty on structural changes and inflammatory mediators in the airways of subjects with severe asthma. *Respir. Med.* **2019**, *150*, 165–172. [CrossRef]
25. Shembade, N.; Harhaj, E.W. Regulation of NF-kB signaling by the A20 deubiquitinase. *Cell. Mol. Immunol.* **2012**, *9*, 123–130. [CrossRef]
26. Ye, H.; Dogan, A.; Karran, L.; Willis, T.G.; Chen, L.; Wlodarska, I.; Dyer, M.J.; Isaacson, P.G.; Du, M.Q. BCL10 expression in normal and neoplastic lymphoid tissue. Nuclear localization in MALT lymphoma. *Am. J. Pathol.* **2000**, *157*, 1147–1154. [CrossRef]
27. Cho, J.S.; Kang, J.H.; Um, J.Y.; Han, I.H.; Park, I.H.; Lee, H.M. Lipopolysaccharide induces pro-inflammatory cytokines and MMP production via TLR4 in nasal polyp-derived fibroblast and organ culture. *PLoS ONE* **2014**, *9*, e90683. [CrossRef]
28. He, Z.; Zhu, Y.; Jiang, H. Toll-like receptor 4 mediates lipopolysaccharide-induced collagen secretion by phosphoinositide3-kinase-Akt pathway in fibroblasts during acute lung injury. *J. Recept. Signal Transduct. Res.* **2009**, *29*, 119–125. [CrossRef]
29. Dong, W.; Liu, Y.; Peng, J.; Chen, L.; Zou, T.; Xiao, H.; Liu, Z.; Li, W.; Bu, Y.; Qi, Y. The IRAK-1-BCL10-MALT1-TRAF6-TAK1 cascade mediates signaling to NF-kB from Toll-like receptor 4. *J. Biol. Chem.* **2006**, *281*, 26029–26040. [CrossRef]
30. Kawai, T.; Akira, S. Signaling to NF-kB by Toll-like receptors. *Trends Mol. Med.* **2007**, *13*, 460–469. [CrossRef]
31. Liu, T.; Zhang, L.; Joo, D.; Sun, S.C. NF-κB signaling in inflammation. *Signal Transduct. Target. Ther.* **2017**, *2*, 17023. [CrossRef] [PubMed]
32. Yum, S.; Li, M.; Fang, Y.; Chen, Z.J. TBK1 recruitment to STING activates both IRF3 and NF-κB that mediate immune defense against tumors and viral infections. *Proc. Natl. Acad. Sci. USA* **2021**, *118*, e2100225118. [CrossRef] [PubMed]
33. Tully, J.E.; Hoffman, S.M.; Lahue, K.G.; Nolin, J.D.; Anathy, V.; Lundblad, L.K.; Daphtary, N.; Aliyeva, M.; Black, K.E.; Dixon, A.E.; et al. Epithelial NF-kB orchestrates house dust mite-induced airway inflammation, hyperresponsiveness, and fibrotic remodeling. *J. Immunol.* **2013**, *191*, 5811–5821. [CrossRef]
34. Edwards, M.R.; Bartlett, N.W.; Clarke, D.; Birrell, M.; Belvisi, M.; Johnston, S.L. Targeting the NF-kB pathway in asthma and chronic obstructive pulmonary disease. *Pharmacol. Ther.* **2009**, *121*, 1–13. [CrossRef] [PubMed]

35. Zhang, Q.; Siebert, R.; Yan, M.; Hinzmann, B.; Cui, X.; Xue, L.; Rakestraw, K.M.; Naeve, C.W.; Beckmann, G.; Weisenburger, D.D.; et al. Inactivating mutations and overexpression of BCL10, a caspase recruitment domain-containing gene, in MALT lymphoma with t(1;14)(p22;q32). *Nat. Genet.* **1999**, *22*, 63–68. [CrossRef] [PubMed]

36. Ramakrishnan, R.K.; Bajbouj, K.; Hachim, M.Y.; Mogas, A.K.; Mahboub, B.; Olivenstein, R.; Hamoudi, R.; Halwani, R.; Hamid, Q. Enhanced mitophagy in bronchial fibroblasts from severe asthmatic patients. *PLoS ONE* **2020**, *15*, e0242695. [CrossRef] [PubMed]

37. Torres, J.M.; Martinez-Barricarte, R.; Garcia-Gomez, S.; Mazariegos, M.S.; Itan, Y.; Boisson, B.; Rholvarez, R.; Jimenez-Reinoso, A.; del Pino, L.; Rodriguez-Pena, R.; et al. Inherited BCL10 deficiency impairs hematopoietic and nonhematopoietic immunity. *J. Clin. Investig.* **2014**, *124*, 5239–5248. [CrossRef]

38. Yan, M.; Lee, J.; Schilbach, S.; Goddard, A.; Dixit, V. mE10, a novel caspase recruitment domain-containing proapoptotic molecule. *J. Biol. Chem.* **1999**, *274*, 10287–10292. [CrossRef]

39. Tian, M.T.; Gonzalez, G.; Scheer, B.; DeFranco, A.L. Bcl10 can promote survival of antigen-stimulated B lymphocytes. *Blood* **2005**, *106*, 2105–2112. [CrossRef]

40. Rueda, D.; Gaide, O.; Ho, L.; Lewkowicz, E.; Niedergang, F.; Hailfinger, S.; Rebeaud, F.; Guzzardi, M.; Conne, B.; Thelen, M.; et al. Bcl10 controls TCR- and FcgammaR-induced actin polymerization. *J. Immunol.* **2007**, *178*, 4373–4384. [CrossRef]

41. Marion, S.; Mazzolini, J.; Herit, F.; Bourdoncle, P.; Kambou-Pene, N.; Hailfinger, S.; Sachse, M.; Ruland, J.; Benmerah, A.; Echard, A.; et al. The NF-kB signaling protein Bcl10 regulates actin dynamics by controlling AP1 and OCRL-bearing vesicles. *Dev. Cell* **2012**, *23*, 954–967. [CrossRef] [PubMed]

42. Symons, M.H.; Mitchison, T.J. Control of actin polymerization in live and permeabilized fibroblasts. *J. Cell Biol.* **1991**, *114*, 503–513. [CrossRef] [PubMed]

43. Lam, D.; Ng, N.; Lee, S.; Batzer, G.; Horner, A.A. Airway house dust extract exposures modify allergen-induced airway hypersensitivity responses by TLR4-dependent and independent pathways. *J. Immunol.* **2008**, *181*, 2925–2932. [CrossRef]

44. Li, X.; Chen, Q.; Chu, C.; You, H.; Jin, M.; Zhao, X.; Zhu, X.; Zhou, W.; Ji, W. Ovalbumin-induced experimental allergic asthma is Toll-like receptor 2 dependent. *Allergy Asthma Proc.* **2014**, *35*, e15–e20. [CrossRef] [PubMed]

45. Paik, Y.H.; Schwabe, R.F.; Bataller, R.; Russo, M.P.; Jobin, C.; Brenner, D.A. Toll-like receptor 4 mediates inflammatory signaling by bacterial lipopolysaccharide in human hepatic stellate cells. *Hepatology* **2003**, *37*, 1043–1055. [CrossRef] [PubMed]

46. Yokoyama, T.; Komori, A.; Nakamura, M.; Takii, Y.; Kamihira, T.; Shimoda, S.; Mori, T.; Fujiwara, S.; Koyabu, M.; Taniguchi, K.; et al. Human intrahepatic biliary epithelial cells function in innate immunity by producing IL-6 and IL-8 via the TLR4-NF-kB and -MAPK signaling pathways. *Liver Int.* **2006**, *26*, 467–476. [CrossRef]

47. Kenyon, N.J.; Ward, R.W.; McGrew, G.; Last, J.A. TGF-beta1 causes airway fibrosis and increased collagen I and III mRNA in mice. *Thorax* **2003**, *58*, 772–777. [CrossRef]

48. Juhl, P.; Bondesen, S.; Hawkins, C.L.; Karsdal, M.A.; Bay-Jensen, A.C.; Davies, M.J.; Siebuhr, A.S. Dermal fibroblasts have different extracellular matrix profiles induced by TGF-β, PDGF and IL-6 in a model for skin fibrosis. *Sci. Rep.* **2020**, *10*, 17300. [CrossRef]

49. Neveu, W.A.; Allard, J.L.; Raymond, D.M.; Bourassa, L.M.; Burns, S.M.; Bunn, J.Y.; Irvin, C.G.; Kaminsky, D.A.; Rincon, M. Elevation of IL-6 in the allergic asthmatic airway is independent of inflammation but associates with loss of central airway function. *Respir. Res.* **2010**, *11*, 28. [CrossRef]

50. Peters, M.C.; Mauger, D.; Ross, K.R.; Phillips, B.; Gaston, B.; Cardet, J.C.; Israel, E.; Levy, B.D.; Phipatanakul, W.; Jarjour, N.N.; et al. Evidence for Exacerbation-Prone Asthma and Predictive Biomarkers of Exacerbation Frequency. *Am. J. Respir. Crit. Care Med.* **2020**, *202*, 973–982. [CrossRef]

51. Kobayashi, T.; Tanaka, K.; Fujita, T.; Umezawa, H.; Amano, H.; Yoshioka, K.; Naito, Y.; Hatano, M.; Kimura, S.; Tatsumi, K.; et al. Bidirectional role of IL-6 signal in pathogenesis of lung fibrosis. *Respir. Res.* **2015**, *16*, 99. [CrossRef] [PubMed]

52. Ordonez, C.L.; Shaughnessy, T.E.; Matthay, M.A.; Fahy, J.V. Increased neutrophil numbers and IL-8 levels in airway secretions in acute severe asthma: Clinical and biologic significance. *Am. J. Respir. Crit. Care Med.* **2000**, *161 Pt 1*, 1185–1190. [CrossRef] [PubMed]

53. Shannon, J.; Ernst, P.; Yamauchi, Y.; Olivenstein, R.; Lemiere, C.; Foley, S.; Cicora, L.; Ludwig, M.; Hamid, Q.; Martin, J.G. Differences in airway cytokine profile in severe asthma compared to moderate asthma. *Chest* **2008**, *133*, 420–426. [CrossRef] [PubMed]

54. Fernando, R.I.; Castillo, M.D.; Litzinger, M.; Hamilton, D.H.; Palena, C. IL-8 signaling plays a critical role in the epithelial-mesenchymal transition of human carcinoma cells. *Cancer Res.* **2011**, *71*, 5296–5306. [CrossRef]

55. Kristan, S.S.; Marc, M.M.; Kern, I.; Flezar, M.; Suskovic, S.; Kosnik, M.; Korosec, P. Airway angiogenesis in stable and exacerbated chronic obstructive pulmonary disease. *Scand. J. Immunol.* **2012**, *75*, 109–114. [CrossRef]

56. Kuo, P.L.; Hsu, Y.L.; Huang, M.S.; Chiang, S.L.; Ko, Y.C. Bronchial epithelium-derived IL-8 and RANTES increased bronchial smooth muscle cell migration and proliferation by Kruppel-like factor 5 in areca nut-mediated airway remodeling. *Toxicol. Sci.* **2011**, *121*, 177–190. [CrossRef]

57. Halwani, R.; Al-Muhsen, S.; Al-Jahdali, H.; Hamid, Q. Role of transforming growth factor-β in airway remodeling in asthma. *Am. J. Respir. Cell Mol. Biol.* **2011**, *44*, 127–133. [CrossRef]

58. Michał, P.; Konrad, S.; Piotr, K. TGF-β gene polimorphisms as risk factors for asthma control among clinic patients. *J. Inflamm.* **2021**, *18*, 28. [CrossRef]

59. Chakir, J.; Shannon, J.; Molet, S.; Fukakusa, M.; Elias, J.; Laviolette, M.; Boulet, L.P.; Hamid, Q. Airway remodeling-associated mediators in moderate to severe asthma: Effect of steroids on TGF-beta, IL-11, IL-17, and type I and type III collagen expression. *J. Allergy Clin. Immunol.* **2003**, *111*, 1293–1298. [CrossRef]
60. Klemm, S.; Zimmermann, S.; Peschel, C.; Mak, T.W.; Ruland, J. Bcl10 and Malt1 control lysophosphatidic acid-induced NF-kB activation and cytokine production. *Proc. Natl. Acad. Sci. USA* **2007**, *104*, 134–138. [CrossRef]
61. Barnes, P.J. Corticosteroid effects on cell signalling. *Eur. Respir. J.* **2006**, *27*, 413–426. [CrossRef] [PubMed]
62. Athari, S.S. Targeting cell signaling in allergic asthma. *Signal Transduct. Target. Ther.* **2019**, *4*, 45. [CrossRef] [PubMed]

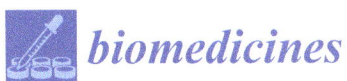

Article

Assessing the Anti-Inflammatory Effects of an Orally Dosed Enzymatically Liberated Fish Oil in a House Dust Model of Allergic Asthma

Crawford Currie [1,*], Bomi Framroze [1], Dave Singh [2,3], Simon Lea [2,3], Christian Bjerknes [1] and Erland Hermansen [1,4]

[1]   Hofseth BioCare, Kipervikgata 13, 6003 Ålesund, Norway
[2]   Division of Infection, Immunity and Respiratory Medicine, School of Biological Sciences, Faculty of Biology, Medicine and Health, Manchester Academic Health Science Centre, The University of Manchester, Manchester M13 9PL, UK
[3]   The Medicines Evaluation Unit, Manchester University NHS Foundation Trust, Manchester M23 9QZ, UK
[4]   Department of Clinical Medicine, University of Bergen, 5007 Bergen, Norway
*   Correspondence: cc@hofsethbiocare.no

Citation: Currie, C.; Framroze, B.; Singh, D.; Lea, S.; Bjerknes, C.; Hermansen, E. Assessing the Anti-Inflammatory Effects of an Orally Dosed Enzymatically Liberated Fish Oil in a House Dust Model of Allergic Asthma. *Biomedicines* 2022, 10, 2574. https://doi.org/10.3390/biomedicines10102574

Academic Editor: Stanisława Bazan-Socha

Received: 28 August 2022
Accepted: 11 October 2022
Published: 14 October 2022

Publisher's Note: MDPI stays neutral with regard to jurisdictional claims in published maps and institutional affiliations.

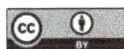

Copyright: © 2022 by the authors. Licensee MDPI, Basel, Switzerland. This article is an open access article distributed under the terms and conditions of the Creative Commons Attribution (CC BY) license (https:// creativecommons.org/licenses/by/ 4.0/).

Abstract: Eosinophils are a major driver of inflammation in a number of human diseases, including asthma. Biologic therapies targeting IL-5 have enabled better control of severe eosinophilic asthma, but no such advances have been made for enhancing the control of moderate asthma. However, a number of moderate asthma sufferers remain troubled by unresolved symptoms, treatment side effects, or both. OmeGo, an enzymatically liberated fish oil, has demonstrated antioxidant and anti-inflammatory properties including the reduction of eosinophilia. A house dust mite model of induced asthma in mice was utilized in this study, and OmeGo showed a significant reduction in eosinophilic lung and systemic inflammation and reduced lung remodelling compared to cod liver oil. The CRTH2 antagonist fevipiprant showed an anti-inflammatory profile similar to that of OmeGo. OmeGo has the potential to be a pragmatic, cost-effective co-treatment for less severe forms of eosinophilic asthma. Proof-of-concept studies are planned.

Keywords: allergy; asthma; eosinophils; immune health; natural therapeutics

1. Introduction

Eosinophils are well recognised as important drivers of a number of inflammatory diseases in humans, including asthma. Biologic therapies targeting cytokines involved in the activation of eosinophils have been a major advance in the management of eosinophilic asthma [1]; however, for milder forms of asthma, there have been no new additions to the treatment armamentarium for a number of years.

Polyunsaturated fatty acids (PUFAs) contained in the oil fraction of fresh fish provide anti-inflammatory and antioxidant benefits important for the maintenance of good health [2]. Observational and epidemiological studies indicate that regular fish consumption can have wide ranging benefits on human health, including the cardiovascular and respiratory systems. Indeed, changing dietary habits have seen a decline in fish consumption and an increase in the prevalence of asthma and allergic disease in Western countries [3–5]. To compensate for this, dietary supplementation with omega-3 fish oil is frequently used to try to attain the health benefits of consuming fresh fish. Fish oil PUFAs are known to be metabolized into specialized pro-resolving mediators (SPMs), which provide broad inflammation-resolving effects [6]. Whilst trials of omega-3 supplementation suggest a potential to reduce airway inflammation and improve lung function, the effects have been variable [7–10]. However, there is evidence that whole fish consumption during pregnancy and in young children can reduce the risk of developing allergic conditions, a benefit likely derived from the range of anti-inflammatory factors naturally contained in fish oil and not just omega-3 [11].

The potential to reduce the burden of asthma via a dietary intervention could be beneficial for sufferers and healthcare systems alike. This trial, therefore, assessed the extent to which oral OmeGo, an intervention more closely related to eating whole fish, could reduce lung inflammation in a standard animal model of induced asthma. OmeGo is minimally processed whole fish oil with low levels of oxidation and free fatty acids and contains all of the polyunsaturated acids found in whole fish, not just omega-3. Previous in vitro work demonstrated OmeGo to significantly reduce eosinophilic effector function, whereas this was not the case for oils containing either omega-3 alone or omega-3 and astaxanthin [12], and a similar comparative profile between OmeGo and omega-3 oils was also demonstrated in animal models of induced eosinophilia [13]. As these previous in vivo studies administered OmeGo by the intraperitoneal route, this paper describes experiments focused now on oral delivery, to provide information that is more relevant to its use in humans. Furthermore, we evaluated lung remodelling as well as inflammation to further assess the potential to improve health outcomes compared to omega-3 supplementation alone [14].

2. Materials and Methods

The study utilized an HDM model of asthma in mice to compare the impact of 7 days of treatment with OmeGo compared to either fevipiprant or cod liver oil on lung and serum inflammatory markers and lung fibrosis.

The study was conducted according to GLP guidelines and in accordance with the laws and regulations of India, where the studies were performed. The study was approved by the Institutional Animal Ethics Committee (proposal number 214429) before the start of the study. The health status of the animals was assessed by a veterinarian, and all were noted to be in good health. The animals were acclimated to the laboratory conditions, and randomisation to the five treatment groups occurred the day before the trial commenced. The five groups were: no treatment (negative control), 0.5 mL of cod liver oil (vehicle control), 18 mg or 32 mg of OmeGo (test item), or 2 mg fevipiprant (positive control), respectively.

As per the experimental procedure shown in Figure 1, the study involved 50 healthy young adult female mice of 10 animals per group.

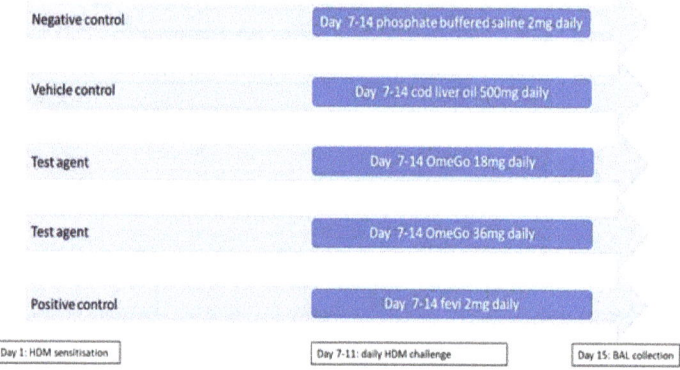

Figure 1. Experimental design. The mice were randomised into five groups of 10 animals per group. On day 1, animals were anaesthetised and sensitised intranasally with 1 μg HDM protein in 40 μL phosphate buffered saline (PBS). Following this, the mice were challenged daily with 10 μg HDM protein intranasally from day 7 to day 11. Oral interventions of PBS, cod liver oil, OmeGo low or high dose, or fevipiprant were given on days 7–14. BAL fluid was collected on day 15.

On day 1, the mice were anaesthetized using ketamine (100 mg/kg) and xylazine (10 mg/kg) given via intraperitoneal injection. HDM sensitisation was achieved with the intranasal application of 1 µg HDM protein in 40 µL phosphate buffered saline (PBS). Subsequently, daily intranasal HDM challenge was performed from day 7 to day 11 using 10 µg HDM protein in 40 µL PBS.

Between days 7 and 14, the mice received either cod liver oil, OmeGo, or fevipiprant treatment, all given orally. The fifth group of mice received no treatment (negative control). On day 15, the mice were anaesthetised and their trachea exposed to enable bronchoalveolar lavage (BAL) fluid collection using 3 mL of PBS containing 1 mM EDTA. The spleen was also removed from each animal, frozen and subsequently assessed for the extent of eosinophilia.

After collection, the BAL fluid was centrifuged ($400 \times g$ at 4 °C for 7 min). The resulting cell pellet was collected, stored at -20 °C and subsequently analysed for total leucocyte cell count and differential cell count to provide eosinophil, neutrophil, lymphocyte and alveolar macrophage levels. A hemocytometer was used to measure total cell counts in the cell pellets and spleen tissue. For total leukocyte counts, the resuspended cell pellets in 50 µL phosphate buffered saline (PBS) were measured using a hemocytometer [15].

Serum HDM-specific IgE was assessed using the antigen-capture ELISA method [16]. Total lung collagen content was assessed using the calorimetric Quickzyme Total Assay Kit. Collagen content was normalized to the weight of each lung to be able to compare the total collagen value across groups.

Further details are contained in Appendix A. All analyses were performed in duplicate.

The animals were observed in the morning and evening to check for morbidity and mortality and were weighed during randomisation and on day 1, day 7 and day 15 of the study.

Necropsy at end of treatment was according to the guidelines of the CPSCEA committee.

The number of animals selected was guided by our previous HDM work, in which OmeGo was dosed intraperitoneally (IP) in five animals per group [12] and showed a significant 42% reduction in serum eosinophil count. To be conservative, in case of greater inter-animal responses with oral OmeGo compared to IP dosing, we chose to double the size to 10 animals per group in the present study. All raw data from this study were analysed using "Sigma Plot" v14 statistical software, and this was used to calculate the mean and standard deviations. All continuous data were checked for their homogeneity using the Shapiro–Wilk test. Once homogeneity was confirmed, the data were analysed using ANOVA, and data showing significance in their variances were subjected to unpaired *t*-test. *p* values ≤ 0.05 were deemed statistically significant.

3. Results

The initial analysis assessed vehicle control (cod liver oil) versus negative control. This showed non-significant, small to negligible numeric differences for total BAL leukocyte count, BAL eosinophil count and percent eosinophil in spleen tissue ($p = 0.638$, 0.382 and 0.314, respectively). All other analyses also showed minimal numeric differences between the two groups (vehicle and negative control). All efficacy analyses were, therefore, based in comparison to vehicle control, cod liver oil, rather than negative control.

At the end of the study, total leukocyte count in the BAL fluid showed a statistically significant decrease in the high-dose OmeGo ($p < 0.05$) and fevipiprant ($p < 0.01$) groups compared to cod liver oil. Analyses of individual cell counts, namely eosinophils, neutrophils, macrophages and lymphocytes, were undertaken and are described below.

None of the animals showed any treatment related ill-effects (morbidity or mortality), and there were no statistically significant differences in body weight in any of the treatment groups compared to the cod liver oil group (vehicle control). There was also no significant change in weight during the trial compared to baseline (day 1).

3.1. Cell Counts

3.1.1. Eosinophils

The impact of OmeGo and fevipiprant on lung and splenic eosinophilia was assessed at the end of the trial. Compared to cod liver oil, a significant 7% ($p \leq 0.05$) and 10% ($p \leq 0.01$) decrease in BAL eosinophils was seen with low- and high-dose OmeGo, respectively, and an 18% ($p \leq 0.001$) decrease with fevipiprant (Figure 2). Splenic eosinophilia was significantly reduced by 16% and 17% (both $p \leq 0.05$) with low- and high-dose OmeGo, respectively, and by 23% ($p \leq 0.01$) with fevipiprant (Figure 3).

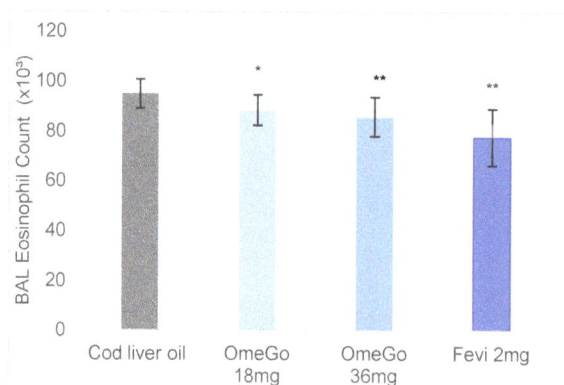

Figure 2. Eosinophil cell count in bronchoalveolar lavage (BAL) fluid of mice at study end, illustrating mean eosinophil count with cod liver oil (vehicle control), two doses of OmeGo, or fevipiprant. Cells were quantified with a hemocytometer. ** denotes $p < 0.01$, * denotes $p < 0.05$.

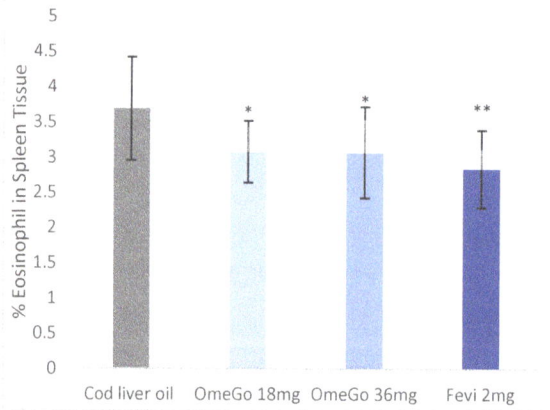

Figure 3. Percentage of eosinophils in spleen tissue of mice at study end with cod liver oil (vehicle control), two doses of OmeGo, or fevipiprant. Cells were quantified with a hemocytometer. ** denotes $p < 0.01$, * denotes $p < 0.05$.

3.1.2. Neutrophils

By the end of the study, HDM sensitisation had resulted in higher lung neutrophils in the cod liver oil group compared to the OmeGo and fevipiprant groups. Low-dose and high-dose OmeGo reduced bronchoalveolar neutrophil count by 9% and 11% (both $p \leq 0.05$), respectively, while in the fevipiprant group there was an 18% reduction ($p = 0.01$) versus cod liver oil (Figure 4).

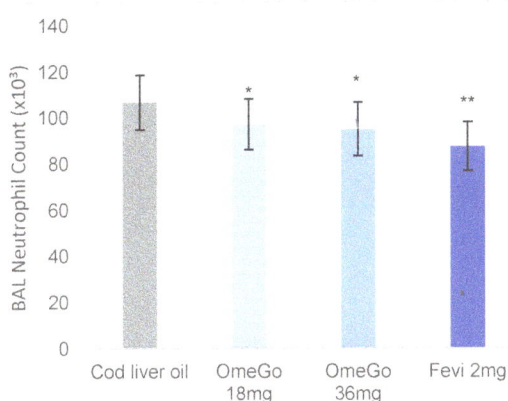

Figure 4. Cell count neutrophils in bronchoalveolar lavage (BAL) fluid of mice at end of study, illustrating mean neutrophil count with cod liver oil, two doses of OmeGo, or fevipiprant. Cells were quantified using a hemocytometer. p values less than 0.01 are summarized using two asterisks, and p values less than 0.05 are summarized with one asterisk.

3.1.3. Macrophages and Lymphocytes

Unfortunately, the HDM sensitisation regimen employed in this study did not induce an increase in lymphocytes in the BAL fluid at study end, with no numeric difference noted between any of the groups, including negative control. OmeGo and fevipiprant showed a numeric reduction in alveolar macrophages of 14%, but this difference was not significant.

3.2. Cytokines

Low-dose OmeGo significantly reduced IL-13 by 11%, and high-dose OmeGo drove a 24% reduction in serum IL-13 levels ($p < 0.01$) and a 17% reduction in IL-4 ($p < 0.05$), all compared to cod liver oil. OmeGo did not significantly impact IL-6, IL-17A or CXCL-1 levels. Fevipiprant significantly reduced CXCL-1 (32%, $p < 0.001$), IL-4 (58%, $p < 0.001$), IL-6 (18%, $p < 0.05$) and IL-13 (63%, $p < 0.001$) but not IL-10 or IL-17A. In terms of changes in serum IgE levels, the 12% reduction with OmeGo and the 6% reduction with fevipiprant were non-significant (Figure 5).

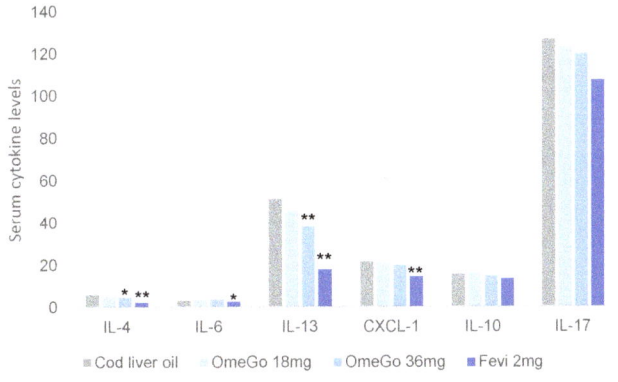

Figure 5. Mean serum cytokine levels at study end with cod liver oil, two doses OmeGo, or fevipiprant. ** denotes $p < 0.01$, * denotes $p < 0.05$.

3.3. Lung Collagen Content

Total lung collagen content was significantly reduced by OmeGo and fevipiprant compared to vehicle control: a 4% and 5% reduction, respectively, with low- and high-dose OmeGo ($p < 0.05$) and an 11% reduction with fevipiprant ($p < 0.01$) at study end (Figure 6). No other histopathological assessments of the lung were undertaken.

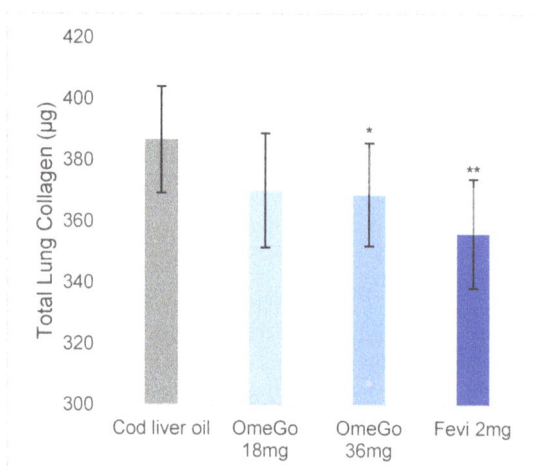

Figure 6. Mean total lung collagen content at the end of the study with cod liver oil, two doses of OmeGo, or fevipiprant, assessed using the calorimetric Quickzyme Total Assay Kit. ** denotes $p < 0.01$, * denotes $p < 0.05$.

4. Discussion

In this study, oral OmeGo significantly reduced lung and splenic eosinophilia compared to cod liver oil (vehicle control) in a house dust mite (HDM) mouse model of asthma. These results are consistent with previous work that assessed OmeGo's modulation of eosinophil function, including in vivo studies with OmeGo dosed via intraperitoneal injection [12] and in vitro work in human eosinophils [13].

This study further characterised OmeGo's modulation of inflammatory mediators relevant to asthma pathophysiology. Beyond eosinophil modulation, oral OmeGo significantly reduced BAL (bronchoalveolar lavage) neutrophil levels and total lung collagen content. Airway remodelling is a typical feature in persistent asthma, contributing to airflow limitation. Collagen deposition occurs early in the natural history of asthma [17,18] and is correlated with disease severity [19]. Allergen exposure causes an increase in airway remodelling markers in patients with asthma [20], with IL-13 an underlying driver of the process. Thus, OmeGo's significant impact on IL-13 provides biologic plausibility to this initial result in assessing OmeGo's potential to reduce lung remodelling [21].

IL-4 is an important driver in the initiation of lung inflammation in asthma, including Th2 cell proliferation and IgE synthesis [22,23], and high-dose OmeGo significantly reduced IL-4 by 17% ($p < 0.05$); however, the numeric reduction in serum IgE did not quite achieve significance.

The house dust mite is a common air-borne allergen, with up to 85% of asthma patients being allergic to HDM [24]. The HDM model of induced asthma is, therefore, commonly used to mimic the inflammatory and allergic milieu found in many asthma patients, namely eosinophilia, raised IgE levels and other inflammatory mediators associated with Type 2 inflammation as well as neutrophilia [24,25]. Consistent with the published literature, HDM sensitisation in our study resulted in a leukocytosis driven by eosinophils and neutrophils. We saw no impact on lymphocyte numbers and only a limited impact on macrophage numbers, and previous work indicates that longer duration HDM models are more likely to induce a significant expansion of macrophage numbers [26] and drive greater fold increases overall in leukocyte recruitment [27,28].

A 5-week HDM mouse model of induced asthma demonstrated a 500-fold increase in BAL eosinophils, equating to 1.5 million eosinophils/mL on flow cytometry [27]. In contrast, a short duration, higher HDM dose (total of 300 μg) in vivo study resulted in a BAL eosinophilia of around 350,000 cells/mL in the saline control group, which was almost totally resolved with intraperitoneal dexamethasone and reduced by approximately 50% with CRTH2 antagonist treatment [29]. We utilized a standard short-exposure HDM model protocol with a total HDM challenge dose of 50 μg; this resulted in an eosinophil count of 97,400 cells/mL in the negative control group (saline). This lower level of induced leukocytosis may explain the smaller magnitude of cell count reductions with CRTH2 antagonism (fevipiprant) in our study, such as a 20% decrease in eosinophilia, compared to previous ex vivo studies with CRTH2 antagonists. This methodological difference may also have influenced the magnitude of effect observed with OmeGo.

The CRTH2 receptor is a well recognised activator of eosinophil-driven inflammation [30,31], hence our choice of the CRTH2 antagonist (fevipiprant) as a positive control. The effects of fevipiprant and OmeGo were generally similar with regard to lung and systemic inflammation, with significant reductions in both eosinophil and neutrophil counts as well as total lung collagen. CRTH2 antagonists are known to inhibit experimental allergen challenge responses in humans [32,33], and the similarity of the effects observed in this in vivo animal model indicates potential for OmeGo to attenuate allergic responses in humans.

Vehicle control, consisting of 0.5 mL cod liver oil, containing DHA (docosahexanoic acid) and EPA (eicosapentaenoic acid) omega-3, did not show an effect on any of the endpoints compared to negative control. This contrasting effect between OmeGo and cod liver oil is consistent with our previous work on the modulation of eosinophil function with OmeGo. This effect appears to be driven by a bioactive fraction not present in highly processed supplements [12,13]. The variable outcomes seen with omega-3 supplementation compared to the consumption of fresh fish [10] suggests that minimal processing helps to retain the full bioactivity of the individual PUFAs to provide health benefits associated with eating fresh fish.

Our study has a number of limitations. By using a shorter-duration HDM exposure model, we did not elicit an elevation in lymphocytes and only a moderate increase in macrophage count, which, therefore, limits the insights on the potential of the interventions to modulate the activity of these immune cells. In addition, analyzing other mediators of inflammation would have been valuable, but there was insufficient serum to analyse changes in IL-5, a cytokine involved in eosinophil activation and recruitment. The elevation of IL-17 was not modulated by OmeGo, and other analyses for inflammatory mediators such as the impact on IL-1β and granulocyte-macrophage colony-stimulating factor (GM-CSF) in the BAL could have provided useful insights into OmeGo's impact on lung barrier function and provided mechanistic explanations for the modulation of lung collagen deposition. Investigation of primary inflammatory pathway mediators, such as nuclear factor kappa B (NFκB), GATA-3, and peroxisome proliferator-activated receptor gamma (PPARγ), would have been valuable to assess the means by which OmeGo reduced lung inflammation. Additionally, further immunohistochemistry work, including assessments of lung damage and collagen deposition, could provide more insights regarding pharmacological effects. Nevertheless, the study builds on previous work and elucidates further the anti-inflammatory action of the whole fish oil, OmeGo.

5. Conclusions

OmeGo, dosed orally, significantly reduced lung and systemic inflammation in an HDM mouse model of induced asthma. Reductions in eosinophils and neutrophils were accompanied by a reduction in total lung collagen, suggesting the potential to moderate airway inflammation and remodelling and help maintain lung function. Human studies are planned in subjects with mild to moderate asthma to assess whether these results can translate into improved asthma control with OmeGo added to standard-of-care treatment.

Author Contributions: Conceptualization, B.F. and C.C.; methodology, B.F.; formal analysis, S.L. and E.H.; data curation, B.F. and C.C.; writing—original draft preparation, C.C. and D.S.; writing—review and editing, B.F., C.B., E.H., D.S. and C.C.; visualization, C.C. and D.S.; infographic, S.L.; project administration, B.F.; funding acquisition, B.F. All authors have read and agreed to the published version of the manuscript.

Funding: This research was funded by Hofseth BioCare, Kipervikgata 13, Ålesund, 6003, Norway, funding number R_21_224_003.

Institutional Review Board Statement: The animal study protocol was approved by the Institutional Animal Ethics Committee (IAEC proposal number SF_21_44_29).

Informed Consent Statement: Not applicable.

Data Availability Statement: The raw data, original Project Plan, original final report and a sample of the test items are retained in the Archives of sa-FORD (Sanctuary for Research and Development). Plot number V-10, MIDC Industrial Area, Taloja, Dist: Raigad 410 208, India for a period of 5 years.

Conflicts of Interest: D.S. and S.L. declare no conflict of interest. C.C., B.F., C.B. and E.H. are employees of Hofseth BioCare.

Appendix A

The animals were allocated to different test groups by a manual randomization method. Individual body weights of allocated animals were within 20% of the group means, and the body weights of the animals were analysed statistically to rule out significant differences between the groups before administration of the HDM extract. Following allocation to the experimental groups, each animal was uniquely identified by turmeric fur marking/micro-toe pad tattooing and colour-coded cage card labelled with project number, project type, test system, sex, dose, group, animal number, date of treatment, and experiment start and completion dates.

The mice were housed in groups of five animals per individually ventilated cages. Corn cob, prepared from pure corn and dried, freed of dust and sterilized, was procured from an approved vendor and used as bedding material. The bedding was replaced as often as necessary to keep the animals and their surroundings clean and dry. The room temperature was maintained between 21 °C to 22.5 °C and relative humidity at 50.9% to 66.8% for the duration of the study. Artificial light was set to give a cycle of 12 h light and 12 h dark. Adequately filtered air was provided with at least 12 changes per hour. The animals were offered a conventional laboratory rodent diet ad libitum supplied by Nutrivet Life Sciences, and Aquaguard filtered drinking water was provided ad libitum.

For the differential leukocyte counts, including eosinophil count, 80 μL of resuspended cell pellets were stained using the HEMA3 stain set (Fisher Scientific), and centrifuged using a StatSpin Cytofuge 2 (Beckman Coulter).

Ninety-six well plates coated with 5 μg HDM in 100 μL coating buffer and incubated for 12 h at 4 °C were blocked with 200 μL/well of assay diluent. Precleared serum samples (Protein G Sepharose beads) were washed with PBS, and a 50 μL aliquot of undiluted serum was added to each well and incubated at 4 °C overnight. The wells were washed with PBS; 100 μL of biotin-anti-mouse IgE (Sigma, Virginia Beach, VA, USA) was added and incubated for 1 h, followed by a 30 min incubation with avidin-horse radish peroxidase. TMB substrate solution (100 μL) was added to each well and incubated in the dark for 30 min. The reaction was stopped with 2 N sulphuric acid. Optical densities, normalized to saline controls, were read at 450 nm using a Varian Cary 50 spectrophotometer.

References

1. McGregor, M.C.; Krings, J.G.; Nair, P.; Castro, M. Role of Biologics in Asthma. *Am. J. Respir. Crit. Care Med.* **2019**, *199*, 433–445. [CrossRef] [PubMed]
2. Calder, P.C. Marine omega-3 fatty acids and inflammatory processes: Effects, mechanisms and clinical relevance. *Biochim. Biophys. Acta* **2015**, *1851*, 469–484. [CrossRef] [PubMed]
3. De Luis, D.A.; Armentia, A.; Aller, R.; Asensio, A.; Sedano, E.; Izaola, O.; Cuellar, L. Dietary intake in patients with asthma: A case control study. *Nutrition* **2005**, *21*, 320–324. [CrossRef]
4. Denny, S.I.; Thompson, R.L.; Margetts, B.M. Dietary factors in the pathogenesis of asthma and chronic obstructive pulmonary disease. *Curr. Allergy Asthma. Rep.* **2003**, *3*, 130–136. [CrossRef] [PubMed]
5. Li, J.; Xun, P.; Zamora, D.; Sood, A.; Liu, K.; Daviglus, M.; Iribarren, C.; Jacobs, D., Jr.; Shikany, J.M.; He, K. Intakes of long-chain omega-3 (n-3) PUFAs and fish in relation to incidence of asthma among American young adults: The CARDIA study. *Am. J. Clin. Nutr.* **2013**, *97*, 173–178. [CrossRef] [PubMed]
6. Regidor, P.A.; Mueller, A.; Sailer, M.; Gonzalez Santos, F.; Rizo, J.M.; Egea, F.M. Chronic Inflammation in PCOS: The Potential Benefits of Specialized Pro-Resolving Lipid Mediators (SPMs) in the Improvement of the Resolutive Response. *Int. J. Mol. Sci.* **2020**, *22*, 384. [CrossRef] [PubMed]
7. Brannan, J.D.; Bood, J.; Alkhabaz, A.; Balgoma, D.; Otis, J.; Delin, I.; Dahlén, B.; Wheelock, C.E.; Nair, P.; Dahlén, S.E.; et al. The effect of omega-3 fatty acids on bronchial hyperresponsiveness, sputum eosinophilia, and mast cell mediators in asthma. *Chest* **2015**, *147*, 397–405. [CrossRef]
8. Mickleborough, T.D.; Lindley, M.R.; Ionescu, A.A.; Fly, A.D. Protective effect of fish oil supplementation on exercise-induced bronchoconstriction in asthma. *Chest* **2006**, *129*, 39–49. [CrossRef] [PubMed]
9. Schubert, R.; Kitz, R.; Beermann, C.; Rose, M.A.; Lieb, A.; Sommerer, P.C.; Moskovits, J.; Alberternst, H.; Böhles, H.J.; Schulze, J.; et al. Effect of n-3 polyunsaturated fatty acids in asthma after low-dose allergen challenge. *Int. Arch. Allergy Immunol.* **2009**, *148*, 321–329. [CrossRef]
10. Hardy, M.S.; Kekic, A.; Graybill, N.L.; Lancaster, Z.R. A systematic review of the association between fish oil supplementation and the development of asthma exacerbations. *SAGE Open Med.* **2016**, *4*, 2050312116666216. [CrossRef]
11. Zhang, G.Q.; Liu, B.; Li, J.; Luo, C.Q.; Zhang, Q.; Chen, J.L.; Sinha, A.; Li, Z.Y. Fish intake during pregnancy or infancy and allergic outcomes in children: A systematic review and meta-analysis. *Pediatr. Allergy Immunol.* **2017**, *28*, 152–161. [CrossRef]
12. Currie, C.; Framroze, B.; Singh, D.P.; Sharma, D.; Bjerknes, C.; Hermansen, E. Pharmacological evaluation of the effects of enzymatically liberated fish oil on eosinophilic inflammation in animal models. *Biotechnol. Appl. Biochem.* **2022**, *69*, 1723–1732. [CrossRef] [PubMed]
13. Framroze, B.; Heggdal, H. An in vitro study to explore the modulation of eosinophil effector function in human allergic peripheral blood eosinophils using enzymatically extracted salmonid oil. *Funct. Foods Health Dis.* **2020**, *10*, 357. [CrossRef]
14. Yang, H.; Xun, P.; He, K. Fish and fish oil intake in relation to risk of asthma: A systematic review and meta-analysis. *PLoS ONE* **2013**, *8*, e80048. [CrossRef]
15. Penton, P.C.; Wang, X.; Amatullah, H.; Cooper, J.; Godri, K.; North, M.L.; Khanna, N.; Scott, J.A.; Chow, C.W. Spleen tyrosine kinase inhibition attenuates airway hyperresponsiveness and pollution-induced enhanced airway response in a chronic mouse model of asthma. *J. Allergy Clin. Immunol.* **2013**, *131*, 512–520.e10. [CrossRef] [PubMed]
16. Salehi, S.; Wang, X.; Juvet, S.; Scott, J.A.; Chow, C.W. Syk Regulates Neutrophilic Airway Hyper-Responsiveness in a Chronic Mouse Model of Allergic Airways Inflammation. *PLoS ONE* **2017**, *12*, e0163614. [CrossRef] [PubMed]
17. Turato, G.; Barbato, A.; Baraldo, S.; Zanin, M.E.; Bazzan, E.; Lokar-Oliani, K.; Calabrese, F.; Panizzolo, C.; Snijders, D.; Maestrelli, P.; et al. Nonatopic children with multitrigger wheezing have airway pathology comparable to atopic asthma. *Am. J. Respir. Crit. Care Med.* **2008**, *178*, 476–482. [CrossRef]
18. Barbato, A.; Turato, G.; Baraldo, S.; Bazzan, E.; Calabrese, F.; Panizzolo, C.; Zanin, M.E.; Zuin, R.; Maestrelli, P.; Fabbri, L.M.; et al. Epithelial damage and angiogenesis in the airways of children with asthma. *Am. J. Respir. Crit. Care Med.* **2006**, *174*, 975–981. [CrossRef] [PubMed]
19. Chetta, A.; Foresi, A.; Del Donno, M.; Bertorelli, G.; Pesci, A.; Olivieri, D. Airways remodeling is a distinctive feature of asthma and is related to severity of disease. *Chest* **1997**, *111*, 852–857. [CrossRef]
20. Grainge, C.L.; Lau, L.C.; Ward, J.A.; Dulay, V.; Lahiff, G.; Wilson, S.; Holgate, S.; Davies, D.E.; Howarth, P.H. Effect of bronchoconstriction on airway remodeling in asthma. *N. Engl. J. Med.* **2011**, *364*, 2006–2015. [CrossRef]
21. Zhu, Z.; Homer, R.J.; Wang, Z.; Chen, Q.; Geba, G.P.; Wang, J.; Zhang, Y.; Elias, J.A. Pulmonary expression of interleukin-13 causes inflammation, mucus hypersecretion, subepithelial fibrosis, physiologic abnormalities, and eotaxin production. *J. Clin. Investig.* **1999**, *103*, 779–788. [CrossRef] [PubMed]
22. Brusselle, G.G.; Maes, T.; Bracke, K.R. Eosinophils in the spotlight: Eosinophilic airway inflammation in nonallergic asthma. *Nat. Med.* **2013**, *19*, 977–979. [CrossRef] [PubMed]
23. Tepper, R.I.; Levinson, D.A.; Stanger, B.Z.; Campos-Torres, J.; Abbas, A.K.; Leder, P. IL-4 induces allergic-like inflammatory disease and alters T cell development in transgenic mice. *Cell* **1990**, *62*, 457–467. [CrossRef]
24. Gregory, L.G.; Lloyd, C.M. Orchestrating house dust mite-associated allergy in the lung. *Trends Immunol.* **2011**, *32*, 402–411. [CrossRef]

25. Plantinga, M.; Guilliams, M.; Vanheerswynghels, M.; Deswarte, K.; Branco-Madeira, F.; Toussaint, W.; Vanhoutte, L.; Neyt, K.; Killeen, N.; Malissen, B.; et al. Conventional and monocyte-derived CD11b(+) dendritic cells initiate and maintain T helper 2 cell-mediated immunity to house dust mite allergen. *Immunity* **2013**, *38*, 322–335. [CrossRef]
26. Woo, L.N.; Guo, W.Y.; Wang, X.; Young, A.; Salehi, S.; Hin, A.; Zhang, Y.; Scott, J.A.; Chow, C.W. A 4-Week Model of House Dust Mite (HDM) Induced Allergic Airways Inflammation with Airway Remodeling. *Sci. Rep.* **2018**, *8*, 6925. [CrossRef] [PubMed]
27. Ulrich, K.; Hincks, J.S.; Walsh, R.; Wetterstrand, E.M.; Fidock, M.D.; Sreckovic, S.; Lamb, D.J.; Douglas, G.J.; Yeadon, M.; Perros-Huguet, C.; et al. Anti-inflammatory modulation of chronic airway inflammation in the murine house dust mite model. *Pulm. Pharmacol. Ther.* **2008**, *21*, 637–647. [CrossRef]
28. Piyadasa, H.; Altieri, A.; Basu, S.; Schwartz, J.; Halayko, A.J.; Mookherjee, N. Biosignature for airway inflammation in a house dust mite-challenged murine model of allergic asthma. *Biol. Open* **2016**, *5*, 112–121. [CrossRef] [PubMed]
29. Kaila, N.; Huang, A.; Moretto, A.; Follows, B.; Janz, K.; Lowe, M.; Thomason, J.; Mansour, T.S.; Hubeau, C.; Page, K.; et al. Diazine indole acetic acids as potent, selective, and orally bioavailable antagonists of chemoattractant receptor homologous molecule expressed on Th2 cells (CRTH2) for the treatment of allergic inflammatory diseases. *J. Med. Chem.* **2012**, *55*, 5088–5109. [CrossRef]
30. Kupczyk, M.; Kuna, P. Targeting the PGD(2)/CRTH2/DP1 Signaling Pathway in Asthma and Allergic Disease: Current Status and Future Perspectives. *Drugs* **2017**, *77*, 1281–1294. [CrossRef]
31. Singh, D.; Ravi, A.; Southworth, T. CRTH2 antagonists in asthma: Current perspectives. *Clin. Pharmacol.* **2017**, *9*, 165–173. [CrossRef] [PubMed]
32. Singh, D.; Cadden, P.; Hunter, M.; Pearce Collins, L.; Perkins, M.; Pettipher, R.; Townsend, E.; Vinall, S.; O'Connor, B. Inhibition of the asthmatic allergen challenge response by the CRTH2 antagonist OC000459. *Eur. Respir. J.* **2012**, *41*, 46–52. [CrossRef] [PubMed]
33. Diamant, Z.; Sidharta, P.N.; Singh, D.; O'Connor, B.J.; Zuiker, R.; Leaker, B.R.; Silkey, M.; Dingemanse, J. Setipiprant, a selective CRTH2 antagonist, reduces allergen-induced airway responses in allergic asthmatics. *Clin. Exp. Allergy* **2014**, *44*, 1044–1052. [CrossRef] [PubMed]

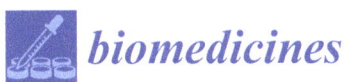

Article

Leukotriene B$_4$ Receptor 2 Mediates the Production of G-CSF That Plays a Critical Role in Steroid-Resistant Neutrophilic Airway Inflammation

Dong-Wook Kwak [1,†], Donghwan Park [1,†] and Jae-Hong Kim [2,*]

1. Department of Biotechnology, College of Life Sciences, Korea University, Seoul 02841, Republic of Korea
2. Department of Life Sciences, College of Life Sciences, Korea University, Seoul 02841, Republic of Korea
* Correspondence: jhongkim@korea.ac.kr; Tel.: +82-2-3290-3452
† These authors contributed equally to this work.

Abstract: Granulocyte colony-stimulating factor (G-CSF) has been suggested to be closely associated with neutrophilic asthma pathogenesis. However, little is known about the factors regulating the production of G-CSF in neutrophilic asthma. We previously reported that a leukotriene B$_4$ receptor 2, BLT2, played an important role in neutrophilic airway inflammation. Therefore, in the current study, we investigated whether BLT2 plays a role in the production of G-CSF in lipopolysaccharide/ovalbumin (LPS/OVA)-induced steroid-resistant neutrophilic asthma. The data showed that BLT2 critically mediated G-CSF production, contributing to the progression of neutrophilic airway inflammation. We also observed that 12-lipoxygenase (12-LO), which catalyzes the synthesis of the BLT2 ligand 12(S)-HETE, was also necessary for G-CSF production. Together, these results suggest that the 12-LO-BLT2-linked signaling network is critical for the production of G-CSF, contributing to the development of neutrophilic airway inflammation. Our findings can provide a potential new target for the therapy of severe neutrophilic asthma.

Keywords: BLT2; G-CSF; 12-LO; neutrophil; airway inflammation

Citation: Kwak, D.-W.; Park, D.; Kim, J.-H. Leukotriene B$_4$ Receptor 2 Mediates the Production of G-CSF That Plays a Critical Role in Steroid-Resistant Neutrophilic Airway Inflammation. *Biomedicines* **2022**, *10*, 2979. https://doi.org/10.3390/biomedicines10112979

Academic Editor: Stanislawa Bazan-Socha

Received: 31 October 2022
Accepted: 17 November 2022
Published: 19 November 2022

Publisher's Note: MDPI stays neutral with regard to jurisdictional claims in published maps and institutional affiliations.

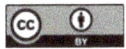

Copyright: © 2022 by the authors. Licensee MDPI, Basel, Switzerland. This article is an open access article distributed under the terms and conditions of the Creative Commons Attribution (CC BY) license (https://creativecommons.org/licenses/by/4.0/).

1. Introduction

Neutrophilic asthma is considered to be a poorly controlled disease, showing severe pathological symptoms [1,2]. While mild and moderate asthma can be treated effectively with glucocorticoids, severe neutrophilic asthma is poorly controlled by steroid treatment [3]. Increased numbers of neutrophils are closely correlated with the severity of the disease, and their presence is suggested to be associated with the exacerbation of asthmatic inflammation [4]. Since there is no effective therapy for neutrophilic asthma, identifying a target for developing an effective therapy for severe asthma is urgently needed.

Colony-stimulating factors (CSFs) were previously defined as regulators of the generation of myeloid populations but were later demonstrated to also regulate the survival, proliferation, and function of myeloid cells, which are functions closely related to inflammation [5]. Among CSFs, granulocyte colony-stimulating factor (G-CSF)/CSF3 is a major regulator of neutrophil differentiation, migration, and recruitment to inflammation sites, as well as survival [6,7]. Various types of cells, including epithelial cells, stromal cells, endothelial cells, and macrophages, produce G-CSF [8]. Recently, G-CSF was reported to be associated with severe neutrophilic asthma development and exacerbation, and increased levels of G-CSF were reported in the sputum of patients with asthma [9,10]. A transcriptomic sputum dataset from patients with severe asthma showed that CSF3 and CSF3R expression levels showed a positive correlation with the severity of the neutrophilic asthma [11]. Also, the neutralization of the G-CSF receptor (G-CSFR) attenuated neutrophilic asthma and mucus secretion in a murine model [11]. Together, these results suggest the role of G-CSF as a critical player in neutrophilic asthma development and exacerbation [12]. Despite the suggested critical roles of G-CSF in neutrophilic asthmatic pathogenesis, little is known about the regulators of the production of G-CSF in severe neutrophilic asthma.

Eicosanoids such as leukotrienes (LTs) and prostaglandins (PGs) are well-defined lipid metabolites that were reported to be associated with asthma pathology [13–15]. Among them, leukotriene B_4 (LTB$_4$) interacts with two distinct receptors, BLT1 and BLT2 [16]. The majority of studies have focused on BLT1, which is the high-affinity receptor for LTB$_4$ and is expressed mainly on immune cells, such as leukocytes [17–19]. On the other hand, BLT2 is a low-affinity receptor for LTB$_4$ and is expressed ubiquitously, including in airway epithelial and mast cells [20,21]. BLT2 is also known to interact with 12(S)-hydroxyeicosatetraenoic acid (12(S)-HETE), a lipid mediator derived from arachidonic acid by the enzymatic action of 12-lipoxygenase (12-LO) [22]. Recently, we observed that BLT2 and its ligand 12(S)-HETE played critical roles in asthmatic airway inflammation [23–28]. Especially, BLT2 was shown to play mediatory roles in the production of IL-17 and IL-1β, eventually contributing to the neutrophilic asthma development in the murine models [29–31]. However, the mediatory role of BLT2 in G-CSF production in neutrophilic asthma has not been elucidated yet.

In the present study, we examined whether BLT2 was involved in G-CSF production in lipopolysaccharide/ovalbumin (LPS/OVA)-induced steroid-resistant severe neutrophilic airway inflammation. The data showed that BLT2 critically mediated the production of G-CSF, thereby contributing to the progression of neutrophilic airway inflammation. We also observed that 12-LO was located upstream of BLT2, mediating G-CSF production. Collectively, our results suggest that a 12-LO-BLT2-linked network mediates the production of G-CSF, thus contributing to neutrophilic airway inflammation. The present study can provide a potential new target for the therapy of severe neutrophilic asthma.

2. Materials and Methods

2.1. Reagents and Chemicals

Dexamethasone, dimethyl sulfoxide (DMSO), LPS (*Escherichia coli* serotype O55:B5), and ovalbumin were purchased from Sigma-Aldrich (St. Louis, MO, USA). The 12-LO inhibitor baicalein and BLT2 antagonist LY255283 were purchased from Enzo Life Sciences, Inc. (Farmingdale, NY, USA) and Cayman Chemical (Ann Arbor, MI, USA), respectively. Antibodies against BLT2, 12-LO, and GAPDH were obtained from Enzo Life Sciences, Inc., Invitrogen (Rockford, IL, USA), and Santa Cruz Biotechnology, Inc. (Dallas, TX, USA), respectively. Neutralizing monoclonal antibodies against G-CSF and the IgG1 isotype control were obtained from R&D Systems (Minneapolis, MN, USA).

2.2. Mice

8-week-old wild-type (WT) female C57BL/6 mice were obtained from Orient Bio (Seongnam, Republic of Korea). BLT2$^{-/-}$ mice used in the experiments were generated and genotyped by analyzing polymerase chain reaction (PCR) as reported previously [26]. Animals used in the experiments were maintained under a 12:12 h light/dark cycle with a density of 4–5 mice per cage on disposable bedding. The mice were provided with rodent chow and water ad libitum. The study was conducted in strict accordance with guidelines approved by Korea University Institutional Animal Care and Use Committee (KU-IACUC). The experimental protocol in the present study was approved by KU-IACUC (approval no. KU-IACUC-2022-0031).

2.3. Animal Model for LPS/OVA-Induced Steroid-Resistant Neutrophilic Airway Inflammation

Mice were anesthetized with 5% isoflurane before the treatment. Then, the mice were sensitized with 10 μg of LPS plus 75 μg of OVA in 20 μL of phosphate-buffered saline (PBS) by intranasal administration. During the challenges, 50 μg of OVA in 20 μL PBS was administered intranasally (i.n.). To test for steroid resistance, dexamethasone (1 mg/kg) was injected intraperitoneally (i.p.) 1 h before each challenge. For the inhibition experiments, 100 μL of LY255283 (10 mg/kg), baicalein (20 mg/kg), or vehicle control (mixture of 8:2 DMSO/PBS) was administered i.p. 1 h before each challenge. For the neutralization of G-CSF, an anti-G-CSF antibody (5 mg/kg) or control IgG antibody in PBS (100 µL) was injected i.p. 1 h before each challenge. Negative control (NC) mice were not injected or treated during the experiment.

2.4. Western Blotting

Western blotting was performed as previously described [30]. Mouse lung tissues were homogenized in buffer containing 150 mM NaCl, 1 mM EDTA, 1 mM EGTA, 0.5% sodium deoxycholate, 1% Triton X-100, 100 mM Tris-HCl (pH 7.4), and proteinase inhibitor cocktail. Lysate proteins were separated by running 10% sodium dodecyl sulfate-polyacrylamide gel electrophoresis, then transferred onto polyvinylidene fluoride membranes. The membranes were then blocked for 1 h in TBS-T containing 5% nonfat dry milk, then incubated with primary antibodies for 1 h at room temperature (RT). After the membranes were washed for 1 h, they were incubated with horseradish peroxidase-conjugated secondary antibodies for 1 h and then washed for 1 h. Then, the bands were detected by enhanced chemiluminescence (Amersham Biosciences, Buckingham, UK).

2.5. Measurements of 12(S)-HETE, G-CSF, and Myeloperoxidase (MPO)

G-CSF and MPO were measured using bronchoalveolar lavage fluid (BALF) by enzyme-linked immunosorbent assay (ELISA) kits (Abcam, Cambridge, UK) in accordance with the manufacturer's instructions. The 12(S)-HETE ELISA kit was purchased from Enzo Life Sciences Inc., and the levels of 12(S)-HETE in BALF were quantified following the manufacturer's instructions.

2.6. Bronchoalveolar Lavage Cell Counting

Bronchoalveolar lavage (BAL) cells were separated from BALF by centrifugation at $1000 \times g$ for 3 min. Then, the supernatants were collected for ELISAs, and the cell pellets were resuspended in PBS. Slides of BAL cells were processed using a CytoSpin (CytoSpin, Hanil Science, Gimpo, Republic of Korea) at 500 rpm for 5 min and stained by a Diff-Quik staining kit (Sysmex, Kobe, Japan).

2.7. Histological Staining and Analysis of Lung Tissues

Lung tissues were fixed in 10% formalin for 10 days and then embedded in paraffin. The sections of lung tissues (4.0–4.5 µm thick) were adhered on Superfrost Plus glass slides (Fisher Scientific, Pittsburgh, PA, USA). After deparaffinization, they were stained with hematoxylin and eosin (H&E) or periodic acid-Schiff (PAS) staining solution. The images were observed through a DP71 digital camera (Olympus, Tokyo, Japan) using a BX51 microscope (Olympus, Tokyo, Japan). A subjective scale from 0 to 3 was used to evaluate the degree of lung inflammation [23]. Briefly, grade 0 indicated no observable inflammation, and grade 1 indicated intermittent cuffing with inflammatory cells. Grade 2 is defined when most vessels or bronchi have slight (1–5 cells thick) layers of inflammatory cells, and grade 3 is defined when most vessels or bronchi have dense (more than 5 cells thick) layers of inflammatory cells. To perform immunofluorescence (IF) staining, the sections of lung tissues (4.0–4.5 µm thick) were precisely adhered on Superfrost™ Plus slides. After deparaffinization, they were rehydrated and then blocked for 1 h with buffer (PBS containing 1% bovine serum albumin) at RT. Then, the slides were incubated with antibodies against BLT2, MPO, and G-CSF conjugated with Alexa Fluor 488, 594, and 647, respectively, using antibody conjugation kits (Abcam, Cambridge, UK) at 4 °C. After washing three times in PBS, they were incubated with 4′,6-diamidino-2-phenylindole (DAPI) (Sigma-Aldrich). The slides were processed with washing in PBS and mounted. The images were observed by confocal laser scanning microscopy (LSM 700, Carl Zeiss, Oberkochen, Germany).

2.8. Statistical Analysis

Statistical analyses were performed with a one-way analysis of variance (ANOVA) followed by Bonferroni's post hoc test. A two-way ANOVA followed by Bonferroni's post hoc test was done to compare the data obtained from BLT2$^{-/-}$ and WT mice. GraphPad Prism 8.0 (GraphPad Software Inc., San Diego, CA, USA) was used for the statistical analyses. The results are presented as the mean $\pm$ SD. A *p*-value of <0.05 indicated statistical significance.

3. Results

3.1. Elevated Levels of G-CSF in the Steroid-Resistant Neutrophilic Airway Inflammation Model

First, we established a murine model for steroid-resistant neutrophilic airway inflammation as described previously with some modifications [10,32]. Mice were intranasally sensitized with 10 µg of LPS and 75 µg of OVA on days 0, 1, 2, and 7, followed by a challenge with 50 µg of OVA on days 14, 15, 21, 22, 28, and 29. The mice were euthanized 6 h after the last challenge. Inhibitors were i.p. injected 1 h before each challenge (Figure 1A). To confirm whether the mouse model was steroid-resistant, we examined the effect of corticosteroid (dexamethasone) treatment. Dexamethasone administration did not significantly reduce the recruitment of immune cells, airway inflammation (H&E), or mucus secretion (PAS) induced by LPS/OVA treatment (Figure 1B,C). Similarly, myeloperoxidase (MPO) and G-CSF levels in BALF were not reduced by dexamethasone treatment (Figure 1D,E). Neither the number of total cells nor neutrophils in BALF were affected by dexamethasone treatment (Figure 1F). Immunofluorescence staining analysis showed that the levels of MPO and G-CSF expression increased by LPS/OVA treatment were not attenuated by dexamethasone treatment (Figure 1G,H). Taken together, our experimental murine model exhibited a steroid-resistant neutrophilic airway inflammation phenotype with elevated G-CSF levels.

3.2. G-CSF Is Critical for Neutrophilic Airway Inflammation

Recent studies showed that G-CSF had a critical role in the recruitment of neutrophils into airways in severe asthma [10]. To investigate the contributory role of G-CSF in our neutrophilic asthma model, a neutralizing monoclonal antibody against G-CSF was i.p. injected 1 h before each challenge. Histopathological analysis by H&E and PAS staining showed that the lung inflammation and mucus secretion induced by LPS/OVA were reduced by anti-G-CSF treatment (Figure 2A,B). We also observed that the increased levels of G-CSF and MPO activity were significantly suppressed by anti-G-CSF treatment (Figure 2C,D). Similarly, increases in the number of total cells and neutrophils infiltrating the airways induced by LPS/OVA administration were reduced to basal levels after anti-G-CSF treatment (Figure 2E). IF staining showed that G-CSF neutralization decreased G-CSF and MPO levels in lung tissue (Figure 2F,G). Together, these results suggest a critical contributory role of G-CSF in neutrophilic airway inflammation.

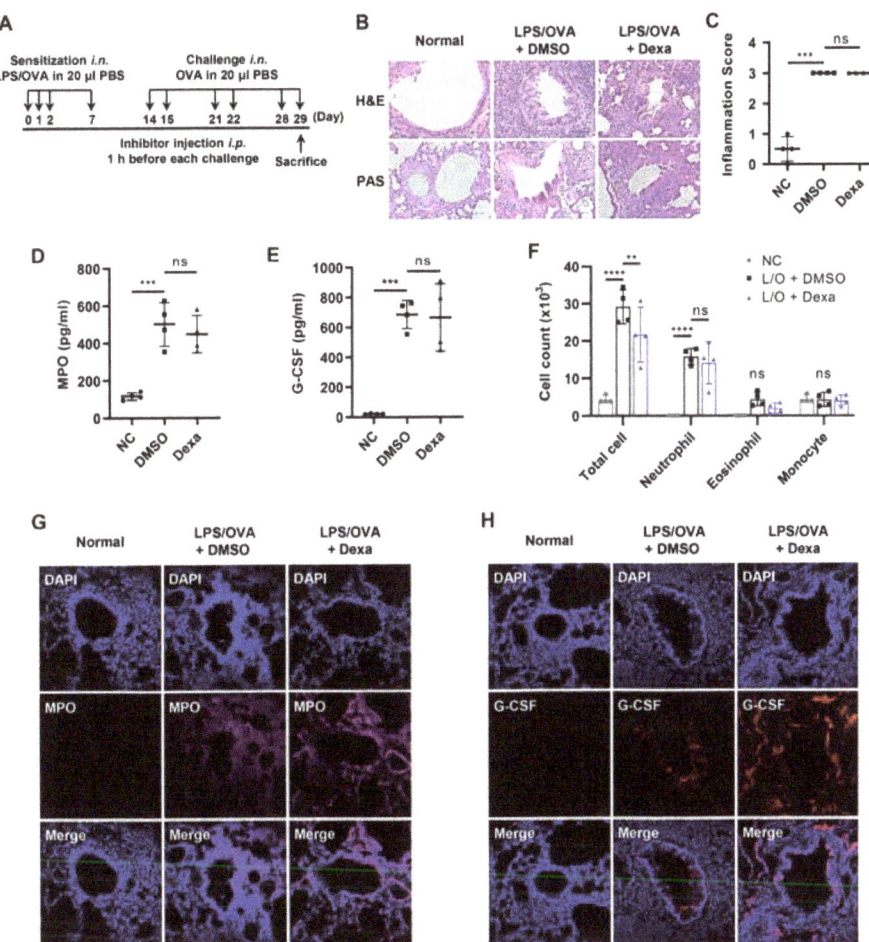

Figure 1. Elevated levels of G-CSF in the steroid-resistant neutrophilic lung airway inflammation model. For the experiment, mice were administered dexamethasone (Dexa; 1 mg/kg) or DMSO by i.p. injection 1 h before each challenge (*n* = 4 per group). The negative controls (NC) were not treated. (**A**) Scheme of the LPS/OVA-induced steroid-resistant neutrophilic airway inflammation model. (**B,C**) H&E and PAS staining of mice lung tissues. Perivascular and peribronchial inflammation, in addition to mucus secretion, was examined and scored (400×). Inflammation scores are shown as the mean ± SD (*n* = 4 per group). (**D,E**) MPO and G-CSF levels in BALF were analyzed by ELISA. (**F**) The number of immune cells in BALF was estimated using a CytoSpin and staining with Diff-Quik. The results are shown as the mean ± SD (*n* = 4 per group). (**G,H**) Immunofluorescence (IF) staining of mice lung tissues for MPO (magenta, Alexa Flour 594) and G-CSF (red, Alexa Flour 647). The nuclei were counterstained with DAPI (blue; 400×). The IF images are representatives of three independent trials with similar results. All experiments were performed in triplicate. ** *p* < 0.01, *** *p* < 0.001, **** *p* < 0.0001, ns: not significant versus each control group.

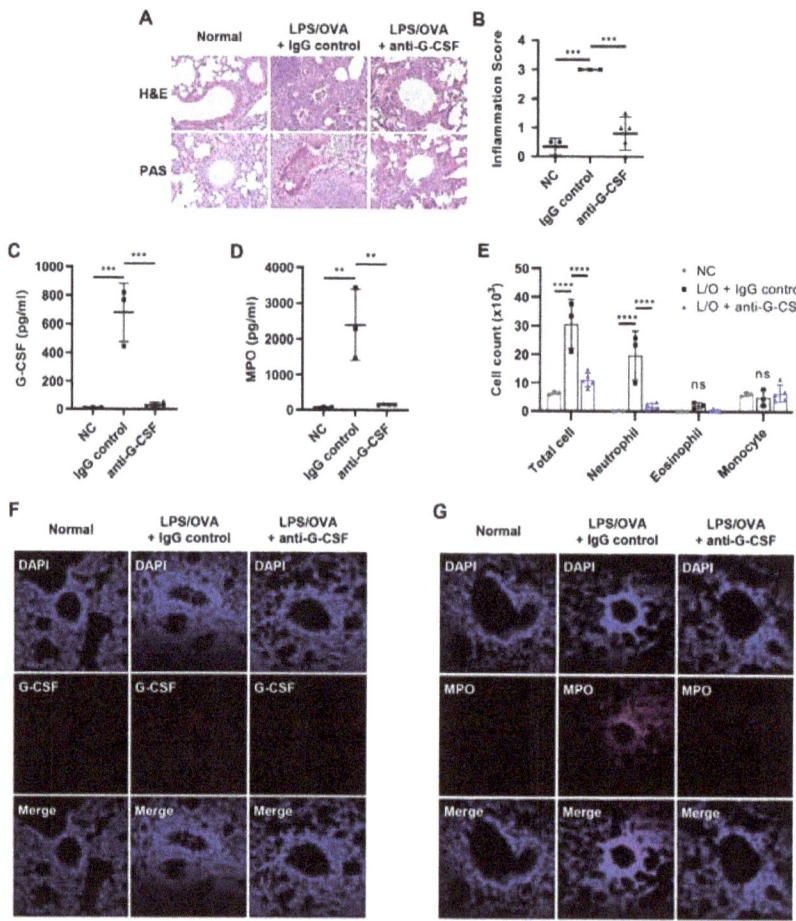

Figure 2. G-CSF is critical for neutrophilic airway inflammation. For the analysis of the effect of anti-G-CSF, mice were administered anti-G-CSF (5 mg/kg) or control IgG1 (5 mg/kg) by i.p. injection 1 h before each challenge (*n* = 3–5 per group). The negative controls (NC) were untreated. (**A,B**) H&E and PAS staining of mice lung tissues. Perivascular and peribronchial inflammation, in addition to mucus secretion, was examined and scored (400×). Inflammation scores are shown as the mean ± SD (*n* = 3–5 per group). (**C,D**) G-CSF and MPO levels in BALF were analyzed by ELISA. (**E**) The number of immune cells in BALF was estimated using a CytoSpin and staining with Diff-Quik. The results are shown as the mean ± SD (*n* = 3–5 per group). (**F,G**) IF staining of mouse lung tissues for G-CSF (red, Alexa Flour 647) and MPO (magenta, Alexa Flour 594). The nuclei were counterstained with DAPI (blue; 400×). The IF images are representatives of three independent trials with similar results. All experiments were performed in triplicate. ** $p < 0.01$, *** $p < 0.001$, **** $p < 0.0001$, ns: not significant versus each control group.

3.3. BLT2 Mediates the Production of G-CSF in Neutrophilic Airway Inflammation

Since previous studies suggested a mediating role of BLT2 in neutrophilic airway inflammation [29–31], we investigated whether BLT2 had any role in the production of G-CSF. Lung inflammation and mucus secretion were markedly suppressed by treatment with the BLT2 antagonist, LY255283 (Figure 3A,B). Under our experimental conditions, the protein level of BLT2 in lung tissue was suppressed by LY255283 (Figure 3C). Clearly, G-CSF, as well as MPO levels increased by LPS/OVA treatment, were alleviated by LY255283 treatment (Figure 3D,E). We also found that the number of total cells and neutrophils in BALF was significantly suppressed by LY255283 (Figure 3F). IF staining also showed that the levels of G-CSF and MPO, as well as that of BLT2, in lung tissue were attenuated by LY255283 treatment (Figure 3F,G). Together, these data suggest that BLT2 is essential for the production of G-CSF, thus contributing to neutrophilic airway inflammation.

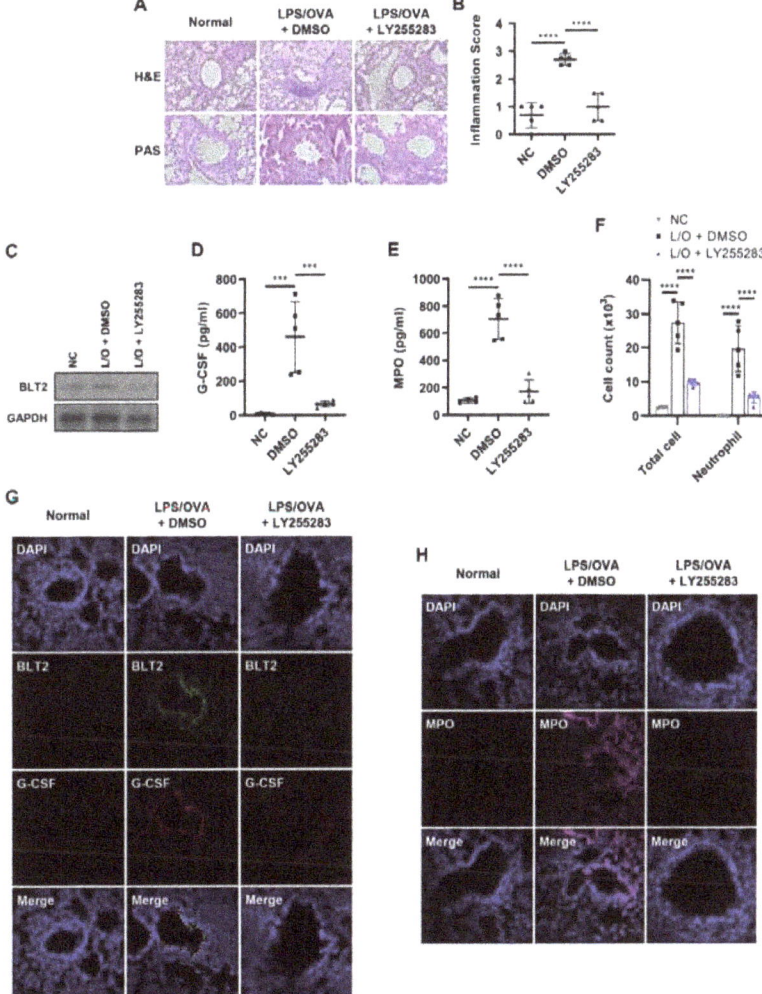

Figure 3. BLT2 mediates the production of G-CSF in neutrophilic airway inflammation. The BLT2 antagonist LY255283 (10 mg/kg) or DMSO was administered by i.p. injection 1 h before each challenge. The negative controls (NC) were untreated. (**A,B**) H&E and PAS staining of mice lung tissues.

Perivascular and peribronchial inflammation in addition to mucus secretion, was examined and scored (400×). Inflammation scores are shown as the mean ± SD (*n* = 5 per group). (**C**) Lung tissue was homogenized, and the protein was isolated to assess the level of BLT2 by Western blotting. (**D,E**) G-CSF and MPO levels in BALF were analyzed by ELISA. (**F**) The number of immune cells in BALF was estimated using a CytoSpin and staining with Diff-Quik. The results are shown as the mean ± SD (*n* = 5 per group). (**G,H**) IF staining of mice lung tissue for BLT2 (green, Alexa Flour 488), G-CSF (red, Alexa Flour 647), and MPO (magenta, Alexa Flour 594). The nuclei were counterstained with DAPI (blue; 400×). The IF images are representatives of three independent trials with similar results. All experiments were performed in triplicate. *** *p* < 0.001, **** *p* < 0.0001 versus each control group.

3.4. BLT2 Knockout Attenuates Both G-CSF Production and Neutrophilic Airway Inflammation

To further investigate the role of BLT2 in neutrophilic airway inflammation, BLT2$^{-/-}$ mice were tested. As expected, we found that BLT2$^{-/-}$ mice showed the suppression of inflammation and mucus secretion in the airways (Figure 4A,B). Clearly, G-CSF, as well as MPO levels after LPS/OVA treatment, were also attenuated in BLT2$^{-/-}$ mice (Figure 4C,D). The numbers of total cells and neutrophils in BLT2$^{-/-}$ mice were reduced compared to those in WT mice (Figure 4E). IF staining showed decreased levels of G-CSF and MPO in the lung tissue of BLT2$^{-/-}$ mice after LPS/OVA treatment compared to the lung tissue of WT mice (Figure 4F,G). These results also suggest that BLT2 mediates the production of G-CSF and neutrophilic airway inflammation.

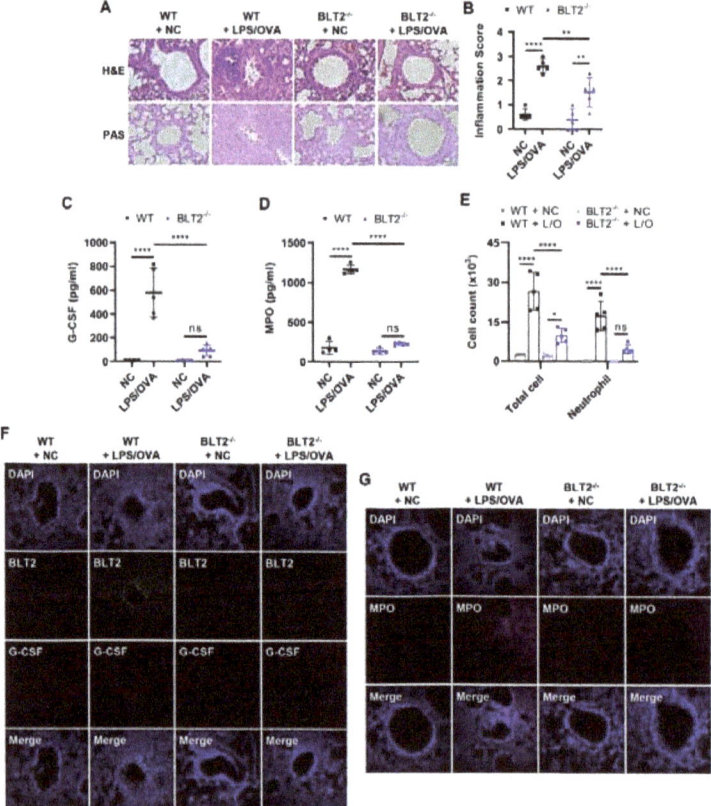

Figure 4. BLT2 knockout attenuates both G-CSF production and neutrophilic airway inflammation. BLT2$^{-/-}$ mice received the same schedule for sensitization and challenge (BLT2$^{-/-}$ + LPS/OVA).

Wild-type negative controls (WT + NC) and BLT2$^{-/-}$ negative controls (BLT2$^{-/-}$ + NC) were not treated. (**A,B**) H&E and PAS staining of mice lung tissues. Perivascular and peribronchial inflammation in addition to mucus secretion, was examined and scored (400×). Inflammation scores are shown as the mean ± SD (*n* = 5 per group). (**C,D**) G-CSF and MPO levels in BALF were analyzed by ELISA. (**E**) The number of immune cells in BALF was estimated using a CytoSpin and staining with Diff-Quik. The results are shown as the mean ± SD (*n* = 5 per group). (**F,G**) IF staining of mice lung tissues for BLT2 (green, Alexa Flour 488), G-CSF (red, Alexa Flour 647), and MPO (magenta, Alexa Flour 594). The nuclei were counterstained with DAPI (blue; 400×). The IF images are representatives of three independent trials with similar results. All experiments were performed in triplicate. * $p < 0.05$, ** $p < 0.01$, **** $p < 0.0001$, ns: not significant versus each control group.

3.5. 12-LO Is Also Necessary for the Production of G-CSF and Contributes to Neutrophilic Airway Inflammation

Since 12-LO is an enzyme that produces 12(*S*)-HETE, which is a ligand for BLT2, we examined whether 12-LO activity was also necessary for the production of G-CSF. The levels of 12(*S*)-HETE in BALF were suppressed by the administration of the 12-LO inhibitor, baicalein (Figure 5A). Histopathological analysis showed that inflammation and mucus secretion in lung tissue were suppressed by baicalein treatment (Figure 5B,C). Under these experimental conditions, the protein level of 12-LO was also suppressed in lung tissue by baicalein (Figure 5D). Clearly, G-CSF, as well as MPO levels in BALF increased by LPS/OVA treatment, were markedly suppressed by baicalein administration (Figure 5E,F). The number of total cells and neutrophils in BALF was also significantly reduced by baicalein treatment (Figure 5G). IF staining also showed that the levels of G-CSF, MPO, and BLT2 in lung tissue were markedly decreased by baicalein treatment (Figure 5H,I). Taken together, these results showed that 12-LO was necessary for the production of G-CSF, thus contributing to neutrophilic airway inflammation.

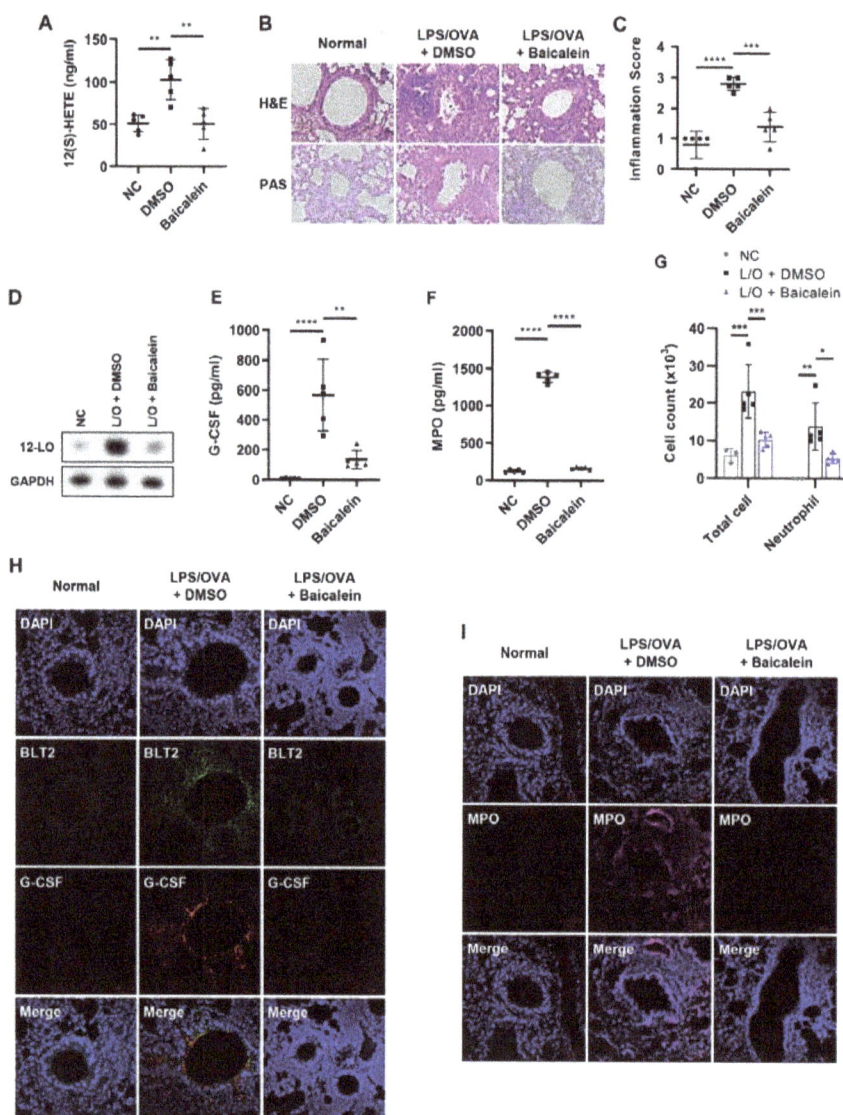

Figure 5. 12-LO is also necessary for the production of G-CSF and contributes to neutrophilic airway inflammation. The 12-LO inhibitor baicalein (20 mg/kg) or DMSO was administered by i.p. injection 1 h before each challenge. The negative controls (NC) were untreated. (**A**) 12(*S*)-HETE levels in BALF were analyzed by ELISA. (**B,C**) H&E and PAS staining of mice lung tissues. Perivascular and peribronchial inflammation in addition to mucus secretion, was examined and scored (400×). Inflammation scores are shown as the mean ± SD (*n* = 5 per group). (**D**) Mouse lung tissue was homogenized, and the protein was isolated to assess the level of 12-LO by Western blotting. (**E,F**) G-CSF and MPO levels in BALF were analyzed by ELISA. (**G**) The number of immune cells in BALF was estimated using a CytoSpin and staining with Diff-Quik. The results are shown as the mean ± SD (*n* = 5 per group). (**H,I**) IF staining of mice lung tissue for BLT2 (green, Alexa Flour 488), G-CSF (red, Alexa Flour 647), and MPO (magenta, Alexa Flour 594). Nuclei were counterstained with DAPI

(blue; 400×). The IF images are representatives of three independent trials with similar results. All experiments were performed in triplicate. * $p < 0.05$, ** $p < 0.01$, *** $p < 0.001$, **** $p < 0.0001$ versus each control group.

4. Discussion

In this study, we demonstrated the critical mediatory role of BLT2 in the production of G-CSF in steroid-resistant neutrophilic airway inflammation. The results showed that the blockade of BLT2 by antagonist treatment or genetic ablation suppressed the production of G-CSF, thus alleviating neutrophilic inflammation in the murine model. We also found that 12-LO, an enzyme that synthesizes 12(*S*)-HETE, which is a ligand for BLT2, was necessary for the production of G-CSF. Taken together, our results point to BLT2 as a potential therapeutic target in G-CSF-associated neutrophilic airway inflammation.

The contributory role of myeloid hematopoietic growth factors such as G-CSF has been reported in a variety of neutrophilic inflammatory diseases. G-CSF was shown to play roles in the pathogenesis of neutrophilic inflammatory diseases such as inflammatory arthritis, allergic encephalomyelitis, and cigarette smoke-induced chronic obstructive pulmonary disease (COPD) [33–36]. In patients with smoke-induced COPD, single nucleotide polymorphisms (SNPs) of G-CSF were suggested to protect against low lung function [37]. Recently, the contributory roles of G-CSF in inducing neutrophilic influx were demonstrated in severe asthma [10,38,39].

In addition to G-CSF, interleukin-17 (IL-17) and interleukin-1β (IL-1β) have been reported to be strongly related to severe neutrophilic asthma [40–44]. Th17 cells secrete inflammatory cytokines such as IL-17 to communicate with other cells in the immune system and were shown to be involved with the neutrophil influx into bronchial airways and asthma severity [45,46]. NLRP3 inflammasome-dependent IL-1β production also acts as a major chemoattractant of neutrophils and contributes to the development of neutrophilic airway inflammation [43,47]. We previously reported the mediating roles of BLT2 in regulating the production of IL-17 and NLRP3-dependent IL-1β in neutrophilic airway inflammation [29–31]. Thus, we were curious about the signaling network linking BLT2-mediated G-CSF production to IL-17 or IL-1β production. To test this, we examined whether G-CSF depletion affected the production of IL-17/IL-1β in neutrophilic airway inflammation. We observed the suppression of IL-17 levels in BALF and IL-1β in lung lysates by anti-G-CSF treatment (Figure S1A,B). These results suggest that G-CSF is necessary for the production of IL-17/IL-1β in the development of neutrophilic airway inflammation.

In addition to BLT2, BLT1 was also reported to play a role in mediating the recruitment of neutrophils in inflammatory responses [48]. Therefore, we investigated whether LTB₄ and its receptor BLT1 played roles in the production of G-CSF in our experimental conditions. Quite interestingly, no reduction in the levels of G-CSF in BALF was detected by treatment with the BLT1 antagonist U75302 (Figure S2A). We also did not observe increases in the levels of LTB₄ in BALF (data not shown). The reason why BLT1 did not mediate the production of G-CSF in the present study is not clear, but we suspect that it may be due to the different cell types targeted by LTB₄-BLT1 and 12(*S*)-HETE-BLT2 signaling. BLT1 is highly expressed in leukocytes [16], whereas BLT2 is broadly expressed in other cell types, including airway epithelial cells [20]. Therefore, we suspect that BLT2 activation in airway epithelial cells mainly mediated the production of G-CSF at the early time point (6 h) following the LPS/OVA challenge in our murine experimental model. Then, G-CSF was, in turn, likely to trigger the production of IL-17 and IL-1β at the delayed time point by activating BLT1 and BLT2 on other cell types (e.g., macrophages) in the asthmatic airway microenvironment. Indeed, the level of G-CSF in BALF was reduced by the antagonist of BLT1 as well as BLT2 at the delayed time point (24 h) following the last challenge (Figure S2B). Further studies are necessary to elucidate the detailed mechanism of how BLT1 contributes to the synthesis of these cytokines in the development of severe neutrophilic asthma.

5. Conclusions

In summary, we have shown that BLT2 played a critical mediating role in the production of G-CSF in steroid-resistant neutrophilic lung airway inflammation. We also found that the blockade of BLT2 suppressed the production of G-CSF, thus alleviating neutrophilic inflammation in the murine model. In support of the mediatory role of BLT2 in the production of G-CSF, the synthesis of its ligands by 12-LO was also shown to be necessary for mediating the production of G-CSF. Together, our results suggest that the 12-LO-BLT2 cascade is critical for the production of G-CSF, thus contributing to the progression of neutrophilic airway inflammation (as summarized in Figure 6). This study was the first to report the mediatory role of BLT2 in the production of G-CSF in neutrophilic asthma. The results provide a new perspective for developing effective therapies for severe neutrophilic asthma.

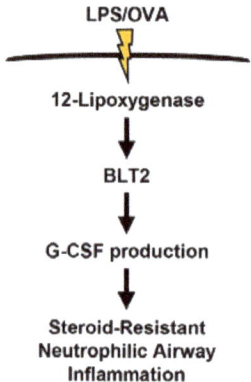

Figure 6. The proposed scheme of the 12-LO-BLT2-G-CSF cascade in LPS/OVA-induced steroid-resistant neutrophilic airway inflammation.

Supplementary Materials: The following supporting information can be downloaded at: https://www.mdpi.com/article/10.3390/biomedicines10112979/s1, Figure S1: G-CSF is critical for IL-17/IL-1β production in steroid-resistant neutrophilic airway inflammation.; Figure S2: BLT1 has no effect on G-CSF production in the early time point following the challenge.

Author Contributions: D.-W.K. and D.P. planned the study, performed the experiments, analyzed data, and wrote the manuscript. J.-H.K. supervised the study and wrote the manuscript. All authors have read and agreed to the published version of the manuscript.

Funding: This work was supported by a Bio and Medical Technology Development Program grant (2017M3A9D8063317) through the National Research Foundation (NRF) funded by the Ministry of Science, Information and Communication Technologies (ICT) and Future Planning of the Republic of Korea. This work was also supported by a Korea University Grant.

Institutional Review Board Statement: All experimental animals used in this study were treated according to guidelines approved by the Institutional Animal Care and Use Committee of Korea University (KU-IACUC), and the experimental protocols were approved by KU-IACUC (Approval no. KU-IACUC-2022-0031).

Informed Consent Statement: Not applicable.

Data Availability Statement: Not applicable.

Conflicts of Interest: The authors declare no conflict of interest.

References

1. Shilovskiy, I.P.; Nikolskii, A.A.; Kurbacheva, O.M.; Khaitov, M.R. Modern View of Neutrophilic Asthma Molecular Mechanisms and Therapy. *Biochemistry* **2020**, *85*, 854–868. [CrossRef] [PubMed]
2. Zhang, X.; Xu, Z.; Wen, X.; Huang, G.; Nian, S.; Li, L.; Guo, X.; Ye, Y.; Yuan, Q. The onset, development and pathogenesis of severe neutrophilic asthma. *Immunol. Cell Biol.* **2022**, *100*, 144–159. [CrossRef]
3. Bruijnzeel, P.L.; Uddin, M.; Koenderman, L. Targeting neutrophilic inflammation in severe neutrophilic asthma: Can we target the disease-relevant neutrophil phenotype? *J. Leukoc. Biol.* **2015**, *98*, 549–556. [CrossRef] [PubMed]
4. Moore, W.C.; Hastie, A.T.; Li, X.; Li, H.; Busse, W.W.; Jarjour, N.N.; Wenzel, S.E.; Peters, S.P.; Meyers, D.A.; Bleecker, E.R.; et al. Sputum neutrophil counts are associated with more severe asthma phenotypes using cluster analysis. *J. Allergy Clin. Immunol.* **2014**, *133*, 1557–1563 e1555. [CrossRef]
5. Hamilton, J.A.; Cook, A.D.; Tak, P.P. Anti-colony-stimulating factor therapies for inflammatory and autoimmune diseases. *Nat. Rev. Drug Discov.* **2016**, *16*, 53–70. [CrossRef]
6. Avalos, B.R. Molecular analysis of the granulocyte colony-stimulating factor receptor. *Blood* **1996**, *88*, 761–777. [CrossRef] [PubMed]
7. Basu, S.; Dunn, A.; Ward, A. G-CSF: Function and modes of action (Review). *Int. J. Mol. Med.* **2002**, *10*, 3–10. [CrossRef]
8. Panopoulos, A.D.; Watowich, S.S. Granulocyte colony-stimulating factor: Molecular mechanisms of action during steady state and 'emergency' hematopoiesis. *Cytokine* **2008**, *42*, 277–288. [CrossRef]
9. Wang, H.; Aloe, C.; McQualter, J.; Papanicolaou, A.; Vlahos, R.; Wilson, N.; Bozinovski, S. G-CSFR antagonism reduces mucosal injury and airways fibrosis in a virus-dependent model of severe asthma. *Br. J. Pharmacol.* **2021**, *178*, 1869–1885. [CrossRef]
10. Kim, Y.M.; Kim, H.; Lee, S.; Kim, S.; Lee, J.U.; Choi, Y.; Park, H.W.; You, G.; Kang, H.; Lee, S.; et al. Airway G-CSF identifies neutrophilic inflammation and contributes to asthma progression. *Eur. Respir. J.* **2020**, *55*, 1900827. [CrossRef] [PubMed]
11. Wang, H.; FitzPatrick, M.; Wilson, N.J.; Anthony, D.; Reading, P.C.; Satzke, C.; Dunne, E.M.; Licciardi, P.V.; Seow, H.J.; Nichol, K.; et al. CSF3R/CD114 mediates infection-dependent transition to severe asthma. *J. Allergy Clin. Immunol.* **2019**, *143*, 785–788 e786. [CrossRef]
12. Papanicolaou, A.; Wang, H.; Satzke, C.; Vlahos, R.; Wilson, N.; Bozinovski, S. Novel Therapies for Pneumonia-Associated Severe Asthma Phenotypes. *Trends Mol. Med.* **2020**, *26*, 1047–1058. [CrossRef] [PubMed]
13. Sanak, M. Eicosanoid Mediators in the Airway Inflammation of Asthmatic Patients: What is New? *Allergy Asthma Immunol. Res.* **2016**, *8*, 481–490. [CrossRef] [PubMed]
14. Peebles, R.S., Jr. Prostaglandins in asthma and allergic diseases. *Pharmacol. Ther.* **2019**, *193*, 1–19. [CrossRef]
15. Mabalirajan, U.; Rehman, R.; Ahmad, T.; Kumar, S.; Leishangthem, G.D.; Singh, S.; Dinda, A.K.; Biswal, S.; Agrawal, A.; Ghosh, B. 12/15-lipoxygenase expressed in non-epithelial cells causes airway epithelial injury in asthma. *Sci. Rep.* **2013**, *3*, 1540. [CrossRef]
16. Tager, A.M.; Luster, A.D. BLT1 and BLT2: The leukotriene B(4) receptors. *Prostaglandins Leukot. Essent. Fatty Acids* **2003**, *69*, 123–134. [CrossRef]
17. Yokomizo, T.; Izumi, T.; Chang, K.; Takuwa, Y.; Shimizu, T. A G-protein-coupled receptor for leukotriene B4 that mediates chemotaxis. *Nature* **1997**, *387*, 620–624. [CrossRef]
18. Islam, S.A.; Thomas, S.Y.; Hess, C.; Medoff, B.D.; Means, T.K.; Brander, C.; Lilly, C.M.; Tager, A.M.; Luster, A.D. The leukotriene B4 lipid chemoattractant receptor BLT1 defines antigen-primed T cells in humans. *Blood* **2006**, *107*, 444–453. [CrossRef]
19. Kim, N.D.; Chou, R.C.; Seung, E.; Tager, A.M.; Luster, A.D. A unique requirement for the leukotriene B4 receptor BLT1 for neutrophil recruitment in inflammatory arthritis. *J. Exp. Med.* **2006**, *203*, 829–835. [CrossRef]
20. Pace, E.; Ferraro, M.; Di Vincenzo, S.; Bruno, A.; Giarratano, A.; Scafidi, V.; Lipari, L.; Di Benedetto, D.V.; Sciarrino, S.; Gjomarkaj, M. Cigarette smoke increases BLT2 receptor functions in bronchial epithelial cells: In vitro and ex vivo evidence. *Immunology* **2013**, *139*, 245–255. [CrossRef] [PubMed]
21. Lundeen, K.A.; Sun, B.; Karlsson, L.; Fourie, A.M. Leukotriene B4 receptors BLT1 and BLT2: Expression and function in human and murine mast cells. *J. Immunol.* **2006**, *177*, 3439–3447. [CrossRef] [PubMed]
22. Okuno, T.; Yokomizo, T. Biological functions of 12(S)-hydroxyheptadecatrienoic acid as a ligand of leukotriene B4 receptor 2. *Inflamm. Regen.* **2018**, *38*, 29. [CrossRef]
23. Cho, K.J.; Seo, J.M.; Shin, Y.; Yoo, M.H.; Park, C.S.; Lee, S.H.; Chang, Y.S.; Cho, S.H.; Kim, J.H. Blockade of airway inflammation and hyperresponsiveness by inhibition of BLT2, a low-affinity leukotriene B4 receptor. *Am. J. Respir. Cell Mol. Biol.* **2010**, *42*, 294–303. [CrossRef] [PubMed]
24. Ro, M.; Lee, A.J.; Kim, J.H. 5-/12-Lipoxygenase-linked cascade contributes to the IL-33-induced synthesis of IL-13 in mast cells, thus promoting asthma development. *Allergy* **2018**, *73*, 350–360. [CrossRef] [PubMed]
25. Cho, K.J.; Seo, J.M.; Lee, M.G.; Kim, J.H. BLT2 Is upregulated in allergen-stimulated mast cells and mediates the synthesis of Th2 cytokines. *J. Immunol.* **2010**, *185*, 6329–6337. [CrossRef]
26. Lee, A.J.; Ro, M.; Kim, J.H. Leukotriene B4 Receptor 2 Is Critical for the Synthesis of Vascular Endothelial Growth Factor in Allergen-Stimulated Mast Cells. *J. Immunol.* **2016**, *197*, 2069–2078. [CrossRef]
27. Park, D.; Kwak, D.W.; Kim, J.H. Leukotriene B4 receptors contribute to house dust mite-induced eosinophilic airway inflammation via TH2 cytokine production. *BMB Rep.* **2021**, *54*, 182–187. [CrossRef]
28. Lee, A.J.; Ro, M.; Cho, K.J.; Kim, J.H. Lipopolysaccharide/TLR4 Stimulates IL-13 Production through a MyD88-BLT2-Linked Cascade in Mast Cells, Potentially Contributing to the Allergic Response. *J. Immunol.* **2017**, *199*, 409–417. [CrossRef] [PubMed]

29. Ro, M.; Kwon, S.Y.; Kim, J.H. Leukotriene B4 receptors mediate the production of IL-17, thus contributing to neutrophil-dominant asthmatic airway inflammation. *Allergy* **2019**, *74*, 1797–1799. [CrossRef]
30. Kwak, D.W.; Park, D.; Kim, J.H. Leukotriene B4 receptors play critical roles in house dust mites-induced neutrophilic airway inflammation and IL-17 production. *Biochem. Biophys. Res. Commun.* **2021**, *534*, 646–652. [CrossRef]
31. Kwak, D.W.; Park, D.; Kim, J.H. Leukotriene B4 Receptors Are Necessary for the Stimulation of NLRP3 Inflammasome and IL-1beta Synthesis in Neutrophil-Dominant Asthmatic Airway Inflammation. *Biomedicines* **2021**, *9*, 535. [CrossRef] [PubMed]
32. Kim, Y.K.; Oh, S.Y.; Jeon, S.G.; Park, H.W.; Lee, S.Y.; Chun, E.Y.; Bang, B.; Lee, H.S.; Oh, M.H.; Kim, Y.S.; et al. Airway exposure levels of lipopolysaccharide determine type 1 versus type 2 experimental asthma. *J. Immunol.* **2007**, *178*, 5375–5382. [CrossRef]
33. Mo, Y.; Chen, J.; Humphrey, D.M., Jr.; Fodah, R.A.; Warawa, J.M.; Hoyle, G.W. Abnormal epithelial structure and chronic lung inflammation after repair of chlorine-induced airway injury. *Am. J. Physiol. Lung Cell Mol. Physiol.* **2015**, *308*, L168–L178. [CrossRef]
34. Lawlor, K.E.; Campbell, I.K.; Metcalf, D.; O'Donnell, K.; van Nieuwenhuijze, A.; Roberts, A.W.; Wicks, I.P. Critical role for granulocyte colony-stimulating factor in inflammatory arthritis. *Proc. Natl. Acad. Sci. USA* **2004**, *101*, 11398–11403. [CrossRef] [PubMed]
35. Tsantikos, E.; Lau, M.; Castelino, C.M.; Maxwell, M.J.; Passey, S.L.; Hansen, M.J.; McGregor, N.E.; Sims, N.A.; Steinfort, D.P.; Irving, L.B.; et al. Granulocyte-CSF links destructive inflammation and comorbidities in obstructive lung disease. *J. Clin. Investig.* **2018**, *128*, 2406–2418. [CrossRef]
36. Rumble, J.M.; Huber, A.K.; Krishnamoorthy, G.; Srinivasan, A.; Giles, D.A.; Zhang, X.; Wang, L.; Segal, B.M. Neutrophil-related factors as biomarkers in EAE and MS. *J. Exp. Med.* **2015**, *212*, 23–35. [CrossRef] [PubMed]
37. He, J.Q.; Shumansky, K.; Connett, J.E.; Anthonisen, N.R.; Pare, P.D.; Sandford, A.J. Association of genetic variations in the CSF2 and CSF3 genes with lung function in smoking-induced COPD. *Eur. Respir. J.* **2008**, *32*, 25–34. [CrossRef]
38. Steinke, J.W.; Lawrence, M.G.; Teague, W.G.; Braciale, T.J.; Patrie, J.T.; Borish, L. Bronchoalveolar lavage cytokine patterns in children with severe neutrophilic and paucigranulocytic asthma. *J. Allergy Clin. Immunol.* **2021**, *147*, 686–693. [CrossRef]
39. Ouyang, S.; Liu, C.; Xiao, J.; Chen, X.; Lui, A.C.; Li, X. Targeting IL-17A/glucocorticoid synergy to CSF3 expression in neutrophilic airway diseases. *JCI Insight* **2020**, *5*, e132836. [CrossRef]
40. Agache, I.; Ciobanu, C.; Agache, C.; Anghel, M. Increased serum IL-17 is an independent risk factor for severe asthma. *Respir. Med.* **2010**, *104*, 1131–1137. [CrossRef]
41. Sun, Y.C.; Zhou, Q.T.; Yao, W.Z. Sputum interleukin-17 is increased and associated with airway neutrophilia in patients with severe asthma. *Chin. Med. J. (Engl.)* **2005**, *118*, 953–956. [PubMed]
42. Chakir, J.; Shannon, J.; Molet, S.; Fukakusa, M.; Elias, J.; Laviolette, M.; Boulet, L.P.; Hamid, Q. Airway remodeling-associated mediators in moderate to severe asthma: Effect of steroids on TGF-beta, IL-11, IL-17, and type I and type III collagen expression. *J. Allergy Clin. Immunol.* **2003**, *111*, 1293–1298. [CrossRef] [PubMed]
43. Simpson, J.L.; Phipps, S.; Baines, K.J.; Oreo, K.M.; Gunawardhana, L.; Gibson, P.G. Elevated expression of the NLRP3 inflammasome in neutrophilic asthma. *Eur. Respir. J.* **2014**, *43*, 1067–1076. [CrossRef]
44. Kim, R.Y.; Pinkerton, J.W.; Essilfie, A.T.; Robertson, A.A.B.; Baines, K.J.; Brown, A.C.; Mayall, J.R.; Ali, M.K.; Starkey, M.R.; Hansbro, N.G.; et al. Role for NLRP3 Inflammasome-mediated, IL-1beta-Dependent Responses in Severe, Steroid-Resistant Asthma. *Am. J. Respir. Crit. Care Med.* **2017**, *196*, 283–297. [CrossRef] [PubMed]
45. Newcomb, D.C.; Peebles, R.S., Jr. Th17-mediated inflammation in asthma. *Curr. Opin. Immunol.* **2013**, *25*, 755–760. [CrossRef]
46. Wei, Q.; Liao, J.; Jiang, M.; Liu, J.; Liang, X.; Nong, G. Relationship between Th17-mediated immunity and airway inflammation in childhood neutrophilic asthma. *Allergy Asthma Clin. Immunol.* **2021**, *17*, 4. [CrossRef] [PubMed]
47. Williams, E.J.; Negewo, N.A.; Baines, K.J. Role of the NLRP3 inflammasome in asthma: Relationship with neutrophilic inflammation, obesity, and therapeutic options. *J. Allergy Clin. Immunol.* **2021**, *147*, 2060–2062. [CrossRef]
48. Gelfand, E.W. Importance of the leukotriene B4-BLT1 and LTB4-BLT2 pathways in asthma. *Semin. Immunol.* **2017**, *33*, 44–51. [CrossRef]

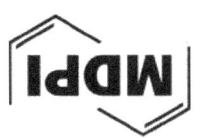

MDPI

St. Alban-Anlage 66

4052 Basel

Switzerland

Tel. +41 61 683 77 34

Fax +41 61 302 89 18

www.mdpi.com

Biomedicines Editorial Office

E-mail: biomedicines@mdpi.com

www.mdpi.com/journal/biomedicines

www.ingramcontent.com/pod-product-compliance
Lightning Source LLC
LaVergne TN
LVHW070632100526
838202LV00012B/791